Waisted

Waisted

The Biology of Body Fat

Nathan Denton *DPhil*
Science Communications Manager,
Gene Therapy Program,
University of Pennsylvania, USA

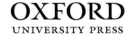

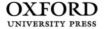

Great Clarendon Street, Oxford, OX2 6DP,
United Kingdom

Oxford University Press is a department of the University of Oxford.
It furthers the University's objective of excellence in research, scholarship,
and education by publishing worldwide. Oxford is a registered trade mark of
Oxford University Press in the UK and in certain other countries

First Edition published in 2022

Impression: 1

Published in the United States of America by Oxford University Press
198 Madison Avenue, New York, NY 10016, United States of America

British Library Cataloguing in Publication Data

Data available

Library of Congress Control Number: 2021944588

ISBN 978–0–19–886527–8

DOI: 10.1093/med/9780198865278.001.0001

Printed and bound by
CPI Group (UK) Ltd, Croydon, CR0 4YY

For Meredith,
For always being there for me

Acknowledgements

Many people played an instrumental role in making this book possible, although not everyone may be aware of their contribution. First, I wish to thank Professor Fredrik Karpe for sharing his inspiring fascination with and knowledge of adipose tissue as it opened my eyes to a biological world to which I had previously little exposure. Those formative years spent in the laboratory for my postgraduate studies with him, Dr Katherine Pinnick, and the many, many brilliant people at the Oxford Centre for Diabetes, Endocrinology, and Metabolism laid the groundwork for this book.

I would like to thank my undergraduate mentors, Dr Richard Boyd, Dr Paul Dennis, Professor William James, and Dr Piers Nye who provided a wonderful, unique learning environment that cultivated a life-long scientific curiosity. I also appreciate the words of encouragement from Professor Russell Foster and Professor Frances Ashcroft to pursue this project and whose science communication efforts act as great sources of inspiration. I also wish to thank my parents, Sue and George, for their support during this substantial task. Finally, I want to thank Meredith, my wonderful wife, for her tireless cheerleading, unending patience, and insightful feedback on multiple drafts.

Contents

Abbreviations   xi

1. Introduction   1

2. A Brief History of Body Shape   7

3. What Does Fat Do?   47

4. I Can Get Fat Where? The Other Types of Fat   91

5. What Shape Is Healthy? Body Composition, Body Shape,
    and Health   121

6. Same but Different: Fat Biology around the Body   161

7. Defining Your Shape: The Determinants of Body Fat
    Distribution   197

8. Conclusion   271

Index   279

Abbreviations

α-MSH	alpha-melanocyte-stimulating hormone
AgRP	agouti-related protein
ATP	adenosine triphosphate
BIA	bioelectrical impedance analysis
BMD	bone mineral density
BMI	body mass index
CGL1	congenital generalized lipodystrophy type 1
CGL2	congenital generalized lipodystrophy type 2
CT	computed tomography
DNL	*de novo* lipogenesis
DNP	2,4-dinitrophenol
DXA	dual-energy X-ray absorptiometry
ER	oestrogen receptor
FH	familial hypercholesterolaemia
fMRI	functional MRI
FPLD	familial partial lipodystrophy of the Dunnigan variety
GWAS	genome-wide association studies
HDL	high-density lipoproteins
HIIT	high-intensity interval training
HRT	hormone replacement therapy
HSL	hormone sensitive lipase
LDL	low-density lipoproteins
LPL	lipoprotein lipase
MCRs	melanocortin receptors
MDP	mandibular dysplasia with deafness and progeroid features syndrome
MHO	metabolically healthy obesity
MRI	magnetic resonance imaging
NAFLD	non-alcoholic fatty liver disease
PCOS	polycystic ovary syndrome
PET	positron emission tomography
PPARG	peroxisome proliferator-activated receptor gamma
SVF	stromovascular fraction
TAG	triacylglycerol

TZDs   thiazolidinediones
UCP-1   uncoupling protein 1
VLDL   very low-density lipoproteins
WHO   World Health Organization
WHR   waist-hip ratio

1
Introduction

Fat, and its associated negative health consequences, garners significant media attention and is a frequent topic of conversation with our doctors, partners, children, friends, and colleagues. The frequency and intensity of such discussions has only grown in recent decades in tandem with the substantial increase in obesity over a breathtakingly short period of time. The global prevalence of adult and childhood obesity has nearly tripled since 1975 and shows little sign of slowing. Major contributing factors in this growing crisis include our increasingly sedentary lifestyles and changing dietary habits, aided in large part by ineffective preventative policies, increasingly industrialized food manufacturing practices, and unhelpful social attitudes and norms. With the global obesity crisis unfolding before our very eyes, wreaking ever-increasing amounts of havoc on individuals, communities, healthcare systems, and economies, now, more than ever, is the time to understand what fat is, what it does, and why.

The current prevalence of overweight and obesity around the world is staggering. In their most recent statistics,[1] the World Health Organization (WHO) estimate that 39% of the world's adult population (i.e., 18 years and older) were overweight and 13% were obese in 2016. This translates to more than two billion overweight adults, of which over 650 million are obese. Such figures should stop any medical doctor, politician, or socially aware citizen in their tracks. Compounding this dire situation is the increase in childhood obesity, with approximately 41 million children under the age of 5 years classified as overweight or obese in 2016. Emerging evidence also suggests that the current generation of children are less active, less fit, and weaker,[2] meaning they are being set up for a shorter life expectancy coupled with more illness. The projections for 2030 onwards make for pretty grim reading as well.[3] The scale of obesity and its associated issues are so vast and far-reaching that obesity has even been deemed a threat to national security.[4]

This list of statistics about how the world is going to collapse under our collective weight should be shocking, but perhaps not entirely surprising. If anything, the scale of the problem is almost too large to comprehend and the numbers have essentially lost their impact and meaning through repetition. But why are these monolithic statistics important? Being overweight or obese puts individuals at significantly increased risk of developing numerous health problems,[3] such as cardiovascular disease (e.g., heart disease and stroke), metabolic disease (e.g., type 2 diabetes), musculoskeletal disorders (particularly increased risk of fracture and osteoarthritis, a disabling degeneration of the joints), certain cancers (e.g., of the breast, endometrium, ovaries, prostate, liver, gallbladder, kidney, and colon), and respiratory problems (e.g., sleep apnoea, in which individuals stop breathing whilst sleeping). Aside from these non-communicable diseases, obesity is complicating the battle against COVID-19 as it is associated with significantly worse outcomes in patients infected with the virus.[5]

Being overweight or obese puts an immense strain on one's body and can accelerate the path to ill health or an untimely demise. What is not so clear, however, is whether obesity itself is a disease; has anyone died as a direct result of being obese? This heated debate boiled over in 2013, when the American Medical Association moved to classify obesity as a disease,[6] thus codifying the century-old medical framing of obesity[7] and associated treatment of numerous diseases caused by obesity. While some still resist such 'medicalization', an abundance of evidence indicates that dysfunctional adipose tissue is a major contributing factor to obesity and obesity-related diseases, such as type 2 diabetes. In 2019, 463 million adults were estimated to have type 2 diabetes worldwide, with projections suggesting it will affect 700 million people by 2040.[8] However, not all overweight or obese people get diabetes, and not all people with diabetes are overweight or obese. This curious situation is an example of the fact that *where* we accumulate fat is actually more important than *how much* we accumulate. The message that we should be watching not only our weight, but where it accrues has been slow to enter the public's consciousness. *Waisted* fills this gap by exploring the biology underlying the relationship between body composition, regional fat distribution, and health.

As we will see throughout the pages of this book, fat affects far more than our health, as its accumulation and striking pattern of distribution through the body makes a significant contribution to the human condition. Fat not only contains the surplus calories that enabled our evolution. It is also laden with myriad social and cultural meanings that vary by place and time. Excessive accumulation of fat in the form of obesity has represented power, respect, and wealth in various societies throughout the ages,[9] as embodied in such striking physiques as the gluttonous Henry VIII to no fewer than five US presidents (William Howard Taft, Grover Cleveland, William McKinley, Zachary Taylor, and Theodore Roosevelt). Obesity can equally be a mark of shame, poverty, immorality, gluttony, and mental weakness, as detractors of the aforementioned Henry VIII stated towards the end of his reign (and life).

Moreover, fat is the vital substance responsible for the distinctive female and male forms that are subject to dynamic, nuanced, and sometimes contradictory meanings that guide and reflect our place and status within society. Whether a woman's figure is deemed slim, petite, shapeless, curvy, voluptuous, or fat, adipose tissue is responsible for the soft feminine curves that have inspired endless debate and artistic expression. These emotive shapes have been represented in art for centuries,[7] from the carved stone Venus of Willendorf statue (estimated date of creation 28,000 – 25,000 BCE), to Peter Paul Ruben's famous paintings of the full-bodied female form during the late 1600s, to contemporary plus-size fashion models such as Tess Holiday adorning the front cover of Cosmopolitan magazine in August 2018.[10] The hard, masculine lines defined by its absence have equally been a source of inspiration (and frustration) for many through the ages, spanning the ancient Roman depiction of Apollo Belvedere to the superlative physiques adorning Hollywood, the Olympic games, and mainstream and social media alike. Simply put, fat has played, and continues to play, a foundational role in shaping our biology, our bodies, and our society.

It is now time to embark on a whistle-stop tour of fat biology, with a focus on white adipose tissue. Certain details might be familiar to some readers, but hopefully much will be new and interesting. As there is a huge breadth of evolving material to cover on many different fronts, *Waisted* aims to present the salient points which draw different academic realms together. As such, the purpose of furnishing *Waisted* with extensive citations serves two purposes; to provide a body of evidence to support its claims and provide numerous jumping-off points to further explore literature for those so inclined.

As a growing proportion of the global population joins the swelling ranks of a demographic that is not only at greater risk of developing all manner of disease, but has often been victim of prejudice and ridicule, understanding fat biology and how it intersects with society is crucial. As such, Chapter 2 considers the origins of fat and the vital role it has played in the evolutionary history of humans, as well as the reasons underpinning its conspicuous distribution pattern in humans. The second part of this chapter examines different sociocultural perspectives on body shape in a bid to understand how the evolutionary origins and biological functions of fat inform the deeply entrenched attitudes towards the social and aesthetic meanings assigned to this tissue and how they vary around the world.

Chapter 3 provides an overview of the various biological functions of (white) adipose tissue in the context of its evolutionary origins, while Chapter 4 explores the biology of some of the more esoteric types of fat, namely brown adipose tissue and bone marrow fat. Chapter 5 then returns to the main white fat story and reviews the different methods used to measure body fat mass and distribution before discussing the evidence indicating that where, rather than how much, fat accumulates plays a crucial role in determining one's health. Additionally, it highlights that the way obesity is evaluated and defined will likely evolve to reflect our increasingly nuanced understanding. Chapter 6 explores the ways in which the biological properties of fat vary around the body before the mechanisms underpinning different fat depots acting 'the same but different' are considered. Finally, Chapter 7 draws upon the previously introduced concepts and information to explore how various important factors such as genetics, hormones, and surgery can influence body fat distribution and health.

Fat played a crucial role in the evolution of modern humanity, but now it occupies an instrumental role in one of the most important existential crises humanity has ever faced. The need to understand the 'enemy within' has never been greater. Exploring the origins and function of fat represents an opportunity to re-evaluate our relationship with an oft-derided part of our body that is actually vital for life. Such consideration is a necessary first step towards forming a new relationship with fat in which we treat it with the respect it deserves and strive to provide it, and therefore ourselves, with what it needs to function properly. Such work will be essential if we are to avert the health crisis unfolding before our very eyes.

References

1. WHO factsheet - overweight and obesity. *World Health Organization* (2018). Available at: www.who.int/mediacentre/factsheets/fs311/en/ .
2. Sandercock, G. R. H. & Cohen, D. D. Temporal trends in muscular fitness of English 10-year-olds 1998–2014: an allometric approach. *J. Sci. Med. Sport* (2018). doi:10.1016/j.jsams.2018.07.020

3. Blüher, M. Obesity: global epidemiology and pathogenesis. *Nat. Rev. Endocrinol.* **15**, 288–98 (2019).

4. Popkin, B. M. Is the obesity epidemic a national security issue around the globe? *Curr. Opin. Endocrinol. Diabetes. Obes.* **18**, 328–31 (2011).

5. Simonnet, A. *et al.* High prevalence of obesity in severe acute respiratory syndrome coronavirus-2 (SARS-CoV-2) requiring invasive mechanical ventilation. *Obesity* **28**, 1195–9 (2020).

6. Fitzpatrick, K. Obesity is now a disease, American Medical Association decides. *Medical News Today* (2013). Available at: www.medicalnewstoday.com/articles/262226.php .

7. Eknoyan, G. A history of obesity, or how what was good became ugly and then bad. *Adv. Chronic Kidney Dis.* **13**, 421–7 (2006).

8. Saeedi, P. *et al.* Global and regional diabetes prevalence estimates for 2019 and projections for 2030 and 2045: results from the International Diabetes Federation Diabetes Atlas, 9th edition. *Diabetes Res. Clin. Pract.* **157**, 107843 (2019).

9. Forth, C. E. *Fat: A Cultural History of the Stuff of Life.* Reaktion Books, 2019.

10. BBC. 'This is what plus-sized women have needed.' *BBC News* (2018). Available at: www.bbc.co.uk/news/newsbeat-45354696.

2
A Brief History of Body Shape

Part 1—Forging the Human Form

 To make sense of the wide-ranging and powerful social meanings assigned to body shape around the world, it is first necessary to turn the clock back to see where it all began. As will become clear, however enlightened the human race may be, or thinks it is, social attitudes towards the body are built upon a deeply rooted evolutionary foundation which likely developed primarily to ensure that the human race survived, even thrived. The evolution of our impressive intellect has also facilitated the development of modern civilization. Building on our primordial foundations, a rich, sophisticated, and dynamic tapestry of social meanings and attitudes has emerged towards our bodies. We begin this chapter by considering the origins of humanity to see how the archetypal male and female body shapes first came into being.

Walking Tall

The emergence of fat tissue represents a crucial step in the evolution of almost all biological life on the planet for it effectively uncouples an organism's energy demands from the amount of calories immediately available in its surrounding environment. This development was a watershed evolutionary moment. When the food supply is unpredictable, perishable, and generally scarce, the ability to hoard calories in internal stores makes it possible to maintain a constant internal environment (i.e., homeostasis). Fat tissue enabled organisms to accumulate an energy supply to keep the metabolic furnace burning between meals and gain a foothold over their harsh environment. This ability not only fostered the development of more sophisticated and energy-demanding organs like the brain, but also made it possible for organisms to migrate to better habitats as a survival strategy.

Simply put, fat played—and continues to play—a highly important and necessary role in evolution.

Another defining event in evolutionary history was the transition of our primate ancestors from being occasionally to fully bipedal. Evolutionary biologists suggest that this change to upright posture could have been to intimidate or threaten, similar to primates. Whatever the impetus, the pressure to literally 'stand up and fight' to survive might have shaped the development of other aspects of our anatomy as well. Our hands, for example, may have evolved not to operate tools, but rather to form fists for primordial fighting.[1] Once our ancestors embarked on the evolutionary path of bipedalism, this new upright posture imposed new demands on the fledgling human form that are relevant to the story of fat and body shape. Adaptations to such demands over time, in turn, resulted in additional biological advances to the upright posture.

A key part of our anatomy that underwent significant evolutionary change was the pelvis.[2] The modern pelvis is an anatomical melting pot of adaptations that emerged to meet locomotive and obstetric demands[3] in a way that allowed humans to evolve and develop greater intelligence. The selective pressure for a permanently upright posture contributed to substantial remodelling of our ancestor's quadrupedal bodies to support bipedal locomotion. Such changes involved modifying the pelvis's structure to accommodate vertically oriented legs, a process which was accompanied by parallel changes in the shape and arrangement of our spine and vertebrae.[2,4] This realignment resulted in a kinking of the pelvis that pushed our primal buttocks backwards, thereby giving rise to one of the more distinctive curves of the human body. In addition to the changed angle, our ancestor's pelvis also shortened considerably, creating a lengthened space between our ribs that would become our waist. From an evolutionary standpoint, these substantial anatomical changes related to bipedalism would only have taken place if they conferred a competitive advantage in the hostile lands our early ancestors roamed. They were not the only helpful adaptations. What other aspects of bipedalism enabled our ancestors to get ahead in the world, securing their ability to survive and thrive?

The switch to bipedalism was a game-changer for it allowed our ancestors to employ new biological and behavioural strategies to survive in the elements and procure food. These approaches were then retained, reinforced, and developed further through descendants of the successful and fertile. In the context of bipedal locomotion, the pelvis and associated musculature evolved to support the ability to traverse long distances with great efficiency.[5] This enabled humans to practise persistence hunting to procure food. Still practised by some tribes living relatively untouched by the modern world, this technique involves chasing animals for hours or days at a time until they become exhausted enough to be easily trapped and killed.[6] The relative importance and timing of persistence hunting and foraging along our evolutionary and migratory timeline remain somewhat unclear, although scholars suggest that the ability to efficiently traverse long distances could also support land-based migration.[7]

While the pelvis was under significant evolutionary pressure to support efficient locomotion so people could literally run with the pack, reproduction imposed a different, competing set of ergonomic demands on pelvic anatomy, particularly for women. Successful pregnancy and birth with minimal complications and harm to the mother favours a wider pelvic structure and birth canal, a pressure which conflicts directly with the narrower pelvic shape required for efficient bipedal locomotion.[3] Selective pressure for such anatomy increased further alongside human's increased dependence on greater intelligence to solve problems threatening their survival. There was thus a need to accommodate babies being born with increasingly large brains (and therefore heads), as well as an accelerated metabolic rate to support such organs. Meeting this increased energy demand involved expanding fat mass, with humans evolving to carry a relatively larger proportion of body fat compared to chimpanzees, bonobos, gorillas, and orangutans.[8]

The disproportionately larger brains, and heads required to support them, however, are thought to have eventually hit an upper limit—one imposed by the physical constraints of the female reproductive anatomy. More specifically, the trajectory of human development and evolution may have been directed by the limited amount of space through which a baby could fit. The success of evolving intelligence was thus jeopardized by the physical constraints of our ancestral mothers' anatomy. Scholars suggest that this biological impasse was overcome by delivering the foetus at an earlier stage in development[9] via a special rotational manoeuvre unique to humans that allows a still relatively large foetal head to pass through the birth canal.[10] This trade-off meant that the development of the increasingly sophisticated human brain would now be delayed to an unusually protracted post-natal period that lasts well into and beyond adolescence.[11] These adaptations proved to be the masterstroke that unstuck the evolutionary log-jam; humans would evolve greater intelligence via larger, more powerful brains while retaining a pelvis that was narrow enough for efficient movement yet wide enough to achieve relatively complication-free birth.

As one might imagine, the pressure that giving birth selectively imposes on women has resulted in sex-specific differences in pelvic anatomy that exert subtle but detectable biomechanical effects on human gait, with men's legs tending to be more parallel and women's slightly angled.[12] The modern pelvic and birth canal anatomy truly walks the fine line necessary for biological success. In addition to these obstetric and locomotive demands, there is mounting evidence that the shape of our pelvis was moulded by the need to regulate our body temperature. While not an obvious function of this strangely shaped array of bones, the pelvis plays a pivotal role in determining the dimensions and surface area of our body.[3] As these physical properties influence how our body retains/loses heat (e.g., a larger pelvis gives rise to a smaller body surface area-to-volume ratio, a feature which reduces heat loss), the pelvis's size and shape may therefore affect one's chances of survival during exposure to harsh conditions in which rudimentary shelter and clothing are the only available protection. Unable to simply dial up the air-conditioning or central heating in ancient times, it has been suggested that the size and shape of our ancestor's pelvises reflect what climatic conditions they were exposed to, which may explain geography-specific variation in pelvis shape[13] (in which natives of hotter climes tend to have elongated, narrower bodies which lose heat more easily). The pelvis's finely honed shape and size thus say a great deal about our collective history, with the female pelvis evolving into the gateway for future generations.

The Changing Face of Reality

Our ancestor's anatomy underwent additional significant sex-specific changes that enabled them to survive in uncompromising environments while their weaker counterparts (and their insufficient biological traits) were culled from the gene pool. The modern human face, for example, lost the prominent bony ridges that distinguished our primate ancestors while the evolution of an increasingly large and sophisticated brain required the development of a suitably sized domed head to accommodate it.[14] It has also been suggested that our faces, particularly those of males, have adopted shapes that were better suited to protect our precious, vulnerable brains during primitive fistfights.[15] Additionally, our teeth and jaw anatomy evolved to accommodate our increasingly omnivorous diet.[16]

Other changes to human anatomy might have been reinforced by the complex emergence of sex-specific roles in society.[17] Although it is almost impossible to know which came first, sex-specific biology and sex-specific social roles engage in a dynamic, reciprocal relationship; they modify and reinforce each other according to the opportunities and constraints imposed by society, as well as the physical attributes and reproductive activities of each sex to both shape and reflect the nature of society.[18] Men and women would have experienced common pressures to reach a minimum level of mobility, strength, and endurance, for instance, to participate in migration and foraging, and to defend oneself as necessary. However, women's reproductive capability would have increased their likelihood of engaging in less dangerous agricultural and domestic roles. Men, in contrast, engaged far more in warfare, hunting, and building—activities which probably contributed to the development of significantly greater upper body strength accordingly.[19]

Despite the immense pressure to survive, however, the evolutionary process can be modified to an extent by *sexual selection*, a type of social selection.[20] This phenomenon refers to the situation in which a biological feature is preferentially selected during reproduction and so becomes more common in future generations as a result of mate selection. Evolutionary biologists suggest that sexual selection might have been particularly important in shaping the modern human's physical form. Certain aspects of our biology might have been removed or exaggerated over the generations, so long as such modifications didn't jeopardize the health, fertility, functionality, or survival of the evolving human race. The evolutionary process is also subject to external factors such as famine (in which women's higher proportional body fat mass is believed to underlie their survival advantage compared to men during total starvation[21]), with such factors constraining the number and filtering the characteristics of the fertile population from which the next generation derives. In other words, the modern human face and body are the products of selection, in part, based on ergonomics and aesthetics.

Some facial arrangements or features might have been preferred as they reinforced visual differences between the emerging modern human from other primate species, or better distinguished men from women.[22] Others might have been chosen as they conveyed specific meanings within society about the perceived longer-term health or fertility of the individual, affecting decisions regarding the choice of mates and other types of social partner.[23] As will be discussed later, whatever the basis of and truth to these associations, their ubiquitous and timeless nature suggests that they are a hard-wired feature of the human condition. Sexual selection ultimately seems to go hand in hand with the emergence of human attraction and the assignation of social meanings to the shapes and sizes of bodies and their features. This phenomenon will continue to be relevant and important throughout the rest of this chapter.

Fat and Fertility

History has seen a deep evolutionary link forged between energy availability, adipose tissue, and reproduction in humans, as well as many other members of the animal kingdom. Pregnancy and lactation are incredibly energy-demanding and time-consuming processes which represent a massive commitment by the prospective parents and their resident society. The substantial amount of energy required to support pregnancy means that numerous biological mechanisms have evolved to maximize the chances of successful reproduction by coupling a woman's energy reserves to her fertility. While other organisms align reproduction to predictable oscillations in energy availability in the *external* environment (e.g., herbivorous animals give birth in the spring when food is plentiful), the evolutionary trajectory of humans relies much more heavily on *internal* energy stores (i.e., adipose tissue). Simply put, on the long, demanding journey that is pregnancy, humans pack their own proverbial lunch while the rest of the animal kingdom coordinates their supply stops to the natural rhythms of the outside world.

If a woman's energy reserves are insufficient to support pregnancy and lactation, a variety of mechanisms kick in which reduce her fertility and prevent her from being able to successfully reproduce.[24] The range of absolute and relative amounts of fat required for a woman to be fertile has been shaped through thousands of years of biological trial and error; the result is that ~17% body fat appears to be required for the onset of puberty while ~22% body fat is required for regular menstruation.[25] Body fat mass below 10–15% is associated with disruption or cessation of menstruation/fertility. This can, however, be reversed when a woman's fat stores become sufficiently replete (discussed in more detail in Chapter 3). Such a mechanism is self-preserving as it allows the demands on a woman's limited energy reserves to be carefully balanced between the conflicting needs of her own short-term survival and the longer-term survival of humanity via reproduction. Perturbation of this ancient link manifests in complex conditions that increase a woman's risk of various negative health consequences beyond fertility issues. Examples include anorexia nervosa, in which women are often amenorrhoeic, and obesity, which increases one's risk of infertility, cardiovascular and metabolic disease, and certain cancers.

The ability to accumulate fat thus marks a milestone in our evolutionary trajectory and survival as a species. On the one hand, the complex integration of numerous competing selection pressures to manage our molecular and social environment helped support everyday existence, reproduction, and the development of increasingly sophisticated cognitive processes and intellectual capacity. It also guided the physical distribution of our fat stores, resulting in phenomena as disparate as pregnancy and lactation, immunity, appetite, mood, attraction, and metabolic health becoming linked via overall and regional fat accumulation.[26] Emerging from humanity's protracted struggle for existence was the archetypal male and female form which exemplify the ultimate fusion of ergonomics and aesthetics, arguably more so than any other organism currently residing on earth.

The ability to accumulate fat thus conferred a critical evolutionary advantage for humans. That said, fat accumulation can be a double-edged sword, as accumulating fat in a disorganized manner might generate situations which conflict with the ability to successfully respond to other evolutionary pressures. Poised at the interface between competing evolutionary pressures and sex-specific patterns of body composition (i.e., muscle mass), regional fat accumulation, and reproductive biology are the sex steroids, with oestrogen evolving to play the starring role in women[27] and testosterone in men.[28]

As part of its role as co-ordinator for female sexual development, oestrogen directs the localized accumulation of fat in the lower body (i.e., thighs and buttocks). This effect may have something to do with the fact that storing the massive amount of energy required to support pregnancy solely in the upper body would raise a woman's centre of gravity and decrease stability while pregnant[29] or carrying an infant.[30] Scholars suggest that social meanings may have also emerged about body shape that reinforced this pattern of lower body fat accumulation. A woman with an ample supply of stored calories (manifesting as rounded buttocks and thighs) conveyed the message that she stood a good chance of staving off starvation and successfully reproducing, thus resulting in curvier lower bodies being deemed sexually attractive features.[31]

Conversely, the testosterone-driven lean, muscular physique of the archetypal male[32] has traditionally come to be associated with the ability to provide and protect.[33] Likely forged by different selection pressures to those women experienced, it is unclear why the male body has a preponderance to store fat in the abdomen; this may reflect the biomechanics required for (bipedal) hand-to-hand combat[1] and subsistence activity,[34] and/or the possible interplay between testosterone's immune-suppressing effects[35] and visceral fat's role in inflammation and immunity.[36] Regardless, acting on such primordial beliefs as they survived and reproduced, our ancestors would have perpetuated this cycle, propagating the underlying biology and associated social messages.

The Mystery of the Mammaries

Human breasts are unique within the animal kingdom. While all mammals have nipples to support the production and feeding of milk to offspring, no other animal has physically discernible breasts that persist throughout their (adult) lifetime, irrespective of reproductive or lactation status. This curious situation means that the origin of the modern human breast is somewhat shrouded in mystery and intrigue, despite the considerable attention they have historically attracted. The majority of a woman's accumulated calories are not stored in the breast, even for women with an ample bosom. That said, breasts represent a prominent anatomical location in women where fat visibly accumulates, thereby prompting the suggestion that permanent breasts evolved as a visible sign of a woman's nutritional stores and reproductive capacity.[31,37] Biomechanically speaking, however, the breast does not represent a particularly comfortable or ergonomic way of storing calories, as many women who play sports will attest.[38,39] Not only getting in the way of rigorous physical activity, breasts can also cause back pain in many women.[40] In some respects, the modern human breast is often a physical hindrance.

Considering the curious anatomy of the human female breast, the emergence of the modern human breast may be the by-product of other evolutionary processes and/or sexual selection. If breasts played the same biological role as buttocks and thighs, then this would suggest that larger permanent breasts would accurately reflect a woman's greater ability to support pregnancy, a phenomenon which would be reinforced if women with larger breasts were more likely to find a mate and reproduce successfully.

Indeed, it has been suggested that breasts convey a visual signal that indicates a woman's reproductive potential[41] or fertility/ovulatory status.[42] This doesn't seem to be the case though, as actual breast size[43] and male preferences for breast size and shape[44,45] vary considerably around the world (along with other non-physiological preferences). Moreover, breast size (according to—admittedly suboptimal—brassiere size data) varies significantly around the world,[46] as does birth rate.[47] While the relationship between reproductive potential and breast size is somewhat unclear, lower body fat distribution appears to represent the most accurate and reliable anthropometric predictor of fertility.[48,49]

In the absence of obvious ergonomic reasons, pronounced and permanent breasts may have evolved to better delineate the physical form of women from men, or humans from other species. It has even been proposed that breasts serve an erotic role[50] and were potentially selected through the act of persistent sexual activity unrelated to reproduction that served to maintain and cultivate long-term parental relationships (i.e., after genes had already been passed on) which play an important role in the nurturing of children through to adulthood.[51] The latter argument is weakened by the observations documented in the landmark 'Patterns of Sexual Behaviour' study published in 1951, however, which highlighted that many cultures outside of the West do not see breasts as sexually significant. This is particularly the case in subsistence societies where women are frequently topless[52] and breasts are usually associated more with notions of maturity and maternity. Given this, breast evolution in human females may simply be the by-product of the subcutaneous fat accumulation required to support human survival and reproduction.[37] So, how did breasts emerge in the first place?

The Land of Milk and Honey
The coincident accumulation of fat in the hips, thighs, and breasts of women is underpinned by oestrogen, the hormone whose actions may also provide the connection to fertility and lactation.[27] Indeed, the structure of the modern human breast may have been shaped considerably by the complex evolution of lactation, a phenomenon believed to have originated in ancient organisms who utilized a specialized multi-cellular structure to provide moisture and nutrients to permeable eggs.[53] This basic structure is believed to have combined with glands capable of secreting substances to the external environment and their associated hair follicles before undergoing extensive modification as mammals emerged and evolved.

The modern human breast, comprised of glandular tissue and a distinct nipple, was thus honed through millennia of biological trial and error in which individuals capable of performing lactation (thereby secreting a complex, nutrient-rich milk that supports infants) reaped the benefits it conferred through stronger and healthier offspring.[54] It is likely that the primitive breast gained sensitivity to the hormone oestrogen during this evolutionary process,[55] a feature which would provide a crucial mechanism linking breast development to lower body fat accumulation, as well as sexual development and fertility.

Lactation is an incredibly energy-demanding task which connects lower body fat accumulation in women with reproduction. Although the energy demand required to support pregnancy is significant, especially when the food supply is unpredictable, it is dwarfed by the much larger energy demand for the production of breast milk after birth.[56] While adipose tissue is present in the breast structure, a substantial proportion of the energy contained within breast milk is actually derived from fatty acids preferentially stored in the hips and thighs,[57,58] some of which derive from the diet while others are produced by the body.[59] This includes polyunsaturated fatty acids (see Chapter 3), such as linoleic acid, that play a crucial role in the development of a newborn's visual system and brain.[60]

When it comes to lactation, fertility, and breasts, is bigger better? While larger breasts may be indicative of larger overall fat stores, particularly lower body stores that could support pregnancy and lactation, milk production actually correlates with the amount of epithelial/glandular tissue within a breast,[61] not its overall size.[62] This means that larger breasts do not necessarily signify a greater capacity to produce milk. On the contrary, overweight or obese women (who typically have larger breasts) often struggle to initiate the production of milk or produce only small amounts[63] due to a disproportionate amount of fat in their breasts that renders their glandular tissue dysfunctional and compromises their ability to produce milk. In the absence of conclusive research on how milk production and reproductive capacity correlate with an accurate index of overall breast and glandular tissue mass, it seems that (breast) quality is more important than size when it comes to lactation.

In terms of attraction, breast shape and size may provide a secondary visual signal that complements or supplements the appearance of a woman's thighs and hips, the biological attributes which provide the most accurate and reliable visual indicator of a woman's nutritional stores and reproductive capacity.[48,49] This common misperception may not be based on an intentionally deceptive strategy to promote the propagation of an individual's genes,[64,65] but could have simply arisen from the secondary role breasts play in the context of reproduction and nutritional capacity. Ultimately, understanding the relationship between body shape and size, perceived attractiveness, and reproductive success[66] (even general health[67]) represents a fertile ground for further detailed investigation.

The process of lactation essentially secured the breast as a permanent structure in the archetypal female form during evolution. Building on this basic structure, however, a wide range of breast sizes and shapes emerged around the world that may actually be the product of primarily sexual selection. Guided by forces constrained and focused by migration and/or social norms, it is possible that breasts of certain shapes and sizes acquired distinct but overlapping social meanings deemed desirable (or not) within certain geographical areas or societies. Indeed, social and cultural beliefs about other body parts—not just breasts—have emerged over time and may have influenced sexual selection—and therefore the evolution—of the modern female form. Exploring the evolutionary origins of our bodies and the social meanings attached to them increases our understanding of the human race and the attitudes towards body shape that pervade modern society.

Part 2—The 'Beautiful' People

Attraction is a complex phenomenon which can be thought to serve a very simple purpose in evolutionary terms; to help us choose the best possible mate. Choosing a mate is not straightforward and involves receiving, decoding, and integrating a variety of different types of information, as well as identifying and navigating deceptive signals that serve a selfish purpose. Although running the risk of being derided as purely superficial, some of the most important factors which inform the phenomenon of attraction are visual, although sounds and smells also contribute.[23] Such biological attributes serve as 'sexual advertising' for an organism to indicate its biological quality and health. They are abundant across the plant and animal kingdoms, and humans are no different.[68] Selective pressures can pertain to 'attractiveness' as well as, and in relation to, functionality. Such pressures might affect something as simple as the physical form of a body part or as complex as the sound of a voice[69] or personality trait.[70] They may also manifest as magnificent anomalies of nature such as the visually stunning yet ergonomically cumbersome peacock's tail. Our planet provides a competitive environment, one in which any step that can promote the likelihood of passing on an organism's genes must be taken. That said, there is often room for some range of variation around the archetype that meets the minimal requirement to survive and reproduce. And where a range exists, a hierarchy will surely follow.

As discussed previously, ample nutritional stores as conveyed by rounded hips, thighs, and breasts would send the visual message that a female is more likely to survive a period of famine and/or support pregnancy. In addition, wider hips and thighs may suggest that a woman is not only more fertile, but also less likely to suffer obstetrical problems.[71] In the face of adversity, such physical features would become attractive, as would the methods of identifying and obtaining the best possible mate. Other physical features convey visual signals of an individual's health and 'biological quality' as well. For instance, the degree of symmetry between body parts provides valuable information about functionality and development. Scholars note that more symmetrical body patterns are not only more functional[72] (e.g., for locomotion), but that they also convey a visual signal that an individual has a strong biological heritage and underwent a healthy developmental process. Although it may be a disheartening and somewhat superficial sentiment, mounting evidence indicates that physically 'attractive' characteristics contribute toward better health and reproductive prospects.[73] Indeed, it appears that a higher degree of symmetry in the face[74] and bilateral body parts (like breasts) has not only traditionally been deemed to be more attractive, but is also associated with greater fertility in women,[75,76] higher sperm counts in men,[77] and better overall health.[72]

In the Eye of the Beholder?

Methods to accurately assess (and possibly just appreciate) a prospective mate's health status and reproductive capacity likely emerged and permeated society similar to mechanisms for helping an individual find and select the best mate. Determining how physically 'attractive' a person is involves assimilating several different types of information, often from distinct but related features. This process rarely relies on a single piece of information in isolation, even if individuals may fixate on a particular aspect. Of all the possible places to look, it appears that men's eyes[78,79] are drawn to the waist and hips when asked to judge the physical attractiveness of a woman. While there are inherent difficulties in studying such a subjective phenomenon, data from various studies indicate that waist-to-hip ratio (see Chapter 5 for details) accurately predicts the perceived physical 'attractiveness' of a woman.[80,81] This should perhaps be unsurprising given that the size and shape of a woman's hips and thighs in proportion to each other conveys the most accurate and reliable visual signal of a woman's fertility.[48,49] Waist-to-hip ratio's influence in determining attractiveness in women has even been reported amongst blind people who have shown a preference, determined by touch, for women with a lower waist-to-hip ratio[82] (i.e., a narrow waist with wider hips).

Despite the apparent fixation of the mass media and many people (particularly Westerners) with breasts, it may be surprising that they do not seem to exert a particularly strong influence on men and women's perceived attractiveness of a woman.[83] Indeed, their effect appears to depend on other factors such as overall fatness and the relative proportionality of the waist and hips.[81] It has been suggested that larger breasts may not necessarily be attractive in isolation, but instead serve to emphasize waist-to-hip proportionality.[84] Moreover, pervading societal views of female body shape have been reinforced in media and pop culture to suggest, not without criticism, that large, symmetrical breasts and narrow hips convey youthfulness, fertility, health, and desirability whereas larger bodies and a high waist-to-hip ratio make the female figure appear older and less attractive.[85] Body proportionality, particularly between the waist and hips, appears to be the most important determinant of female attractiveness (often peaking at an ideal waist-to-hip ratio of 0.7^{78}), with overall fatness playing a crucial, albeit secondary, role. This is most clearly illustrated in studies in which waist-to-hip ratio has been repeatedly found to represent the main variable that predicts perceived female physical attractiveness, regardless of whether women are slim or reside on the heavier end of the BMI spectrum.[86]

Research suggests that body size and proportionality are only part of the attractiveness equation though; a high degree of body symmetry has also been found to be desirable.[87] The desire for minimal body asymmetry has been shown to be relevant to many different parts of the (female) body, but it is particularly so for bilateral anatomical features such as the breasts.[88] Additionally, the degree of facial symmetry (using the distance between the eyes and nose shape as reference points) heavily influences the perception of a person's attractiveness.[89] These associations between health and physical appearance reportedly reflect reality (at least for judging the attractiveness of women[90]), although many gaps in our understanding of the nature and evolution of human attraction remain.[91]

Loved around the World

Preferences around the male and female form are undoubtedly shaped by a combination of evolutionary biology and sociocultural factors. For example, what constitutes the ideal male body varies around the world according to a number of aforementioned evolutionary factors (e.g., related to strength) as well as sociocultural factors (e.g., social expectations related to socioeconomic status), although there is a growing trend in which the lean, muscular physique deemed the most desirable in the West is increasingly spreading around the world.[92] Given the beneficial effects that fat accumulation, particularly in the lower body, has on a woman's reproductive and survival capacity, it should not be particularly surprising that shapely hips and thighs (i.e., hips and thighs that are proportionately larger than one's waist) are revered almost universally around the world.[93,94] This preference for lower body fat accumulation is shared by distinct populations from locales as diverse as the US,[95] New Zealand,[95] Papua New Guinea,[96] China,[97] and Cameroon.[98]

Despite compelling evidence that curvaceous hips and thighs in women have broad appeal, exceptions have been found. For instance, some studies have found that waist-to-hip ratio does not predict female attractiveness in Japan[99] and South Africa,[100] whereas other factors such as overall fatness (according to BMI) and breast size do. Such inconsistent results may be due to the study design or participants sampled, or they may represent genuinely different sociocultural preferences. As body fatness and body shape are inextricably linked, designing studies that clearly identify which is more important can be difficult, a situation exacerbated further by language differences. Some intrepid researchers have, however, managed to overcome considerable obstacles to gain insights into the meanings of bodies that have emerged from our evolutionary heritage by trekking across the world to study tribes which remain relatively undisturbed by modernity. The Hadza tribe of Tanzania has proven to be particularly informative in this regard. Consistent with expectations, this tribe appears to find women with a lower waist-to-hip ratio more attractive. Their preferred waist-to-hip ratio is notably smaller than that in the West though, as they express a preference for particularly protruding buttocks in conjunction with a narrow waist.[101]

Attitudes around the actual size and shape of the body vary more considerably than those around body proportions, underscoring a complex array of factors involved in shaping meanings around the human form more generally. For instance, intertwined with our evolutionary tendencies toward attraction, the development of human intelligence and society has resulted in highly complex social meanings being ascribed to the female form that manifest in a geography-, culture-, and ethnicity-specific manner; the same is true for the male body.[102] In essence, the physical form is a biological, social, economic, and political barometer whose meanings have enraptured the minds of many for millennia and shows no sign of ceasing any time soon. Humanity's fascination with these factors is grounded, in part, by the evolution and development of a species that could not only survive and reproduce, but also thrive—in general, and within and between social strata that have emerged.

To use an economic analogy, if body shape and physical appearance are a key form of social capital,[103] there is a strong incentive to get the best return on one's investment (in finding a partner), as this can translate to factors such as material wealth, health, and security.[104] As we know, however, humans do not always act rationally in their preferences, which adds complexity to our already compelling evolution as a species. What constitutes a person's ideal body can be affected by a number of inter-related factors ranging from food availability and public health to a country's politics, history, and economics, with various types of media playing an increasingly important role. Indeed, a person's preferences comprise a complex synthesis of local and global as well as traditional and contemporary social meanings about body shapes and sizes that are integrated with our innate primal preferences. Societies are highly dynamic structures subject to various undulating forces, so it should be unsurprising that there does not seem to be a single, universal conception of the ideal body that has withstood the test of time; rather, the ideal form is more likely to be the product of a society's dynamic hive-mind. The following section briefly reviews and highlights examples of the myriad factors which can underpin and influence what constitutes the ideal female[105] and male[102] form in several different ethnicities and cultures. Research on these and other contexts is ongoing and informed by work in academic fields such as sociology and anthropology.

China

China's society, economy, and culture have undergone substantial transformations in a relatively short period of time, with such changes typically following fast on the heels of political revolutions. It appears that social attitudes to the female body have been influenced heavily by significant political events and that they vary between urban and rural settings. China has historically preferred tall, slim women with a slightly rounded belly[106] which has traditional associations with a plentiful store of 'qi' that signalled health, fertility, and strength.[105] Until recent decades, this shape was difficult to attain for many as communist policies resulted in more limited resources, meaning there were not always sufficient calories available for most women to develop such a curvaceous shape. Rather than dwelling on being under- or malnourished, however, the lack of a distinctly feminine shape was often interpreted as being equivalent to a man, as well as being emblematic of hard work and uniformity, features which would have pleased the ruling communist party.[107]

In stark contrast to the older generations who participated in the Cultural Revolution (1966–1976), however, the younger (urban) generation have experienced different political and economic conditions. These conditions have led to their increasing adoption of Westernized attitudes toward their physical appearance, in which thinness is primarily associated with health and beauty whereas fatness is viewed negatively.[108] With the government loosening its control over society to permit the 'acceptable' adoption of Western economics and culture, the introduction of capitalism to China has facilitated the commodification of its citizen's bodies to an arguably greater extent than that achieved in the West. Such a situation appears to have prompted a race for social advancement amongst women who are striving to get the best return on their investment of social capital, often using whatever economic power they have at their disposal to enhance their physical form. Many Chinese women under 30 see beauty not as a luxury, but as a necessity[109] required to succeed in the brutally competitive job market[110] and modern Chinese society more generally.[111] Such a shift amongst the younger generation who wish to leave the societal constraints of the Cultural Revolution behind has been accompanied by a surge in the popularity of cosmetic surgery,[112] particularly abdominal liposuction but also facial procedures such as the increasingly controversial double-eyelid surgery.[113] Cosmetic surgery has become so widespread and normalized that China has even hosted a beauty pageant exclusively for artificially enhanced individuals.[114]

What constitutes the ideal Chinese male form is also subject to complex social and cultural factors, with traditional values competing against and interacting with modern, increasingly Western, notions. Compared to their Caucasian counterparts, Chinese men are generally shorter and of smaller build, something which can be a source of body dissatisfaction.[115]

The degree to which the Western ideal may be assimilated can be influenced by factors such as socio-economic status,[116] with the desire to succeed in a Western nation (e.g., the US) amongst recent immigrants favouring this,[117] while traditional cultural values that do not equate masculinity with muscularity offer some resistance.[118] Perfectionism is also prevalent amongst Chinese men and women living in highly economically developed and rapidly developing nations[119] such as the US and Hong Kong, with this manifesting as higher body dissatisfaction that can drive pathological exercise and dieting behaviours.[120] Clearly the Chinese conception of the ideal body has undergone a radical transformation within the space of only a few generations, with this evolutionary process showing no sign of abating any time soon.

Japan

Beliefs in modesty, simplicity, and discipline have profoundly influenced the traditional Japanese conception of beauty, all of which are epitomized by the kimono. This traditional garment is defined by simple, distinctive straight lines that give women a tubular shape. Far from celebrating and accentuating the undulating curves which define femininity in some other cultures, Japanese women often wore padding (known as 'obi') to conceal their curves under the kimono. Breasts are primarily discussed in the context of maternity in Japan, and do not seem to feature heavily in any discussion about the traditional Japanese notion of beauty, sexuality, or eroticism. This contrasts considerably with many Western countries, although changes occurred post-World War II, largely in response to American influences.[121] Just as in China, however, Japan's generational shift is influencing what constitutes the purportedly ideal female body shape.

Shedding the attitudes of the more conservative older generation, young professional women increasingly wish to convey the image of being strong, fit, and independent through a lean, busty, and toned physique.[105] Japanese women seem to have assimilated some aspects of the Western notion of beauty and the methods to attain it (i.e., exercise, diet, and/or surgery) in their quest for social and economic success, although they appear to hold themselves to their own unique standards.[122] For example, Japanese women tend to be far thinner than Western women, largely because they have a smaller frame which permits them to achieve far smaller bodily proportions. Japanese women are not, however, immune from feeling dissatisfied with their bodies.[123] Indeed, Japanese women tend to report generally lower body esteem than women from other countries, with this potentially stemming from a culture which promotes self-effacement and generates social anxiety to a greater extent than in the West.[124,125] Additionally, Japanese men are proving similar to other Asian (including Chinese) men who wish for a larger body to attain the increasingly Western ideal,[126] although the social and cultural reasons underpinning this complex process are incompletely understood.[122]

As in China, it can be argued that modern Japanese women's attitudes towards their bodies represent their opportunity to break free from traditional conservative values and the associated constraints—particularly gender roles, family ties, and social expectations. It has even been speculated that the pursuit of extreme thinness by some Japanese women represents a way of avoiding the curves which signify biological maturity and the associated maternal expectations and responsibilities, thus potentially representing a mechanism to pursue career goals.[105] Japan not only exemplifies how the defining features of the ideal body change in accordance with the social and economic reality of the current generation, it also highlights how the further widening of generational differences may change social meanings about the body beyond recognition.

South Africa

The ideal female body shape in South Africa represents a true melting pot of several potent social, political, and environmental forces. Owing to its historically inconsistent food supply, a fuller figure is preferred by South African men and women because thinner people have generally been less likely to lead a long and healthy life there compared to their heavier counterparts. The full female shape has been celebrated throughout South Africa's extensive tribal history, with the lower body being the focus of female beauty and fashion. Indeed, large beads and hoops known as 'Golwani' are worn by the Nbedele tribe to adorn and accentuate the waist, buttocks, and legs.[127] Tribal dancing also emphasizes the lower body, particularly the buttocks and thighs. Heavier women have traditionally been associated with high status in society as they indicate their husband's economic power and ability to provide for his family; a similar attitude prevails among certain groups in Nepal and Bangladesh.[128]

In addition to a number of tropical diseases, South Africa's population continues to struggle with a high prevalence of HIV/AIDS. This public health issue was greatly exacerbated by policies based on the AIDS denialism stance of Thabo Mbeki's government during the 2000s that resulted in many avoidable deaths.[129] While there was no official recognition of a health crisis, the general population, particularly rural and poor urban-dwelling people, soon began to associate thin and pale bodies with sickness.[130] Meanwhile, overweight and obese bodies continued to be synonymous with health and wealth amongst women from various tribal groups. The connection between health and weight has become so deeply engrained that many obese individuals who are well aware of the associated health risks often claim to have no desire to lose weight.[131] Simply put, big is beautiful for many South Africans—regardless of the potential health consequences.

In addition to such pressures which have influenced what constitutes the most desirable female body shape, South Africa continues to struggle with the deeply damaging social consequences of apartheid on the relationship between the majority, predominantly poor black and minority, mainly rich white populations. Broadly speaking, the conception of the ideal female body has fluctuated in parallel with substantial political upheavals. Before and during apartheid, black females generally subscribed to the attitudes of their forebears who associated overweight with wealth, power, and high status in (tribal or urban) society. Once apartheid ceased, however, many black women found they had to compete with white women in a historically white-dominated professional workplace and society. Many black women therefore felt they 'needed' to look like their white counterparts in order to succeed; this situation is thought to have precipitated a surge in eating disorders amongst black women.[132,133] However, both black and white females in South Africa appear to be susceptible to developing body image issues and eating disorders.[134]

With time, the balance of power has shifted in favour of the black majority, with the South African conception of the ideal female figure morphing in tandem. The latest incarnation appears to merge the modern feeling of 'Black pride'—which embraces the historical admiration of curvier women—with contemporary Western fashion sensibilities. This has been most clearly highlighted by the runaway global success of Levi's range of 'Eva' jeans which originated from South Africa and built upon the notion that 'stars like Beyoncé, Shakira, and J-Lo have destigmatized curvy bodies and popularized "bootyliciousness"' in mainstream society.[135] Evidently what constitutes the ideal female body differs between black and white South Africans, with such conceptions being affected to different extents by a number of overlapping yet distinct factors related to culture, socioeconomic status, and ethnicity.[136] This is also true for men in South Africa, with studies suggesting that this group provides a relatively clear example of how exposure to Western influences and urbanization affect the conception of the ideal male body. Less educated Black men from more rural areas reportedly show lower rates of body dissatisfaction and eating disorders.[137] However, these phenomena occur at higher rates in more educated, urban men who reject traditional values[138] and are modified further by the complex issues of social status, marginalization, and economic development.[139] The case of South Africa truly exemplifies how the body acts as a social, cultural, and political barometer.

Jamaica

A fuller figure is traditionally revered in Jamaica, just as in South Africa, albeit for slightly different reasons. Afflicted by tropical disease and an inconsistent food supply, thin or slim bodies are thought to be undesirable and are often scorned and pitied in both countries. In Jamaica, however, thinness is often deemed to be a sign of self or familial neglect which can also serve as a distressing reminder of Jamaica's history as a victim of the slave trade. On the other end of the spectrum, Jamaican society has a historical preference for voluptuous female figures who are believed to be 'ripe' with 'vital fluids' that are required for health and fertility; it follows that heavier women are typically considered to be more attractive, wealthier, and higher status.[105] This deep admiration of the fuller female figure, and its lower body curves in particular, is celebrated in Jamaican culture, particularly through dancing to calypso music in dance halls.

While Jamaican society prefers larger women, there is a firm emphasis on body proportionality. Women of various sizes are deemed attractive so long as they are 'properly' proportioned and do not 'lose their shape.' Put bluntly, overweight or obese women who are 'rounder' and have lost what is considered to be a more feminine proportionality are often deemed less desirable in Jamaican society. The emphasis on body shape and size has resulted in a situation in which many young women have resorted to abusing appetite enhancers (i.e., peritol) and 'chicken pills' (i.e., livestock hormones used to fatten chickens) to obtain the curves they want;[140] such a situation is far less common elsewhere, such as in parts of North America or in Europe. However, increased globalization and interaction with outside countries and cultures means that the traditional Jamaican preferences for a fuller figure now jostle alongside preferences for slimmer female bodies;[141] such contradictory messages are undoubtedly sowing seeds of confusion about what constitutes a beautiful body for future generations.

Example Cases from the Middle East

Given the conservative nature of Afghanistan's politics and social attitudes towards women, what constitutes the ideal Afghan female body doesn't seem to have been investigated or discussed much before, especially from the female perspective. Based on Julia Savacool's account,[105] it seems as though such a question has barely crossed the mind of many women in Afghanistan. This may stem from the social expectation to conceal their bodies in public under the burka (the long, black head-to-foot garment), coupled with the general absence of outside media images portraying body types deemed to be ideal. That said, Afghans reportedly favour 'chubby' or 'rounded' bodies, echoing similar traditional associations between shapely bodies with health and fertility as those espoused in countries like South Africa, Jamaica, and China.

Amongst the small population of wealthy Afghan women, some have become increasingly Westernized as highlighted by their use of make-up and gyms, although this is not representative or relevant for the female population at large. Given the constraints imposed by the burka, it appears that Afghan women instead tend to think about their entire presentation rather than individual body parts, with some even stating that 'obsessing about your body size is not a luxury that Afghan women have time for.'[105] Given Afghanistan's constrained political atmosphere and social norms toward women, more thought seems to be given to what women can or cannot do rather than what they look like. This is highlighted by one study which found that women who are willing and able to undergo cosmetic surgery in Afghanistan seem far more concerned with exercising their power to make choices as an individual than trying to achieve some beauty ideal.[142] But despite covering themselves with the burka, women still think about their physical appearance. While a seemingly simple garment, the burka reflects a great deal of highly complex political, social, and cultural attitudes that remain largely unstudied.

In a similar context, Iranians have reported higher degrees of body satisfaction compared to their American counterparts in an era when Western media was banned,[143] although Iran seems to be following world trends in which the ideal male form continues to be muscular while the ideal female body is becoming increasingly thin.[144] A number of complex factors contribute to this reshaping of gender-specific body ideals, with traditional values (which do not place significant importance on physical appearance[145]) wrestling with the (obesogenic) economic and nutritional effects of globalization and its associated Western influences. Potent social forces such as religious attitudes and attire (e.g., the hijab[146]) and marital status also play a role.[147] Growing body dissatisfaction is driving a variety of extreme behaviours, with increasing numbers of Iranian women undergoing cosmetic surgery while men turn to substances (e.g., anabolic steroids) in an effort to attain the desired ideal.[148]

A diametrically opposite Middle Eastern country is Israel, whose society has assimilated many Western values into its culture.[149] The ideal male body in Israel is muscular, something which is likely informed by the compulsory military service.[150] On the other hand, the conception of the ideal female body in Israel appears to be subject to a not-insignificant religious influence, with studies of different groups highlighting how strength of religious belief can shape the type and magnitude of effect that media exposure exerts. For example, culturally insulated ultra-Orthodox Jewish women reportedly have a more positive body image and higher degree of body satisfaction compared to their less religious modern-Orthodox or secular counterparts;[151] this greater religiosity also protects them from succumbing to the pervasive social pressure to be thin and the associated risk of developing an eating disorder.[152]

Fiji and other Pacific Islands

Fijian culture has historically displayed a deep reverence for voluptuous body shapes, with native dancing emphasizing women's bellies and hips. This admiration is built upon time-honoured associations between curvy and robust figures with better health and fertility, as well as higher social status. Traditional religious values which promote eating practices and the reverence of large bodies[153] are embodied in the saying 'kana, mo urouro' ('eat, so you will become fat[154']). Life can be difficult on this relatively isolated Pacific island and larger women have enjoyed a historical preference as they are typically better able to perform physically demanding jobs and generally stand a better chance of living a longer, healthier life. This positive attitude toward larger bodies is shared by men and women from other Pacific Islands, including Tonga[155] and Hawaii.[115] Until only recently, most Fijian women did not care about their body size (but did care about having a curvy shape), even though many women tend to be overweight or obese according to BMI.[156] However, the attitude towards what constitutes the ideal female Pacific Islander body shape has undergone a radical transformation in a relatively short period of time, particularly in Fiji.

Rather than political upheaval or the desire to break free from traditional conservative social attitudes, such a change seems to have been prompted by the invasion of technology and mass media, with such changes being cemented by a shift in the nature of Fiji's economy. The arrival of TV and the Internet on this historically isolated island during the 1990s seems to have turned the long-standing notion that 'big is beautiful' on its head. Generations who had been used to watching Bollywood films starring curvy actresses suddenly found themselves being continually bombarded with (Western) images and TV shows depicting 'attractive,' skinny women who were socially and economically successful. Within a short period of time, a country which didn't have a word to describe the concept of eating disorders suddenly had to contend with a wave of body anxiety[157] and eating disorders,[158] something that continues to ravage the young female population as they scramble to adhere to shifting social meanings about the body.[159] Emerging evidence indicates that this crisis of confidence, often manifesting as disordered eating patterns, is being exacerbated by the use of social media.[160] Men are not immune either, as there is evidence that they are increasingly pursuing the lean, muscular physique that constitutes the Western ideal which has become synonymous with health, dominance, strength, and sporting prowess.[161]

It's not entirely clear why Fiji has proven to be particularly sensitive to the introduction of Western mass media, especially when other countries (e.g., China, Japan, and Jamaica) have been relatively resistant, or at least discriminating, in their assimilation of Western attitudes. It has been suggested that, while the introduction of Western media set the wheels in motion, it was the shift in the Fijian economy to accommodate Western money and wealthy Western tourists that cemented the changing conception of the ideal Fijian body. Many young natives work in the tourism industry and are constantly surrounded by slim, wealthy Western women, a situation which likely reinforces the idealized/warped reality that they see on TV, meaning younger generations probably feel significant pressure to adopt a similar look. The penetration of Western media and money have resulted in Fiji's traditional attitudes being largely replaced with ideals that run antithetical to what would have historically been biologically necessary for a long and healthy existence on this island. The seismic shift in social attitudes towards body shape and the associated fallout evidently represent the tangible costs that Fijian society will continue to pay as it morphs to enjoy the economic benefits conferred by relationships with other countries. This process is complicated further by the particularly high rates of obesity among this Pacific Island population and the associated public health messages promoting healthy lifestyles and body sizes.[162]

United States and United Kingdom

It would be an understatement to say that there is more than a little confusion over what constitutes the ideal body, particularly the female body, in the US and UK (or the 'West' more generally). Trying to pin down such an esoteric, shifting definition is made even more difficult by increasing globalization which enables various conceptions of beauty to subtly and overtly influence each other in a reciprocal relationship. Mass migration has also introduced additional layers of complexity with which to contend; country of origin, race,[163] and ethnicity[164] can all influence how an individual responds upon exposure to images of mainstream beauty standards according to various social and cultural factors, all of which may vary between societies and generations.

Given the increasingly multi-cultural nature of the US and UK, and other industrialized countries, it seems unlikely for a single beauty ideal to exist. With so many different perspectives to consider, this section does not aim to be exhaustive or comprehensive, but merely highlight some of the more prominent factors which may influence certain attitudes towards ideal bodies. A related issue to consider is the thorny matter of how such a body can be attained. Moreover, while the substance of these debates has changed over time, *how* such debates are conducted has changed considerably too. Indeed, mass media and advertising have played an influential role for many decades in portraying images of supposedly ideal female bodies. However, their effect arguably pales in comparison to that of the Internet, with social media (e.g., Facebook, Instagram, Twitter, YouTube) proving to be a particularly potent force that has increased both the speed and polarization of debates. As if this fraught situation weren't already complex enough, the spectre of the global obesity pandemic looms increasingly large, casting a dark shadow across the entire debate and its participants.

Unlike traditional South African, Fijian, or Jamaican societies, for example, North America and Europe don't hold the same deep reverence for the fuller female figure with a rounded lower body to define what constitutes the ideal female body. Contrary to many other cultures, overweight and obese women, regardless of whether they have distinctly feminine proportions, have become synonymous with poor health, reduced fertility, and low socioeconomic status in many Western countries.[165,166] Conversely, slimness and the desire to be slim is strongly related to higher social class.[167] The complex attitude towards obesity emanates from a long history of fluctuating meanings associated with fatness—particularly fatness in male authority figures—ranging from a symbol of immense power and wealth to corrupted softness and effeminate, infertile, and idiotic feebleness.[168] Now, however, the slim ideal for women and lean, muscular ideal for men are most pervasive,[169] despite an increasing proportion of the Western populations falling into the overweight/obese category. And as the general population gets heavier, the gulf between the supposed ideal body and the realistically achievable body size and shape grows wider, stoking increasing levels of anxiety in both men and women.[170]

Images broadcast in the media of what supposedly constitutes the ideal body shape can vary considerably, particularly in recent years, owing to the surging popularity of phenomena such as 'body positivity.' This movement aims to 'challenge prevailing societal views of bodies, address unrealistic body standards, and help people build confidence and acceptance of their own bodies.'[171] The highly popular and influential Western fashion world is dominated with images of impossibly slim individuals whose figure is often attained and maintained through an unhealthy, even dangerous, attitude to eating and exercise. In recent years, however, the dominance of such models has been challenged by the increasing popularity of 'plus-size' models, an unhelpfully broad catch-all term that refers to women[172] and men[173] that range from an otherwise normal/healthy weight through to individuals who are morbidly obese.

Clothes are a powerful way to amplify, mask, or modify the social signals conveyed by certain body shapes. From hiding in loose fitting clothes to trying to show off one's shape with a figure-hugging outfit, clothes send important and powerful social meanings in a variety of contexts.[174,175] Numerous Western clothing trends through the ages have emphasized certain sexually defining body parts, much like traditional or tribal garments or adornments, with attention often being drawn to what have traditionally been deemed 'feminine' curves of the lower body by garments ranging from the Victorian bustle to the mini-skirts, hot-pants, and skin-tight yoga pants that have dominated contemporary society.[176]

Discerning what images and physiques are real or fake (i.e., airbrushed or surgically altered) represents a tortuous minefield for anyone to navigate; even when we know what is fake or impossible to achieve on our own, it can be difficult to resist comparisons between one's body and its artificially enhanced counterparts.[177] While the effect these images have on an individual vary according to many factors such as age, social class, and ethnicity, mounting evidence suggests that persistent exposure to images of unattainable and improbably proportioned bodies on the TV, in magazines, and on the Internet and social media is making us think differently about our own body[178] or that of an actual or potential partner.[179] Developing a distorted image of our bodies can precipitate anxiety, depression, and perfectionism which often manifest as eating disorders in women[180] or muscle dysmorphia in men.[181] In the latter, people often devote extensive amounts of time and energy to activities such as exercise/bodybuilding, shopping for and eating specific foods and supplements, and even taking certain drugs (e.g., anabolic steroids) in a manner that essentially resembles an addiction to crafting and maintaining their body according to an extreme ideal image.[182]

Crossing the Line

The ideal Western (female) body's proportions, size, and shape arguably only become apparent when the poorly defined limits of an essentially unspecified range are crossed in a distinctly individual basis. There is weight to the insightful, if vague, words of the influential ancient Roman physician and philosopher Galen (129–216 A.D.) who favoured bodily constitutions that sat 'midway between thin and corpulent.' What's more, conflicting and confusing dialogue about the body often means that those who may have actually attained an ideal body shape in others' eyes may nonetheless be pre-occupied with their own anxiety over what their body is not, according to their own distorted standards and perceptions.[183] It is tempting to cynically suggest that the constantly shifting standards and attitude to always strive to be something we are not are tools to keep a number of industries ticking (e.g., cosmetics, fashion, and weight loss industries). However, this phenomenon may simply reflect, in part, the natural consequence of our innate desire to strive for social dominance in whatever social group we occupy, albeit manifesting according to the mercurial profit- and novelty-seeking principles that underpin the industrialized, globalized, and market-driven Western society.

Speaking of the economy, the onward march in which almost everything has been commodified has resulted in citizens of Westernized countries increasingly thinking of their bodies as a series of items that can be chopped and changed if they don't meet their own, or other people's, standards. Indeed, cosmetic procedures to sculpt, shape, or slice almost any part of our bodies have become largely normalized in mainstream culture, helped in large part by numerous celebrities and television shows, with this industry continuing to boom in the US and UK.[184] The attitudes towards cosmetic surgery are not straightforward, however, as the physical appearance of the body is often heavily moralized.[185] For example, people are often labelled fat and lazy, whereas those who are slim 'must have worked really hard.' The French lawyer, politician, and gastronome Jean Anthelme Brillat-Savarin (1755–1826) summarized this sentiment in his famous treatise, 'The Physiology of Taste'[186] (published in December 1825, two months before his death), stating that 'it appears that if obesity be not a disease, it is at least a very troublesome predisposition, into which we fall from our own fault.' When it's difficult to escape the images, attitudes, even reality, that constantly reinforce the notion that certain body shapes and sizes are associated with, or even necessary for, social and economic success, taking the shortcut can be incredibly tempting. However, there is growing appreciation for the reality that the development of obesity is a complex, multi-faceted process in which individual responsibility is but one component that interacts with (at least) social and economic circumstances (e.g., education, employment, marital status) and childhood experiences,[187] as well as environmental factors[188] (e.g., available food choices).

Women's bodies in Western society represent a particularly complex social, economic, and political barometer that has arguably become overloaded under the pressure of trying to meet too many conflicting expectations; be thin but curvy, eat but not too much, exercise but not too much, and be confident with your body but strive to be better. With such contradictory expectations, it is easy to see how anxiety, eating disorders, and self-loathing (i.e., body dysmorphic disorder) are increasingly common.[189] The rise of neoliberalism since the 1970s has played a key role in leading

Western and Westernized societies to this point, in which the paradox of consumption butts heads against notions of self-discipline and willpower, with the manifestation of willpower often involving the purchase of fitness products and services that are part of the same obesogenic consumer society.[190] But going under the knife and 'cheating' runs counter to the puritanical, protestant work ethic which the UK and US have a history of instilling in their populations, meaning that undertaking such procedures can result in complex feelings of guilt for those who partake or even consider it. It follows that the most popular cosmetic surgery options principally involve modifying regional fat mass to achieve the feminine shape synonymous with health, fertility, and social success; the most common procedures involve removing abdominal fat via liposuction while breasts and buttocks are typically augmented, enhanced, and shaped. Equally, none of these approaches address the broader structural and cultural elements of society that could facilitate good health and positive, healthy notions of the body in far more effective, population-based ways.

Cosmetic surgery is not the only way in which the West's consumerist attitudes towards our bodies manifest, as highlighted by the widespread popularity of fad diets, quick fixes, and radical (largely unsustainable) life changes exemplified in TV shows such as 'The Biggest Loser' and 'Celebrity Fat Camp.' While these shows are primarily focused on the arduous task of reversing obesity in their participants, they juxtapose socially unacceptable fat bodies against their diametric opposite; the sculpted, toned, and lean— yet curvy—female bodies of the trainers and presenters that we are expected to aspire towards which supposedly signify discipline and mastery of life. This view accompanies the recent trend in favour of 'strong' women (e.g., female athletes) who manage to walk the fine line between being lean and muscular yet retaining distinctly feminine curves.

The 'lean and strong' ideal is undoubtedly healthier than simply being skinny, but it may simply represent another physique that is equally difficult for many to attain and maintain. Moreover, women pursuing such a physique run the risk of being deemed 'too muscular' or even 'masculine.' In parallel, the widespread images of extremely muscular male bodies in the media, far more developed than the lean physique embodied in the ancient *Apollo Belvedere* sculpture from 120–140 C.E. and celebrated during the eighteenth century Enlightenment by the pioneering German art historian and archaeologist Johann Joachim Winckelmann, are combining with the current fascination with health to whip up a wave of body anxiety and a hidden epidemic of steroid abuse.[191] Evidently much work is required in contexts throughout the world to promote truly healthy body shapes and weights in ways that do not inspire pathological behaviour or normalize harmful extremes.

Overall, the human body exemplifies a number of biological strategies which neatly dovetail together in an evolutionarily honed form that can not only support reproduction and stave off starvation, traverse long distances, and provide offspring with nourishing breast milk, but also look 'good' doing it. These processes have played instrumental roles in facilitating the development, evolution, and survival of modern humanity, and they each derive, in part, from harnessing the ability to accumulate fat.

References

1. Morgan, M. H. & Carrier, D. R. Protective buttressing of the human fist and the evolution of hominin hands. *J. Exp. Biol.* **216**, 236–44 (2013).
2. Tardieu, C., Hasegawa, K., & Haeusler, M. How did the pelvis and vertebral column become a functional unit during the transition from occasional to permanent bipedalism? *Anat. Rec. (Hoboken)* **300**, 912–31 (2017).
3. Gruss, L. T. & Schmitt, D. The evolution of the human pelvis: changing adaptations to bipedalism, obstetrics and thermoregulation. *Philos. Trans. R. Soc. Lond. B. Biol. Sci.* **370**, 20140063 (2015).
4. Lovejoy, C. O. The natural history of human gait and posture. Part 1. Spine and pelvis. *Gait Posture* **21**, 95–112 (2005).
5. Bramble, D. M. & Lieberman, D. E. Endurance running and the evolution of Homo. *Nature* **432**, 345–52 (2004).
6. Liebenberg, L. Persistence hunting by modern hunter-gatherers. *Curr. Anthropol.* **47**, 1017–1026 (2006).
7. Marlowe, F. W. Hunter-gatherers and human evolution. *Evol. Anthropol. Issues, News, Rev.* **14**, 54–67 (2005).
8. Pontzer, H. *et al.* Metabolic acceleration and the evolution of human brain size and life history. *Nature* **533**, 390–2 (2016).
9. Rosenberg, K. & Trevathan, W. Bipedalism and human birth: the obstetrical dilemma revisited. *Evol. Anthropol. Issues, News, Rev.* **4**, 161–8 (2005).
10. Franciscus, R. G. When did the modern human pattern of childbirth arise? New insights from an old Neandertal pelvis. *Proc. Natl. Acad. Sci. U. S. A.* **106**, 9125–6 (2009).
11. Stiles, J. & Jernigan, T. L. The basics of brain development. *Neuropsychol. Rev.* **20**, 327–48 (2010).
12. Lewis, C. L., Laudicina, N. M., Khuu, A., & Loverro, K. L. The human pelvis: variation in structure and function during gait. *Anat. Rec. (Hoboken)* **300**, 633–42 (2017).

13. Betti, L. & Manica, A. Human variation in the shape of the birth canal is significant and geographically structured. *Proc. R. Soc. B Biol. Sci.* (2018). doi:10.1098/rspb.2018.1807

14. Zollikofer, C. P. E. Evolution of hominin cranial ontogeny. *Prog. Brain Res.* **195**, 273–92 (2012).

15. Carrier, D. R. & Morgan, M. H. Protective buttressing of the hominin face. *Biol. Rev. Camb. Philos. Soc.* **90**, 330–46 (2015).

16. Scott, G. R. & Turner, C. G. *The Anthropology of Modern Human Teeth.* Cambridge University Press, 1997. doi:10.1017/CBO9781316529843

17. Zhu, N. & Chang, L. Evolved but not fixed: a life history account of gender roles and gender inequality. *Front. Psychol.* **10**, 1709 (2019).

18. Wood, W. & Eagly, A. H. A cross-cultural analysis of the behavior of women and men: implications for the origins of sex differences. *Psychol. Bull.* **128**, 699–727 (2002).

19. Morris, J. S., Link, J., Martin, J. C., & Carrier, D. R. Sexual dimorphism in human arm power and force: implications for sexual selection on fighting ability. *J. Exp. Biol.* **223**, jeb212365 (2020).

20. Lyon, B. E. & Montgomerie, R. Sexual selection is a form of social selection. *Philos. Trans. R. Soc. Lond. B. Biol. Sci.* **367**, 2266–73 (2012).

21. Speakman, J. R. Sex- and age-related mortality profiles during famine: testing the 'body fat' hypothesis. *J. Biosoc. Sci.* **45**, 823–40 (2013).

22. Weston, E. M., Friday, A. E., & Liò, P. Biometric evidence that sexual selection has shaped the hominin face. *PLoS One* **2**, e710 (2007).

23. Little, A. C., Jones, B. C., & DeBruine, L. M. Facial attractiveness: evolutionary based research. *Philos. Trans. R. Soc. Lond. B. Biol. Sci.* **366**, 1638–59 (2011).

24. Caro, T. M. & Sellen, D. W. The reproductive advantages of fat in women. *Ethol. Sociobiol.* **11**, 51–66 (1990).

25. Frisch, R. E. Fatness, menarche, and female fertility. *Perspect. Biol. Med.* **28**, 611–33 (1985).

26. Wells, J. C. K. The evolution of human adiposity and obesity: where did it all go wrong? *Dis. Model. Mech.* **5**, 595–607 (2012).

27. Lange, I. G., Hartel, A., & Meyer, H. H. D. Evolution of oestrogen functions in vertebrates. *J. Steroid Biochem. Mol. Biol.* **83**, 219–26 (2002).

28. Monks, D. A. & Holmes, M. M. Androgen receptors and muscle: a key mechanism underlying life history trade-offs. *J. Comp. Physiol. A* **204**, 51–60 (2018).

29. Pawlowski, B. The evolution of gluteal/femoral fat deposits and balance during pregnancy in bipedal Homo 1. *Curr. Anthropol.* **42**, 572–75 (2001).

30. Pawłowski, B. & Grabarczyk, M. Center of body mass and the evolution of female body shape. *Am. J. Hum. Biol.* **15**, 144–50 (2003).

31. Cant, J. G. H. Hypothesis for the evolution of human breasts and buttocks. *Am. Nat.* **117**, 199–204 (1981).

32. Lassek, W. D. & Gaulin, S. J. C. Costs and benefits of fat-free muscle mass in men: relationship to mating success, dietary requirements, and native immunity. *Evol. Hum. Behav.* **30**, 322–8 (2009).

33. Frederick, D. A. & Haselton, M. G. Why is muscularity sexy? Tests of the Fitness Indicator Hypothesis. *Personal. Soc. Psychol. Bull.* **33**, 1167–83 (2007).

34. Longman, D. P., Wells, J. C. K., & Stock, J. T. Human athletic paleobiology: using sport as a model to investigate human evolutionary adaptation. *Am. J. Phys. Anthropol.* **171**, 42–59 (2020).
35. Foo, Y. Z., Nakagawa, S., Rhodes, G., & Simmons, L. W. The effects of sex hormones on immune function: a meta-analysis. *Biol. Rev. Camb. Philos. Soc.* **92**, 551–71 (2017).
36. West-Eberhard, M. J. Nutrition, the visceral immune system, and the evolutionary origins of pathogenic obesity. *Proc. Natl. Acad. Sci.* **116**, 723–31 (2019).
37. Mascia-Lees, F. E., Relethford, J. H., & Sorger, T. Evolutionary perspectives on permanent breast enlargement in human females. *Am. Anthropol.* **88**, 423–8 (1986).
38. Scurr, J. *et al.* The influence of the breast on sport and exercise participation in school girls in the United Kingdom. *J. Adolesc. Health* **58**, 167–73 (2016).
39. Burnett, E., White, J., & Scurr, J. The influence of the breast on physical activity participation in females. *J. Phys. Act. Health* **12**, 588–94 (2015).
40. Spencer, L. & Briffa, K. Breast size, thoracic kyphosis & thoracic spine pain – association & relevance of bra fitting in post-menopausal women: a correlational study. *Chiropr. Man. Therap.* **21**, 20 (2013).
41. Marlowe, F. The nubility hypothesis: the human breast as an honest signal. *Hum. Nat.* **9**, 263–71 (1998).
42. Gallup, G. G. Permanent breast enlargement in human females: a sociobiological analysis. *J. Hum. Evol.* **11**, 597–601 (1982).
43. Maskarinec, G., Nagata, C., Shimizu, H., & Kashiki, Y. Comparison of mammographic densities and their determinants in women from Japan and Hawaii. *Int. J. Cancer* **102**, 29–33 (2002).
44. Dixson, B. J. *et al.* Men's preferences for women's breast morphology in New Zealand, Samoa, and Papua New Guinea. *Arch. Sex. Behav.* **40**, 1271–9 (2011).
45. Havlíček, J. *et al.* Men's preferences for women's breast size and shape in four cultures. *Evol. Hum. Behav.* **38**, 217–26 (2017).
46. Breast size chart by country. *AverageHeight.com* (2018). Available at: www.averageheight.co/breast-cup-size-by-country.
47. OECD. Fertility rates (indicator). *OECD Data* (2020). doi:10.1787/8272fb01-en
48. Butovskaya, M. *et al.* Waist-to-hip ratio, body-mass index, age and number of children in seven traditional societies. *Sci. Rep.* **7**, 1622 (2017).
49. Zaadstra, B. M. *et al.* Fat and female fecundity: prospective study of effect of body fat distribution on conception rates. *BMJ* **306**, 484–7 (1993).
50. Kościński, K., Makarewicz, R., & Bartoszewicz, Z. Stereotypical and actual associations of breast size with mating-relevant traits. *Arch. Sex. Behav.* (2019). doi:10.1007/s10508-019-1464-z
51. Anderson, P. The reproductive role of the human breast. *Curr. Anthropol.* **24**, 25 (1983).
52. Clellan, F. & Beach, F. *Patterns of Sexual Behavior.* Harper & Row, 1951.
53. Oftedal, O. T. The mammary gland and its origin during synapsid evolution. *J. Mammary Gland Biol. Neoplasia* **7**, 225–52 (2002).
54. Oftedal, O. T. The evolution of milk secretion and its ancient origins. *Animal* **6**, 355–68 (2012).

55. Pawlowski, B. Permanent breasts as a side effect of subcutaneous fat tissue increase in human evolution. *Homo* **50**, 149–62 (1999).

56. Butte, N. F. & King, J. C. Energy requirements during pregnancy and lactation. *Public Health Nutr.* **8**, 1010–27 (2005).

57. Lassek, W. D. & Gaulin, S. J. C. Waist-hip ratio and cognitive ability: is gluteofemoral fat a privileged store of neurodevelopmental resources? *Evol. Hum. Behav.* **29**, 26–34 (2008).

58. Phinney, S. D. *et al.* Human subcutaneous adipose tissue shows site-specific differences in fatty acid composition. *Am. J. Clin. Nutr.* **60**, 725–9 (1994).

59. Del Prado, M. *et al.* Contribution of dietary and newly formed arachidonic acid to milk secretion in women on low fat diets. *Adv. Exp. Med. Biol.* **478**, 407–8 (2000).

60. Innis, S. M. Human milk: maternal dietary lipids and infant development. *Proc. Nutr. Soc.* **66**, 397–404 (2007).

61. Neifert, M. R., Seacat, J. M., & Jobe, W. E. Lactation failure due to insufficient glandular development of the breast. *Pediatrics* **76**, 823–8 (1985).

62. Kent, J. C., Mitoulas, L., Cox, D. B., Owens, R. A., & Hartmann, P. E. Breast volume and milk production during extended lactation in women. *Exp. Physiol.* **84**, 435–47 (1999).

63. Liu, J., Smith, M. G., Dobre, M. A., & Ferguson, J. E. Maternal obesity and breast-feeding practices among white and black women. *Obesity (Silver Spring)* **18**, 175–82 (2010).

64. Low, B. S., Alexander, R. D., & Noonan, K. M. Human hips, breasts and buttocks: is fat deceptive? *Ethol. Sociobiol.* **8**, 249–57 (1987).

65. Anderson, J. L. Breast, hips, and buttocks revisited. Honest fatness for honest fitness. *Ethol. Sociobiol.* **9**, 319–24 (1988).

66. Lassek, W. D. & Gaulin, S. J. C. Do the low WHRs and BMIs judged most attractive indicate higher fertility? *Evol. Psychol.* **16**, 1474704918800063 (2018).

67. Lassek, W. D. & Gaulin, S. J. C. Do the low WHRs and BMIs judged most attractive indicate better health? *Evol. Psychol.* **16**, 1474704918803998 (2018).

68. Grammer, K., Fink, B., Møller, A. P., & Thornhill, R. Darwinian aesthetics: sexual selection and the biology of beauty. *Biol. Rev. Camb. Philos. Soc.* **78**, 385–407 (2003).

69. Puts, D. A., Jones, B. C., & DeBruine, L. M. Sexual selection on human faces and voices. *J. Sex Res.* **49**, 227–43 (2012).

70. Montag, C. & Panksepp, J. Primary emotional systems and personality: an evolutionary perspective. *Front. Psychol.* **8**, 464 (2017).

71. Singh, D. & Singh, D. Shape and significance of feminine beauty: an evolutionary perspective. *Sex Roles* **64**, 723–31 (2011).

72. Møller, A. P. Asymmetry as a predictor of growth, fecundity and survival. *Ecol. Lett.* **2**, 149–56 (1999).

73. Wade, T. J. The relationships between symmetry and attractiveness and mating relevant decisions and behavior: a review. *Symmetry* (2010). doi:10.3390/sym2021081

74. Gangestad, S. W., Thornhill, R., & Yeo, R. A. Facial attractiveness, developmental stability, and fluctuating asymmetry. *Ethol. Sociobiol.* **15**, 73–85 (1994).

75. Møller, A. P., Soler, M., & Thornhill, R. Breast asymmetry, sexual selection, and human reproductive success. *Ethol. Sociobiol.* **16**, 207–19 (1995).
76. Møller, A. P. & Thornhill, R. Bilateral symmetry and sexual selection: a meta-analysis. *Am. Nat.* **151**, 174–92 (1998).
77. Manning, J. T., Scutt, D., & Lewis-Jones, D. I. Developmental stability, ejaculate size, and sperm quality in men. *Evol. Hum. Behav.* (1998). doi:10.1016/S1090-5138(98)00024-5
78. Dixson, B. J., Grimshaw, G. M., Linklater, W. L., & Dixson, A. F. Watching the hourglass: eye tracking reveals men's appreciation of the female form. *Hum. Nat.* **21**, 355–70 (2010).
79. Dixson, B. J., Grimshaw, G. M., Linklater, W. L., & Dixson, A. F. Eye-tracking of men's preferences for waist-to-hip ratio and breast size of women. *Arch. Sex. Behav.* **40**, 43–50 (2011).
80. Singh, D. Body shape and women's attractiveness: the critical role of waist-to-hip ratio. *Hum. Nat.* **4**, 297–321 (1993).
81. Furnham, A., Swami, V., & Shah, K. Body weight, waist-to-hip ratio and breast size correlates of ratings of attractiveness and health. *Pers. Individ. Dif.* **41**, 443–54 (2006).
82. Karremans, J. C., Frankenhuis, W. E., & Arons, S. Blind men prefer a low waist-to-hip ratio. *Evol. Hum. Behav.* **31**, 182–6 (2010).
83. Furnham, A., Melanie, D., McClelland, A., & Dias, M. The role of body weight, waist-to-hip ratio, and breast size in judgments of female attractiveness. *Sex Roles* **39**, 311–26 (1998).
84. Jasieńska, G., Ziomkiewicz, A., Ellison, P. T., Lipson, S. F., & Thune, I. Large breasts and narrow waists indicate high reproductive potential in women. *Proceedings. Biol. Sci.* **271**, 1213–17 (2004).
85. Singh, D. & Young, R. K. Body weight, waist-to-hip ratio, breasts, and hips: role in judgments of female attractiveness and desirability for relationships. *Ethol. Sociobiol.* **16**, 483–507 (1995).
86. Singh, D. Is thin really beautiful and good? Relationship between waist-to-hip ratio (WHR) and female attractiveness. *Pers. Individ. Dif.* **16**, 123–32 (1994).
87. Perilloux, H. K., Webster, G. D., & Gaulin, S. J. C. Signals of genetic quality and maternal investment capacity: the dynamic effects of fluctuating asymmetry and waist-to-hip ratio on men's ratings of women's attractiveness. *Soc. Psychol. Personal. Sci.* **1**, 34–42 (2010).
88. Singh, D. Female health, attractiveness, and desirability for relationships: role of breast asymmetry and waist-to-hip ratio. *Ethol. Sociobiol.* **16**, 465–81 (1995).
89. Zhang, Y., Wang, X., Wang, J., Zhang, L., & Xiang, Y. Patterns of eye movements when observers judge female facial attractiveness. *Front. Psychol.* **8**, (2017). www.frontiersin.org/articles/10.3389/fpsyg.2017.01909/full
90. Weeden, J. & Sabini, J. Physical attractiveness and health in Western societies: a review. *Psychol. Bull.* **131**, 635–53 (2005).
91. Bovet, J. Evolutionary theories and men's preferences for women's waist-to-hip ratio: which hypotheses remain? A systematic review. *Front. Psychol.* **10**, 1221 (2019).

92. Thornborrow, T., Onwuegbusi, T., Mohamed, S., Boothroyd, L. G., & Tovée, M. J. Muscles and the media: a natural experiment across cultures in men's body image. *Front. Psychol.* **11**, 495 (2020).

93. Cunningham, M. R., Roberts, A. R., Barbee, A. P., Druen, P. B., *et al.* 'Their ideas of beauty are, on the whole, the same as ours': consistency and variability in the cross-cultural perception of female physical attractiveness. *J. Pers. Soc. Psychol.* **68**, 261–79 (1995).

94. Singh, D., Dixson, B. J., Jessop, T. S., Morgan, B., & Dixson, A. F. Cross-cultural consensus for waist-hip ratio and women's attractiveness. *Evol. Hum. Behav.* **31**, 176–81 (2010).

95. Dixson, B. J., Dixson, A. F., Bishop, P. J., & Parish, A. Human physique and sexual attractiveness in men and women: a New Zealand–U.S. comparative study. *Arch. Sex. Behav.* **39**, 798–806 (2010).

96. Dixson, B. J., Sagata, K., Linklater, W. L., & Dixson, A. F. Male preferences for female waist-to-hip ratio and body mass index in the highlands of Papua New Guinea. *Am. J. Phys. Anthropol.* **141**, 620–5 (2010).

97. Dixson, B. J., Li, B., & Dixson, A. F. Female waist-to-hip ratio, body mass index and sexual attractiveness in China. *Curr. Zool.* **56**, 175–82 (2010).

98. Dixson, B. J., Dixson, A. F., Morgan, B., & Anderson, M. J. Human physique and sexual attractiveness: sexual preferences of men and women in Bakossiland, Cameroon. *Arch. Sex. Behav.* **36**, 369–75 (2007).

99. Swami, V., Caprario, C., Tovée, M. J., & Furnham, A. Female physical attractiveness in Britain and Japan: a cross-cultural study. *Eur. J. Pers.* **20**, 69–81 (2006).

100. Swami, V., Jones, J., Einon, D., & Furnham, A. Men's preferences for women's profile waist-to-hip ratio, breast size, and ethnic group in Britain and South Africa. *Br. J. Psychol.* **100**, 313–25 (2009).

101. Marlowe, F., Apicella, C., & Reed, D. Men's preferences for women's profile waist-to-hip ratio in two societies. *Evol. Hum. Behav.* **26**, 458–68 (2005).

102. Ricciardelli, L. A., McCabe, M. P., Williams, R. J., & Thompson, J. K. The role of ethnicity and culture in body image and disordered eating among males. *Clin. Psychol. Rev.* **27**, 582–606 (2007).

103. Bainbridge, D. *Curvology: The Origins and Power of Female Body Shape.* Portobello Books, 2015.

104. O'Connor, K. M. & Gladstone, E. Beauty and social capital: being attractive shapes social networks. *Soc. Networks* **52**, 42–7 (2018).

105. Savacool, J. *The World Has Curves.* Rodale, 2009.

106. Zhang, M. A Chinese beauty story: how college women in China negotiate beauty, body image, and mass media. *Chinese J. Commun.* **5**, 437–54 (2012).

107. Ip, H.-Y. Fashioning appearances: feminine beauty in Chinese communist revolutionary culture. *Mod. China* **29**, 329–61 (2003).

108. Xu, H. Developmental idealism, body weight and shape, and marriage entry in transitional China. *Chinese J. Sociol.* **2**, 235–58 (2016).

109. Hua, W. *Buying Beauty.* Hong Kong University Press, 2013.

110. Shao, G. China's plastic surgery market: how far are you willing to go for a job? *CTGN* (2017). Available at: https://news.cgtn.com/news/7749544e7a557a6333566d54/share_p.html.

111. Lindridge, A. M. & Wang, C. Saving "face" in China: modernization, parental pressure, and plastic surgery. *J. Consum. Behav.* **7**, 496–508 (2008).

112. China now world's fastest growing plastic surgery market. *ECNS* (2017). Available at: www.ecns.cn/business/2017/08-11/268998.shtml.

113. Zhou, V. Why double eyelid surgery is on the rise in Asia: rising incomes and acceptance, and star power of Fan Bingbing, Angelababy. *South China Morning Post* (2017). Available at: www.scmp.com/lifestyle/health-beauty/article/2093921/why-double-eyelid-surgery-rise-asia-rising-incomes-and.

114. China's 'artificial beauty' show. *BBC News* (2004). Available at: http://news.bbc.co.uk/1/hi/world/asia-pacific/4090741.stm.

115. Yates, A., Edman, J., & Aruguete, M. Ethnic differences in BMI and body/self-dissatisfaction among Whites, Asian subgroups, Pacific Islanders, and African-Americans. *J. Adolesc. Health* **34**, 300–7 (2004).

116. Brown, P. J. & Konner, M. An anthropological perspective on obesity. *Ann. N. Y. Acad. Sci.* **499**, 29–46 (1987).

117. Irving, L. M., Wall, M., Neumark-Sztainer, D., & Story, M. Steroid use among adolescents: findings from Project EAT. *J. Adolesc. Health* **30**, 243–52 (2002).

118. Liao, K. Y.-H. *et al.* Asian American men's body image concerns: a focus group study. *Psychol. Men Masculinities* **21**, 333–44 (2020).

119. Davis, C. & Katzman, M. A. Perfection as acculturation: psychological correlates of eating problems in Chinese male and female students living in the United States. *Int. J. Eat. Disord.* **25**, 65–70 (1999).

120. Davis, C. & Katzman, M. A. Chinese men and women in the United States and Hong Kong: body and self-esteem ratings as a prelude to dieting and exercise. *Int. J. Eat. Disord.* **23**, 99–102 (1998).

121. Miller, L. Mammary mania in Japan. *Positions* (2003). doi:10.1215/10679847-11-2-271

122. Chisuwa, N. & O'Dea, J. A. Body image and eating disorders amongst Japanese adolescents. A review of the literature. *Appetite* **54**, 5–15 (2010).

123. Brockhoff, M. *et al.* Cultural differences in body dissatisfaction: Japanese adolescents compared with adolescents from China, Malaysia, Australia, Tonga, and Fiji. *Asian J. Soc. Psychol.* **19**, 385–94 (2016).

124. Kowner, R. Japanese body image: structure and esteem scores in a cross-cultural perspective. *Int. J. Psychol.* **37**, 149–59 (2002).

125. Kowner, R. When ideals are too 'far off': physical self-ideal discrepancy and body dissatisfaction in Japan. *Genet. Soc. Gen. Psychol. Monogr.* **130**, 333–61 (2004).

126. Kagawa, M. *et al.* A comparison of body perceptions in relation to measured body composition in young Japanese males and females. *Body Image* **4**, 372–80 (2007).

127. Beckwith, C. & Fisher, A. *African Ceremonies.* Harry N. Abrams, 1999.

128. Bishwajit, G. Household wealth status and overweight and obesity among adult women in Bangladesh and Nepal. *Obes. Sci. Pract.* **3**, 185–92 (2017).

129. Boseley, S. Mbeki Aids denial 'caused 300,000 deaths'. *The Guardian* (2008). Available at: www.theguardian.com/world/2008/nov/26/aids-south-africa.

130. Clark, R. A., Niccolai, L., Kissinger, P. J., Peterson, Y., & Bouvier, V. Ethnic differences in body image attitudes and perceptions among women infected with human immunodeficiency virus. *J. Am. Diet. Assoc.* **99**, 735–7 (1999).
131. Mvo, Z., Dick, J., & Steyn, K. Perceptions of overweight African women about acceptable body size of women and children. *Curationis* **22**, 27–31 (1999).
132. Duguid, S. The body politic. *Telegraph* (2004).
133. Szabo, C. P. & Allwood, C. W. A cross-cultural study of eating attitudes in adolescent South African females. *World Psychiatry* **3**, 41–4 (2004).
134. Caradas, A. A., Lambert, E. V., & Charlton, K. E. An ethnic comparison of eating attitudes and associated body image concerns in adolescent South African schoolgirls. *J. Hum. Nutr. Diet.* **14**, 111–20 (2001).
135. Curvy SA jeans takes US by storm. *www.bizcommunity.com* (2008). Available at: www.bizcommunity.com/Article/196/87/21983.html.
136. Mwaba, K. & Roman, N. V. Body image satisfaction among a sample of black female South African students. *Soc. Behav. Personal. an Int. J.* **37**, 905–9 (2009).
137. Edwards, D. & Moldan, S. Bulimic pathology in black students in South Africa: some unexpected findings. *South African J. Psychol.* **34**, 191–205 (2004).
138. Marais, D. L., Wassenaar, D. R., & Kramers, A. L. Acculturation and eating disorder symptomatology in Black men and women. *Eat. Weight Disord.* **8**, 44–54 (2003).
139. le Grange, D., Telch, C. F., & Tibbs, J. Eating attitudes and behaviors in 1,435 South African Caucasian and non-Caucasian college students. *Am. J. Psychiatry* **155**, 250–4 (1998).
140. Nelson, D. & Silva, N. Taking surprising risks for the ideal body. *NPR* (2010). Available at: www.npr.org/templates/story/story.php?storyId=124700865&t=1538045099849.
141. Gray, P. B. & Frederick, D. A. Body image and body type preferences in St. Kitts, Caribbean: a cross-cultural comparison with U.S. samples regarding attitudes towards muscularity, body fat, and breast size. *Evol. Psychol.* **10**, 147470491201000 (2012).
142. Hatef, A. From under the veil to under the knife: women, cosmetic surgery, and the politics of choice in Afghanistan. *Fem. Media Stud.* **18**, 842–58 (2018).
143. Akiba, D. Cultural variations in body esteem: how young adults in Iran and the United States view their own appearances. *J. Soc. Psychol.* **138**, 539–40 (1998).
144. Shoraka, H., Amirkafi, A., & Garrusi, B. Review of body image and some of the contributing factors in the Iranian population. *Int. J. Prev. Med.* **10**, 19 (2019).
145. Coakley, S. *Religion and the Body.* Cambridge University Press, 2000.
146. Bahaadinbeigy, K., Garrusi, B., & Etminan, A. Contributing factors affecting body satisfaction among pregnant women with an emphasis on self-esteem and depression. *Psychology* (2014). www.semanticscholar.org/paper/Contributing-Factors-Affecting-Body-Satisfaction-an-Bahaadinbeigy-Garrusi/04fe06dc365de5646fd8a0e9305e7ab06e4fd83b

147. Garrusi, B. & Baneshi, M. R. Body dissatisfaction among Iranian youth and adults. *Cad. Saude Publica* **33**, (2017) [Epub]. www.scielo.br/scielo. php?script=sci_arttext&pid=S0102-311X2017000905008

148. Garrusi, B., Garousi, S., & Baneshi, M. R. Body image and body change: predictive factors in an Iranian population. *Int. J. Prev. Med.* **4**, 940–8 (2013).

149. Rebhun, A. P. H. A. H. I. C. J. U. *et al. Jews in Israel: Contemporary Social and Cultural Patterns.* Brandeis University Press, 2004.

150. Barak, Y., Sirota, P., Tessler, M., Achiron, A., & Lampl, Y. Body esteem in Israeli university students. *Isr. J. Psychiatry Relat. Sci.* **31**, 292–5 (1994).

151. Geller, S. *et al.* Exploring body image, strength of faith, and media exposure among three denominations of Jewish women. *Curr. Psychol.* (2018). doi:10.1007/s12144-018-9876-9

152. Gluck, M. E. & Geliebter, A. Body image and eating behaviors in Orthodox and Secular Jewish women. *J. Gend. Specif. Med.* **5**, 19–24 (2001).

153. McCabe, M. P., Waqa, G., Dev, A., Cama, T., & Swinburn, B. A. The role of cultural values and religion on views of body size and eating practices among adolescents from Fiji, Tonga, and Australia. *Br. J. Health Psychol.* **18**, 383–94 (2013).

154. Becker, A. E. *Body, Self, and Society: The View from Fiji.* University of Pennsylvania Press, Incorporated, 1995.

155. Craig, P., Halavatau, V., Comino, E., & Caterson, I. Perception of body size in the Tongan community: differences from and similarities to an Australian sample. *Int. J. Obes. Relat. Metab. Disord.* **23**, 1288–94 (1999).

156. Di Cesare, M. *et al.* Trends in adult body-mass index in 200 countries from 1975 to 2014: a pooled analysis of 1698 population-based measurement studies with 19.2 million participants. *Lancet* (2016). doi:10.1016/S0140-6736(16)30054-X

157. Williams, L. K., Ricciardelli, L. A., McCabe, M. P., Waqa, G. G., & Bavadra, K. Body image attitudes and concerns among indigenous Fijian and European Australian adolescent girls. *Body Image* **3**, 275–87 (2006).

158. Becker, A. E., Burwell, R. A., Gilman, S. E., Herzog, D. B., & Hamburg, P. Eating behaviours and attitudes following prolonged exposure to television among ethnic Fijian adolescent girls. *Br. J. Psychiatry* **180**, 509–14 (2002).

159. Becker, A. E. Television, disordered eating, and young women in Fiji: negotiating body image and identity during rapid social change. *Cult. Med. Psychiatry* **28**, 533–59 (2004).

160. Becker, A. E. *et al.* Social network media exposure and adolescent eating pathology in Fiji. *Br. J. Psychiatry* **198**, 43–50 (2011).

161. Ricciardelli, L. A. *et al.* The pursuit of muscularity among adolescent boys in Fiji and Tonga. *Body Image* **4**, 361–71 (2007).

162. Mavoa, H. M. & McCabe, M. Sociocultural factors relating to Tongans' and Indigenous Fijians' patterns of eating, physical activity and body size. *Asia Pac. J. Clin. Nutr.* **17**, 375–84 (2008).

163. Chin Evans, P. & McConnell, A. R. Do racial minorities respond in the same way to mainstream beauty standards? Social comparison processes in Asian, Black, and White women. *Self Identity* **2**, 153–67 (2003).

164. Rakhkovskaya, L. M. & Warren, C. S. Sociocultural and identity predictors of body dissatisfaction in ethnically diverse college women. *Body Image* **16**, 32–40 (2016).
165. McLaren, L. Socioeconomic status and obesity. *Epidemiol. Rev.* **29**, 29–48 (2007).
166. Sobal, J. & Stunkard, A. J. Socioeconomic status and obesity: a review of the literature. *Psychol. Bull.* **105**, 260–75 (1989).
167. Dornbusch, S. M. *et al.* Sexual maturation, social class, and the desire to be thin among adolescent females. *J. Dev. Behav. Pediatr.* 5, 308–14 (1984).
168. Forth, C. E. *Fat: A Cultural History of the Stuff of Life.* Reaktion Books, 2019.
169. McCabe, M. P. & Ricciardelli, L. A. The structure of the perceived sociocultural influences on body image and body change questionnaire. *Int. J. Behav. Med.* **8**, 19–41 (2001).
170. Elia, C. *et al.* Weight misperception and psychological symptoms from adolescence to young adulthood: longitudinal study of an ethnically diverse UK cohort. *BMC Public Health* **20**, 712 (2020).
171. Cherry, K. What is body positivity? *VeryWell Mind* (2020). Available at: www.verywellmind.com/what-is-body-positivity-4773402.
172. Capon, L. Best plus size models and accounts to follow on Instagram. *Cosmopolitan* (2020). Available at: www.cosmopolitan.com/uk/fashion/a49364/curvy-plus-size-model-instagram/.
173. Capon, L. 11 plus size male models you need to get to know. *Cosmopolitan* (2017). Available at: www.cosmopolitan.com/uk/fashion/g12157785/plus-size-male-model/.
174. Feinberg, R. A., Mataro, L., & Burroughs, W. J. Clothing and social identity. *Cloth. Text. Res. J.* **11**, 18–23 (1992).
175. Damhorst, M. L. Meanings of clothing cues in social context. *Cloth. Text. Res. J.* **3**, 39–48 (1985).
176. Pauline, T. & Thomas, G. Fashion era. (2019). Available at: www.fashion-era.com/.
177. MacCallum, F. & Widdows, H. Altered images: understanding the influence of unrealistic images and beauty aspirations. *Heal. Care Anal.* (2018). doi:10.1007/s10728-016-0327-1
178. Hendrickse, J., Clayton, R. B., Ray, E. C., Ridgway, J. L., & Secharan, R. Experimental effects of viewing thin and plus-size models in objectifying and empowering contexts on Instagram. *Health Commun.* 1–9 (2020). doi:10.1080/10410236.2020.1761077
179. Brooks, K. R. *et al.* Looking at the figures: visual adaptation as a mechanism for body-size and -shape misperception. *Perspect. Psychol. Sci.* **15**, 133–49 (2020).
180. McLean, S. A. & Paxton, S. J. Body image in the context of eating disorders. *Psychiatr. Clin. North Am.* **42**, 145–56 (2019).
181. Mitchell, L. *et al.* Muscle dysmorphia symptomatology and associated psychological features in bodybuilders and non-bodybuilder resistance trainers: a systematic review and meta-analysis. *Sports Med.* **47**, 233–59 (2017).

182. Foster, A. C., Shorter, G. W., & Griffiths, M. D. Muscle dysmorphia: could it be classified as an addiction to body image? *J. Behav. Addict.* **4**, 1–5 (2015).

183. Hosseini, S. A. & Padhy, R. K. *Body Image Distortion. StatPearls* (2020).

184. New statistics reveal the shape of plastic surgery (2017). *American Association of Plastic Surgeons* (2018). Available at: www.plasticsurgery.org/news/press-releases/new-statistics-reveal-the-shape-of-plastic-surgery.

185. Townend, L. The moralizing of obesity: a new name for an old sin? *Crit. Soc. Policy* **29**, 171–90 (2009).

186. Brillat-Savarin, J. A. & Drayton, A. *The Physiology of Taste.* Penguin Books Limited, 2004.

187. Asahara, S., Miura, H., Ogawa, W., & Tamori, Y. Sex difference in the association of obesity with personal or social background among urban residents in Japan. *PLoS One* **15**, e0242105 (2020).

188. Congdon, P. Obesity and urban environments. *Int. J. Environ. Res. Public Health* **16**, 464 (2019).

189. Krebs, G., Fernández de la Cruz, L., & Mataix-Cols, D. Recent advances in understanding and managing body dysmorphic disorder. *Evid. Based. Ment. Health* **20**, 71–5 (2017).

190. Guthman, J. & DuPuis, M. Embodying neoliberalism: economy, culture, and the politics of fat. *Environ. Plan. D Soc. Sp.* **24**, 427–48 (2006).

191. Goldman, A. L., Pope, H. G., & Bhasin, S. The health threat posed by the hidden epidemic of anabolic steroid use and body image disorders among young men. *J. Clin. Endocrinol. Metab.* **104**, 1069–74 (2019).

3
What Does Fat Do?

Part 1—The Metabolic Marketplace

Simply put, fat is a long-term energy store. However, fat doesn't wait lethargically until the body's fuel supply runs low, only to awake in a panic and dish out packets of energy at the last moment. Ever-vigilant and industrious, fat acts dynamically to ensure the body's energy needs are met[1] over the short-, medium-, and long-term, a tremendous feat that is achieved through extensive co-ordination with various other organs, particularly the liver and brain[2] (see reference 2 for an accessible, integrative overview of human metabolism in health and disease). Before discussing fat's role though, it is important to consider what is meant by 'energy metabolism.' The body's metabolism (i.e., energy intake and expenditure) is similar to a country's economy comprising highly integrated but distinct sectors working in conjunction with and depending on each other. While each sector performs different functions and uses different raw materials, all of the transactions within and between sectors utilize a universal currency; money. When it comes to the body's metabolism, money represents the cellular energy unit, adenosine triphosphate (ATP; discussed in greater detail in Chapter 4), which powers all of the biological processes within our body, be they 'services' (e.g., muscle contraction and neuronal activity) or 'manufactured goods' (e.g., organ growth and repair).

Extending this analogy further, the different raw materials like oil, gas, or steel represent biological molecules such as carbohydrate, fatty acids, and amino acids. Each commodity has distinct properties suited for specific purposes; amino acids are used to build muscle, bone, and collagen whereas carbohydrates and fat are primarily used as metabolic fuels, although they play important structural and signalling roles too.[3,4] Just like an economy, there is a constant flow in which commodities are bought, sold, and used to manufacture goods or as a fuel source. If the supply of commodities or money dries up, the economy grinds to a halt, often with disastrous consequences. This biological 'economic activity' is perpetual throughout life, but the demands can shift any second, minute, or hour for days, months, and years. Ensuring the fluctuating demand for biological commodities and currency is met with an adequate supply is the essence of metabolic 'homeostasis' (i.e., the phenomenon of maintaining constant conditions by changing).

As in real-life, a fine balance has to be struck to ensure there is a suffi-cient supply of commodities and money without flooding the marketplace and/or emptying reserves; meeting the body's energy needs is a logis-tical nightmare! Achieving and maintaining optimal conditions involves knowing how much of each commodity is required at any one time and properly managing reserves to ensure that the appropriate amount of each commodity is mobilized to meet the acute demand, all the while accumu-lating and protecting manageable reserves. In addition to the fact that our energy demands can change drastically in the short term, the metabolic marketplace is not supplied at a constant rate throughout the day. Instead, our biological commodity-containing meals are consumed in a periodic fashion over the course of the day. Keeping the wheels of the economy turning seamlessly involves masterfully integrating reserve mobilization and replenishment.

Within this metabolic marketplace, carbohydrates would be low de-nomination currency (e.g., coins) used to pay the majority of small trans-actions, whereas fatty acids would be higher denomination paper money (Figure 3.1). As in real-life, we store the majority of our money in the bank but have some on-hand for everyday use; our body distributes its energy

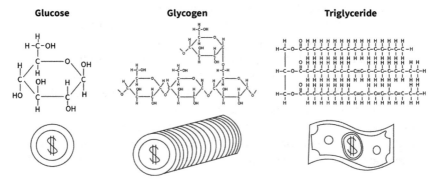

Figure 3.1 Chemical structure of glucose, glycogen, and triglyceride.

reserves in a similar manner. We might have a coin purse in our pocket (e.g., a small carbohydrate store within a cell) to pay immediate bills, replenishing this with coins from our piggy bank (e.g., a carbohydrate store in the liver). These low-value, bulky coins are supplemented with some high-value, space-efficient paper money in our pocket (e.g., a fat droplet within a cell), although the vast majority is kept in the bank (e.g., white adipose tissue). And within the bank, we split our money between a frequently used current account and a savings account that gets left alone for that financial rainy day.

Various mechanisms and warning systems will monitor the size of the bank reserves to prevent their collapse and protect the broader economy. But while their shrinkage is vigorously defended, there appears to be little or no upper limit on how big a bank account can become. By thinking about white adipose tissue as playing the crucial role of the bank in a free-flowing economy, it suddenly becomes clear that fat plays a much more dynamic role than the simplistic phrase 'long-term energy store' would suggest. Indeed, fat works tirelessly with the liver to ensure our dynamically shifting energy demands are met every second of every day, from the relatively low levels required to keep our body ticking over while we sleep to the massive demands required to support exercise. Let's next consider the different types of fuel that the body uses, how they are stored, and the mechanisms used to ensure their supply is kept constant.

Fuelling the Metabolic Fire—Carbohydrates

The human body is powered by flexible engines that can run on various metabolic fuels. Carbohydrates (containing carbon, hydrogen, and oxygen arranged in a ring) represent a key fuel for many organs, particularly glucose which our brains use exclusively. Free glucose circulates in the blood but is stored in the liver and muscle as glycogen, a long, branching structure comprising many glucose molecules joined side by side that coil up and interlock with other glycogen molecules. However, glucose's structure attracts lots of water which bulks it out, thus restricting the number of molecules that can fit in a given space. Although not optimal for storing vast amounts of energy, glucose is crucial for our survival and so a number of a mechanisms have evolved to ensure the body's glucose supply is kept constant.

Circulating glucose levels are controlled in the same way that room temperature is held constant by a thermostat controlling a heater and air-conditioner (Figure 3.2). Moreover, the way glucose is handled by the body has many important lessons applicable to energy metabolism more generally. Blood glucose levels increase after a meal (i.e., the room temperature increases) and stimulate the release of insulin from beta cells in the pancreas. Insulin is the master storage signal and is released in response to an abundance of nutrients. Insulin acts on organs like the liver and muscle, instructing them to extract the nutrients from the bloodstream to reduce the raised circulating level of glucose back to normal (i.e., the raised temperature is sensed by the thermostat, which then activates the air-conditioner to cool the room down).

To stop glucose levels from going too low, this removal is counterbalanced by the release of glucose into the bloodstream from the liver (i.e., a heater is turned on to stop the temperature from dropping too low); this process is controlled by the hormone glucagon secreted by alpha cells in the pancreas. The liver can also make more glucose from other carbohydrates

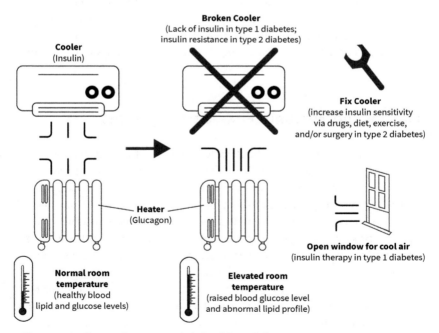

Figure 3.2 Glucose homeostasis in health and disease.

or amino acids via 'gluconeogenesis.' The tight coupling between the addition and removal of glucose from the blood requires a lot of energy to sustain. However, this tension means that changes in demand can be met very rapidly and that deviations from the normal level are minimized in both duration and extent, something which can mean the difference between life and death.

Type 1 Diabetes

Using the thermostat analogy, it is easy to see how the breakdown of this exquisitely sensitive regulatory system can quickly result in disaster. In type 1 diabetes, the pancreas gets damaged by the person's own immune system,[5] meaning too little or no insulin is released in response to glucose (i.e., the air-conditioner is unable to cool the warm room down). The absence of a storage signal means that nutrients absorbed by the gut remain circulating in the blood; prolonged exposure to excessively high levels of glucose results in damage to the blood vessels, kidneys, nerves, and eyes.[6] The lack of insulin is also interpreted by the body as a starvation signal, so the already-high levels of circulating glucose are exacerbated by the release of additional glucose into the bloodstream from the liver (i.e., the thermostat mistakenly thinks the room is colder than it is and turns the heater up). Indeed, blood glucose levels can get so high that they exceed the reabsorption capacity of the kidney, meaning some glucose ends up in the urine; it's no coincidence that *diabetes mellitus* means 'sweet urine' in Latin. Diabetes can be thought of as the body 'starving in the midst of plenty.'

The primary approach for treating type 1 diabetes involves injecting insulin (or insulin-like drugs) at the appropriate time around meals.[5] This is analogous to opening a window to cool down a hot room; such a crude strategy makes precise control difficult to achieve. Injecting too little insulin means glucose levels can remain elevated and cause damage, whereas injecting too much insulin runs the risk of causing excessive removal of glucose from the blood (i.e., hypoglycaemia). The latter situation can starve the patient's brain and put them at risk of slipping into a diabetic coma from which they might not wake. Properly managing type 1 diabetes requires careful planning, vigilance, and discipline.

Type 2 Diabetes

Although similar in name, type 2 diabetes results not from a lack of insulin, but a blunting in the response of its targets, otherwise known as 'insulin resistance'; this means more insulin is required to get the same biological response. While the precise cause of this state is unknown, numerous molecular mechanisms (which may act independently or in concert) have been implicated[7]; the insulin signalling machinery may be damaged by highly reactive free radicals, possibly due to dysfunctional mitochondria; altered levels of inflammatory signals and/or adipokines may activate signalling pathways that dampen insulin sensitivity; reduced numbers of insulin receptors may be present on the cell surface—the list goes on. The pancreas can somewhat compensate for this by pumping out more insulin, although this evidently doesn't address the underlying issue of insulin resistance in the liver, muscle, and/or adipose tissue (AT). Impaired insulin action results in inefficient clearance of nutrients after a meal that, when coupled with inadequate suppression of glucose generation and release from the liver due to inappropriate glucagon release, manifests as persistently high blood glucose levels that can damage the blood vessels and various organs. Think of a hot room in which the air-conditioner is clogged up and needs to work harder to provide cool air while the heater continues running. Insulin resistance and type 2 diabetes are commonly associated with obesity and will be discussed at various times throughout this book.

Fuelling the Metabolic Fire—Fatty Acids

Carbohydrates are an essential metabolic fuel, but they aren't ideal for storing large quantities of energy in a space-efficient manner; instead, this task is handled by fat, or more specifically *fatty acids*. These molecules contain long carbon and hydrogen chains with oxygen atoms at the end of their 'tails.' These fatty acid tails can vary in length and contain none, one, or more 'double-bonds' between carbon atoms, rendering them saturated, mono-unsaturated, or poly-unsaturated, respectively (Figure 3.3); the relevance of fatty acid structure to adipose biology, diet, and health is discussed in Chapters 6 and 7. In their most space-efficient form, fatty acids combine with glycerol to make triacylglycerol (TAG). TAG molecules self-segregate and coalesce to form highly energy-dense droplets which exclude water (imagine oil droplets in water). As organisms have to carry their

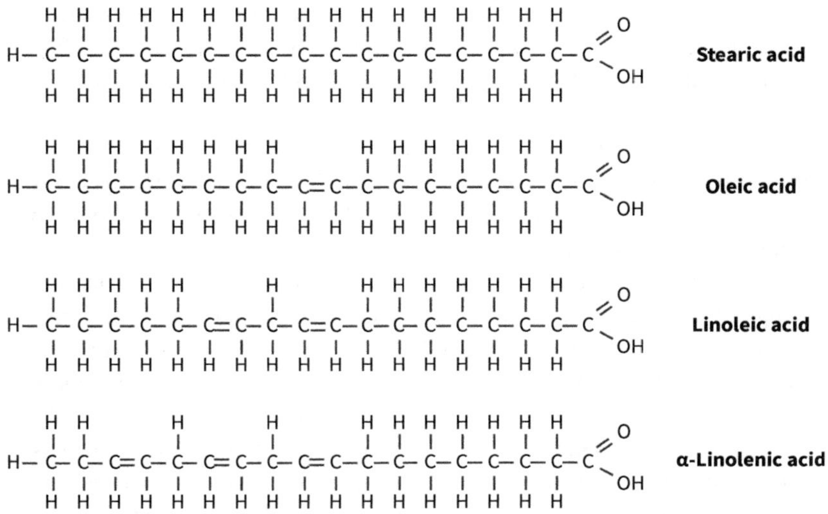

Figure 3.3 Chemical structure of saturated and unsaturated fatty acids.

energy reserves around and still be able to move to their next meal, it's easy to see why evolution has favoured fat as the energy store of choice. Indeed, nearly every type of organism in the world, including archaic bacteria and yeast, and most cells in our body (particularly in muscle and the liver), have the capacity to generate fat droplets and use the constituent fatty acids for energy.[8]

In addition to convenient fat droplets within cells, evolution has provided specially adapted cells which act as remote energy stores that support increasingly complex organisms. These specialized cells are known as *adipocytes* (the main cellular constituent of adipose tissue) and contain a fat droplet so large it fills the cell almost entirely, pushing structures like the nucleus to the periphery. Adipocytes represent the largest population of cells within white adipose tissue, constituting approximately 97% of its weight.[9] The remaining cells—known as the stromovascular fraction (SVF)— include adipocyte precursors (i.e., preadipocytes), stem cells, cells that contribute to the blood supply's structure (i.e., endothelial and smooth muscle cells), and cells from the immune system.[10] Apart from preadipocytes, most SVF cells don't usually participate in fat metabolism but instead play a supporting role. Additionally, the fibrous network in which all of these cells are embedded (known as the extracellular matrix) organizes their physical arrangement and blood supply, protects the fragile adipocytes from mechanical forces, and co-ordinates the maturation of precursor cells into fully fledged adipocytes.[11] Fat's simple appearance under the microscope belies its complex biology.

White fat is distributed throughout the body in stores under the skin (i.e., subcutaneous), around internal organs (i.e., visceral), and in breast tissue (see Figure 3.4). In a healthy individual, approximately 80–90% of total body fat is stored just underneath the skin surrounding the abdominal (waist), sub-scapular (upper back), gluteal (buttock), and femoral (thigh) areas.[12] Conversely, visceral AT comprises the omental and mesenteric depots that surround the digestive organs and accounts for 6–20% of total body fat.[13] Carbohydrate and fat metabolism handled by the liver and (white) adipose tissue are deeply integrated to ensure that our body's shifting energy demands can be rapidly met in a manner that can be sustained for hours, days, or even weeks without replenishment if necessary. To build a cohesive, unified picture of how these different component parts work together, the next few sections will explore fat, carbohydrate, and protein metabolism in a variety of real-life situations. First stop: mealtime.

Part 2—Deconstructing Digestion, Analyzing Absorption, and Scrutinizing Storage

Fat can transform even the blandest morsel into a calorific treat for the palate by giving food a thick, full, rich taste and texture that's difficult to resist.[14] In conjunction with sugar, fat-containing palatable foods have the potential to essentially be addictive,[15,16] something well-known by the hugely successful snack and fast food industries. Our appetite and tastes have become finely honed indicators that direct what we need to eat and when to ensure we meet our body's nutritional requirements while avoiding noxious substances.[17]

Fat Digestion

Have you ever sat back after a greasy meal, satisfied, and wondered if and how the fat actually gets from the dish to your waist and thighs? As you enjoy a meal containing fat, each mouthful of food is broken down mechanically via chewing. These food fragments are swallowed and enter the

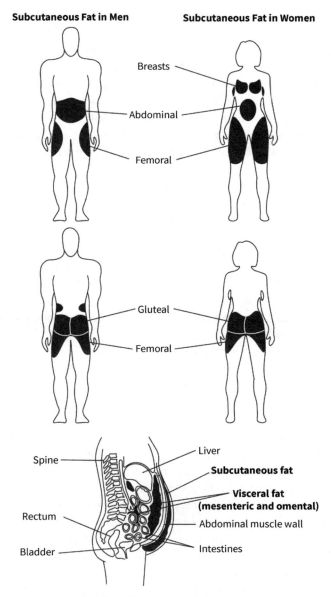

Figure 3.4 Anatomy of white adipose tissue in humans.

stomach where they are digested further by the addition of hydrochloric acid and the churning action of the stomach's muscular walls. Eventually this slurry (known as chyme) is carefully released into the small intestine. The chyme is moved along the small intestine via peristalsis (the muscular equivalent of squeezing toothpaste from a tube) and gets mixed with an alkaline digestive juice (which neutralizes the stomach acid) released from the pancreas. This juice contains enzymes that facilitate the breakdown of proteins, carbohydrates, and fats into their constituent amino acids, mono- or di-saccharides, and free fatty acids, respectively, which are able to be absorbed.

Fatty acids tend to coalesce and form droplets which can be difficult to breakdown. To aid in their digestion, the gall bladder releases bile into the small intestine. Bile contains cholesterol and salts which act as a detergent (akin to washing-up liquid) that disperses large fat droplets into several smaller ones. This effectively increases the surface area for the pancreatic enzymes to work on, thereby making the digestion process much more efficient. If cholesterol accumulates in the gall bladder because there are not enough bile salts present to dissolve it, painful gallstones can form. These need to be removed or shattered before they cause blockages or even infections[18]—ouch!

As digestion proceeds, free fatty acids and glycerol are released from TAG by the enzyme pancreatic lipase acting in the small intestine (Figure 3.5). Before considering fat absorption, it is worth noting that this enzyme can be inhibited by *orlistat*, a drug which is taken orally before a meal.[19] Orlistat is sold as a weight loss aid as it disrupts fat digestion to reduce the amount of fat—and therefore caloric energy—absorbed by the small intestine following a meal. Reducing fat absorption certainly represents one way of reducing calorie intake, but it isn't necessarily the most pleasant approach to bring about weight loss. That's because any ingested fat that isn't being absorbed has to go somewhere, which means into the toilet. Given its mode of action, it is perhaps unsurprising orlistat can also cause abdominal pains and flatulence. Having the most pleasant and effective experience with orlistat involves switching to a low-fat diet, which probably won't entail the most flavoursome foods, but might save you from unpleasant side effects. It should also be considered that many vitamins dissolve in fat, so orlistat can inadvertently affect vitamin absorption, which can be problematic. Despite these side effects, orlistat has been shown to be a moderately effective weight loss tool[20] that should ideally be used under a doctor's supervision. *Olestra*, a fat substitute used

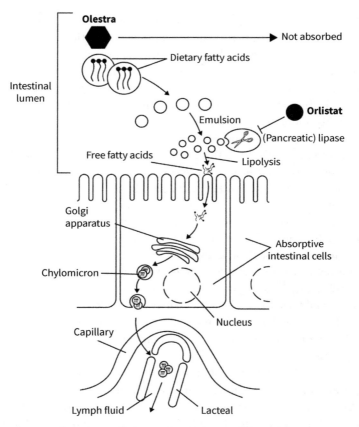

Figure 3.5 Fat digestion and absorption in the small intestine.

in crisps, has similar bowel-churning effects due to its chemical structure that mean it cannot be absorbed by the body.

Fat Absorption

Returning to the small intestine, physical and chemical digestion leave ingested fat's constituent parts (i.e., free fatty acids and glycerol) sitting in the gut ready for absorption. Just like their carbohydrate and protein counterparts, the liberated fatty acids, glycerol, and cholesterol are carried into the cells lining the small intestine by specific transporter proteins. The amino acids from protein and mono-/disaccharides from carbohydrates then travel across the cell and enter the *hepatic portal vein*, the major nutrient highway to the body which drains from the gut directly to the liver. Like a perpetually vigilant traffic controller, the pancreas samples the nutrient-rich blood as it flows past, releasing insulin into the hepatic portal vein in response to the increased levels of glucose, amino acids, and fatty acids after a meal while suppressing glucagon secretion. The insulin joins the nutrients from the small intestine and flows directly to the liver where it instructs liver cells to extract the lion's share of the recently absorbed carbohydrates and amino acids. Blood leaving the liver then enters the general circulation, with the remaining nutrients being absorbed by other organs (e.g., skeletal and cardiac muscle as well as adipose tissue) under the control of insulin.

Fatty acids and cholesterol absorbed by the gut cells don't just run for the door and dive into the bloodstream like everyone else (i.e., carbohydrates and amino acids) though. In a slightly counter-intuitive move, the gut cells take the recently absorbed fatty acids that the body has just spent significant time and energy breaking down and re-assembles them into TAG, which coalesces and forms a droplet. Other fat-related molecules such as cholesterol join this droplet before a protein 'tag' called an *apolipoprotein* is inserted; this combination of fat (i.e., lipid), cholesterol, and protein is known as a *lipoprotein*.

There are different types of lipoprotein that each serve various biological purposes. Numerous apolipoproteins exist that act as an 'identity card' for the different types of lipoprotein. Insertion of a specific apolipoprotein tag into the TAG and cholesterol droplet by the gut cell identifies this lipoprotein as a *chylomicron* to the rest of the body. Chylomicrons are such large particles that they scatter light and give plasma taken after a meal a milky, turbid appearance. Rather than entering the bloodstream with everything else though, the chylomicrons enter the lymphatic system, a distinct circulatory system which forms an important part of our immune system. The chylomicrons flow through the lymphatic system and join the general circulation through a vessel near the heart known as the thoracic duct. This anatomical arrangement means that recently eaten fat enters the bloodstream *without* going through the liver first, unlike carbohydrates and amino acids. It's not entirely clear why this anatomical arrangement exists, but it is possible that it represents an evolutionary mechanism which protects the liver from being swamped with fat while it handles the glut of carbohydrates and amino acids flowing through it directly from the gut after a meal. Now that the fat from our food is now in our bloodstream, what happens next?

Special Delivery

Recall the apolipoprotein tag inserted into the TAG and cholesterol droplet; as well as an identity card, it also serves as a 'grab-handle' for the crucial enzyme *lipoprotein lipase* (LPL).[21] Imagine a sushi bar where organs like fat tissue and muscle are the customers sitting and watching the food (i.e., lipoproteins) move around on a conveyor belt (i.e., the circulatory system). In this scenario, the apolipoprotein tags act as different coloured plates that identify each type of food. Once a customer has picked up the appropriate plate, LPL would be the cutlery used to consume the meal.

Blood flowing through the capillaries supplying muscle and fat after a meal contains chylomicrons and the hormone insulin. Previously mentioned in the context of promoting glucose storage, insulin also promotes LPL molecules to sit on the lining of the capillaries within muscle and fat tissue.[22] As the chylomicrons float through, LPL molecules grab the apolipoprotein handle and break down the TAG molecules contained within the ensnared chylomicron. The free fatty acids cross through the capillary wall, enter the fat or muscle tissue, and are taken up by the constituent cells. While muscle captures nearly all of the fatty acids that are released by LPL, some of them get away from fat tissue and enter the general circulation.[23] The muscle or fat cells then re-assemble (again!) the free fatty acids with glycerol to form TAG molecules[24] which join pre-existing fat droplets and thereby complete dietary fat's journey from the plate to our cells. Stuck outside, the chylomicron shrinks as LPL breaks down the TAG until it becomes the biological equivalent of a deflated balloon, or a 'remnant'. This chylomicron remnant then detaches from the capillary wall and re-joins the general circulation until it is eventually taken up by the liver which cannibalizes it for parts.

One in a Million

The system for extracting and storing fat is complex and remarkably robust, but not infallible. There are a handful of individuals around the world afflicted by genetic mutations that render the enzyme LPL non-functional, thereby bringing the storage of dietary fat to a dangerous standstill. Affecting approximately one person in a million, LPL mutations result in the massive accumulation of TAG-containing lipoproteins (including chylomicrons) in the blood.[25] Imagine the sushi bar again, only this time the customers have their hands tied so they can't take any plates while the chef keeps making food and eventually overloads the conveyor belt. Disabling the mechanism responsible for clearing TAG from the blood into fat and muscle results in extensive fat accumulation in places where it shouldn't, with this situation usually resulting in severe pancreatitis (i.e., inflammation of the pancreas), swelling of the liver, and fat nodules developing under the skin.[25] LPL deficiency can be life-threatening.

The standard approach to treating these patients primarily involves restricting their consumption of fat, although adherence can be difficult owing to the very limited food choices. Dietary modification is typically supplemented with other blood-fat lowering agents such as statins and fibrates. The fortune of these patients seemed to have turned in 2012, however, when a pioneering gene therapy known as *Glybera* that treated the core pathophysiology of LPL deficiency was approved by the EU Commission.[26] This treatment involves injecting a carefully engineered virus that delivers a fully functional version of the LPL gene into fat and muscle, thereby restoring these tissues' ability to extract circulating TAG in LPL-deficient patients. The therapy has proven to be well-tolerated and effective at improving the health of the people who have received it (i.e., clinically significant reductions in the incidence of pancreatitis and abdominal pain over a six-year follow-up period), even though plasma triglyceride levels returned to pre-treatment levels after 16 weeks post-injection.[27] If the drug worked, what could possibly have gone wrong?

Simply put, the inherent problem with rare diseases is that only a relatively small number of people have them, meaning the potential number of customers is limited before even considering who could afford to pay. This lack of a particularly strong financial incentive has resulted in many hotly contested debates between patient advocacy groups and drug companies over which diseases can and should be addressed. Despite becoming famous in 2012 as the first gene therapy approved in Europe, Glybera garnered more attention for being the world's most expensive medicine at the time. With a price tag of $1.6 million per course in 2012,[26] it soon became clear that Glybera would be beyond most patients' reach. With only one person being treated with Glybera in Europe by the end of 2016 (and a total of 31 globally by 2018), it is unsurprising that the manufacturer, UniQure, did not apply to renew their license to continue selling the pioneering treatment.[28] The combination of a lack of adequate demand (from the manufacturer's perspective) and exorbitant price tag sealed Glybera's fate, whilst also showcasing the difficulties in developing medicines for rare diseases. Lessons have undoubtedly been learned from this medical breakthrough's commercial failure[29]; it would be unacceptable if the only options moving forward involve either new therapies not being developed for rare diseases or ground-breaking therapies being shelved because of impossibly high price tags. As the field of gene therapy undergoes an explosion of interest and technological development,[30] it's possible that patients with LPL deficiency (amongst many others) may get a second, even better, chance to obtain a curative solution. Watch this space …

As we can see, the seemingly simple task of digesting and storing fat is actually surprisingly complex. But once the fat has been stored, how do we get it back out when we need it? And under what conditions?

Part 3—Unleashing the Feast

In meeting our body's energy demands, our organs don't exhaust their internal energy stores and then put activities on hold, wait for the next delivery of nutrients, and then continue. Stopping the flow of nutrients to the brain or heart for even a few moments could be fatal. Because survival requires the metabolic furnace burning at all times, our bodies have evolved numerous interlocking mechanisms that ensure its organs are provided with a constant stream of energy so their operations can proceed uninterrupted around the clock. Furthermore, such a system can respond dynamically to fluctuations in both metabolic supply and demand, enabling our bodies to go from almost nil (e.g., grazing on snacks while sitting in front of the TV) to very high (e.g., sprinting to catch a bus) in a short space of time. This distribution network may be highly complex, but it operates from a simple principle; the drawing of nutrients from the circulation and local stores within cells acts as a signal to the supplying organ(s). The capacity to carry around an energy source and mobilize it accordingly frees us from the shackles imposed by food availability and the act of eating; we don't actually need to eat all day long to function, despite what food advertisements might suggest.

Thinking of the body in terms of running a factory can highlight the impressively robust and nuanced biological logistical solutions that have evolved to ensure the metabolic furnace never stops burning, come what may. This factory uses raw materials (with protein acting as steel) and energy sources (with glucose and fatty acids acting as gas and coal) to make products at a rate that precisely matches demand. The cars are made from raw materials and energy sources stored on-site as well as those being delivered regularly. During periods of low demand, the factory can draw more heavily from on-site stores and less on deliveries, with the latter being used to replenish the former. However, a sudden upswing in demand for cars will rapidly deplete the on-site stores and make deliveries essential for keeping the factory operational. During periods of prolonged heavy demand, the remote supply depot will take measures to ensure its own supply is sufficient. In the case that one energy supply runs out, the factory might shift from burning its usual mixture of gas and coal to whichever one is available to keep the factory working. If the steel supply slows sufficiently, the factory might cannibalize older cars to make new ones. Once the demand eventually decreases, however, the factory's on-site and remote supply stores can be replenished.

The metabolic furnace doesn't burn the same in every organ though; different organs have distinct energy demands and reserves, and the fuel mix that feeds the fire needs to change dynamically. For instance, neurons require a constant supply of glucose as they have little or no glycogen; if the glucose supply stops, neurons die, the brain dies, and disability or death follow. The heart also has a high consistent energy demand as it pumps blood all day, every day, with this demand increasing during exercise. The heart's flame is kept burning by fatty acids with glucose making a lesser contribution. Interrupting the heart's demand for nutrients and oxygen, even momentarily, can cause a searing pain at best (i.e., angina) to irreversible tissue damage or death at worse (i.e., a heart attack). The liver also has a high energy demand which is met flexibly by fat, glucose, and amino acids, all of whose availability can fluctuate in accordance to meals.

Skeletal muscle comprises different fibre types that prefer glucose and/or fat as a metabolic fuel supplied by the circulation and/or internal glycogen and TAG stores.[31] There are muscle fibres specially adapted for fast-twitch contraction (e.g., 100m sprint) which prefer glucose, some are slightly slower fast-twitch fibres that use glucose and fatty acids (e.g., 400m/800m running), whereas others are slow twitch and prefer fat to support endurance exercise (e.g., long-distance running).[32] The kidney also has a consistently high energy requirement, but its unique anatomy means that this demand has to be met in different ways depending on the cell's location. For instance, cells near the outside (i.e., renal cortex) have a very good blood supply and can use fatty acids, glucose, and amino acids as fuel, whereas cells in the inner-most part (i.e., renal medulla) need to use glucose due to a lack of oxygen.

Clearly each organ has unique energy demands that are met with different metabolic fuel combinations, with these needs changing as their activity fluctuates. These energy demands are lowest when we're asleep, during which time our last meal/snack will get digested and stored, leaving several hours before the next meal and influx of nutrients. To ensure we wake safely in the morning, a number of vital functions continue to tick over; our heart beats, our chest muscles contract rhythmically to keep us breathing, and our kidneys filter our blood (even if that results in the annoying need to visit the restroom in the middle of the night!), all the while our brain hums away, consolidating information. Mobilization of glycogen from the liver coupled with gluconeogenesis is sufficient to supply our brain with the glucose it requires to get through the night,[33] while the remainder of our organs tend to increase their fat utilization during sleep.[34]

The phenomenon of 'metabolic flexibility' refers to the ability to respond or adapt to fluctuating metabolic demand and has been used to explain the mechanisms governing fuel selection between glucose and fatty acids under various conditions.[35] Obesity and type 2 diabetes are insulin-resistant, metabolically inflexible states in which exercise is made difficult by the body's inability to efficiently and effectively switch between metabolic fuels to meet its energy demands. So, after running the gauntlet to safely store fatty acids away, how do we get them back out again?

Freeing Fat

Fat mobilization during sleep is largely driven by the decreasing concentration of circulating insulin. As the nutrients from the last meal are cleared from the bloodstream under the control of insulin, the level of this hormone drops. As well as increasing LPL activity to promote TAG storage in fat and muscle, insulin inhibits the cellular machinery in adipocytes used to mobilize fatty acids to shift the overall balance towards fat deposition.[36] As sleep progresses, however, falling insulin levels release this brake on fatty acid mobilization. Fatty acid liberation from an adipocyte's TAG droplet is a closely co-ordinated, multi-step process,[37] just like withdrawing money from the bank to pay a bill. This tight control helps to protect fat reserves and minimize wastage when trying to meet the body's energy demands.

The TAG droplet which essentially fills an adipocyte is coated with a variety of proteins that organize its structure, a bit like security staff surrounding a crowd, letting people in or out. Among these fat droplet-associated proteins are the *perilipins*, which act as gatekeepers that control the flow of fatty acids into and out of the TAG droplet.[38] Fatty acid mobilization from a TAG droplet involves the same series of sequential reactions that occur in the gut for fat digestion, albeit catalyzed by different enzymes. The three fatty acid tails of TAG are sequentially snipped off the glycerol backbone by adipose triacylglycerol lipase,[39] hormone-sensitive lipase (HSL),[40] and then monoacylglycerol lipase.[41]

Once deconstructed and released into the circulation, the glycerol goes to the liver to be recycled. However, the fatty acids may be in the right place (i.e., the bloodstream), but they don't dissolve in water and would coalesce into blood flow-disrupting droplets if left unchaperoned. Free fatty acids are made safe to transport by binding instantaneously to albumin, an abundant, multi-functional protein made by the liver. As the fatty acid-laden albumin rushes around the body in the blood, the organs that need it (i.e., the heart, liver, muscle, and kidneys) simply grab them from the albumin and move them across their cell membrane using a transporter protein.

While diminishing insulin levels remove the brake to allow the wheel of fatty acid mobilization to start turning at a speed that will sustain our bodies through a short period of fasting (e.g., a few hours of sleep), such a rate would be insufficient to meet the energy demands required to sustain energy-intensive activity. Rather than just let the fat mobilization machinery roll forward, we can also hit the accelerator to spin the wheels faster when the energy demand increases.

Pushing the Limits

Our body is primed to support exercise in a number of ways, with the response playing out like a carefully coordinated symphony. Physical and metabolic sensors within skeletal muscle co-ordinate a localized response to exercise, while nervous and hormonal signals prepare our body to meet the demands imposed by exercise. As muscles draw upon local energy stores, the liver mobilizes its glycogen stores to keep circulating levels of glucose stable. If the liver's glycogen stores get depleted, which typically occurs during extreme endurance exercise like marathon running, individuals often experience a potentially incapacitating wave of fatigue known as 'hitting the wall.' The liver also takes the lactic acid produced from the incomplete breakdown of glucose[42] that occurs when oxygen is in short supply and converts it back into glucose. Lactic acid accumulation also contributes to the burning sensation in fatigued muscle or the painful 'stitch' in your side upon exercising.

Additionally, nerve impulses to adipose tissue stimulate fatty acid release.[43] Sympathetic nervous system neurons (which co-ordinate our evolutionarily honed 'fight-or-flight' response) release the neurotransmitter noradrenaline/norepinephrine onto adipocytes which activates receptors (more specifically, beta-adrenoceptors) on the cell surface. This activates HSL, via droplet-associated perilipins,[44] which results in TAG breakdown and free fatty acids being released into the bloodstream. The activation of beta-adrenoceptors also increases blood flow to adipose tissue,[45] thus enhancing fatty acid delivery. As our heart beats faster and harder, increased stretching of its chambers can stimulate the release of hormones like atrial natriuretic peptide[46] that acts on adipocytes to further promote fatty acid mobilization.[47] The response to exercise involves the vastly complex co-ordination of organ biology on many levels, across numerous organs.

While keeping the metabolic furnace burning in contracting muscles is certainly important, exercise also forces our body to keep a number of biological plates spinning even faster than normal to stop our bodies from coming apart at the seams. In addition to matching our breathing and heart rate to the intensity of exercise to ensure nutrient delivery and gas exchange, various sophisticated compensatory mechanisms kick into high gear to maintain our body temperature as well as the salt levels, volume, and acidity of our blood.[48] Exercise is the most common form of physiological stress that our body can—and indeed should—be routinely exposed to. Aside from the muscles being worked, exercise has wide-ranging benefits due to the integrated response of numerous organs. Regular aerobic exercise and/or resistance training is a cornerstone of healthy living that exerts well-documented benefits such as increased longevity, reduced disease risk, and enhanced mobility[49]; it also improves the prognosis and symptoms of many chronic diseases.[50] It's no wonder that exercise has been termed the closest thing to a wonder-drug![51]

When Hunger Strikes

With a greater understanding of energy metabolism, let us now consider the role of fat that comes to mind when we first think of our controversial blubber. Imagine waking from an overnight fast only to discover that there is nothing to eat in the house and, worse still, the nearby shops, cafes, and restaurants are empty. If this nightmarish situation persists, then the temporary overnight fast will soon become a period of prolonged starvation. To survive this increasingly hostile nutritional environment, our body undergoes a series of co-ordinated metabolic changes[52] in which we raid our energy reserves while increasing our fuel efficiency. Surviving starvation involves walking along a knife-edge. The body has to balance cannibalizing itself to feed the brain (so we can think of an escape plan) with maintaining sufficient muscle mass and energy reserves (to execute a plan and obtain food). A large fat reserve might mean your body may be powered for a long time, but if you're too unfit or heavy to move yourself out of the dangerous 'food-free zone' and obtain resources, that extra fuel might be more of a burden than a life-saver.[53]

Glucose becomes even more precious than normal during starvation. To preserve this valuable commodity for our brain, the majority of our organs switch from running on their typical fuel mixture to something slightly different. During the early phase of starvation, many organs use the fatty acids from fat as their primary metabolic fuel. However, as fatty acids are not optimal for many organs, the liver instead turns them into *ketone bodies*, molecules which essentially act as a substitute for glucose. This process is known as 'ketogenesis' and involves chopping the long fatty acid tails into small chunks and tweaking their chemical structure before releasing them into the bloodstream. The level of circulating ketone bodies steadily rises until a plateau is reached when the body's energy demands are met; organs like the muscle and kidney adapt to using ketone bodies, meaning the overall demand for fatty acids declines, thus making our fat stores go further. However, the brain is a bit of a fussy eater and takes time to make the switch, a process which is elongated by gluconeogenesis (as glucose may be made from the amino acids derived from muscle breakdown). However, after switching to ketone bodies, the brain becomes dependent on the far greater reserves of energy stored in fat tissue, thus bolstering the chances of prolonging one's existence.

Ketone bodies play a crucial role in the adaptation to starvation, but are actually made by the liver every day, albeit in small amounts that make a modest contribution to the metabolic fuel mixture used by most organs. The production of ketone bodies is primarily determined by insulin (i.e., the master storage signal), or more specifically, its absence.[42] Indeed, the persistent low levels of insulin during starvation release the brake on ketogenesis, thus allowing ketone body production to climb. However, the complete absence of insulin which can occur in patients with type 1 diabetes who don't take their insulin can precipitate an extreme starvation response in which ketogenesis runs amok.[54] The massive accumulation of ketone bodies can cause the blood to become acidic, thereby putting the person at great risk of brain damage, coma, and even death if left untreated. This dangerous situation is known as 'diabetic ketoacidosis' and is accompanied by dizziness, confusion, excessive thirst, frequent urination, nausea/vomiting, and shortness of breath, while the high circulating levels of ketone bodies give the patient distinctly fruity-smelling breath.

Ketogenesis, or more specifically ketogenic ('keto') diets, entered the public's consciousness during the early 2000s as a result of the surging popularity of the Atkins diet. Devised by the late Robert Atkin, an American physician and cardiologist, the Atkins diet is a commercial weight-loss programme which revolves around the highly contentious claim that carbohydrate restriction is the 'key' to weight loss.[55] The low carbohydrate content of the Atkins diet typically induces a certain degree of fat mobilization and ketogenesis, with the ketone bodies also acting as an appetite suppressant.[56]

Like most other (fad) diets, the Atkins nutritional approach usually brings about rapid weight loss that doesn't tend to be sustained over the long-term, although this is typically determined by diet adherence.[57] It has been proposed that the precipitous early weight loss principally arises from the loss of water weight as the body's carbohydrate stores are emptied, with this weight being quickly regained if/when the diet ends and carbohydrate consumption resumes.[58] It is currently unclear what the long-term health implications of the Atkins diet are given reports that suggest it may increase the risk of developing heart disease[59,60] or have no effect.[61] While the Atkins diet may not represent a particularly effective or sustainable long-term intervention to address obesity or metabolic disease for many people, there is mounting evidence indicating that individuals who experience frequent epileptic seizures, particularly children, can benefit from a ketogenic diet,[62] although the mechanisms underpinning this phenomenon remain unclear. There is also growing interest in the role of ketone bodies as signalling molecules that may be relevant to cancer biology as well as the heart, liver, and nervous system in health and disease.[63]

Carb Converter

The liver and adipose tissue are a tremendous double act that not only keep our body's metabolic furnace burning, but also co-ordinate the logistics involved in maintaining replete energy stores. But what happens if our diet provides too much of one nutrient and not enough of another? Just like a good chef will use, rather than waste, surplus ingredients, the liver within our incredibly frugal body makes the shrewd move of converting excess carbohydrates (and amino acids) into fatty acids via 'de novo lipo-genesis' (DNL)[64] under the auspices of insulin. As one might expect, DNL has been found to increase in response to the consistent consumption of a high carbohydrate diet[65] as well as overfeeding.[66] While the liver is the pri-mary site for DNL, this process can also occur in adipose tissue, although this contribution ranges from minor[67] to negligible.[68] Moreover, the im-portance of this process to health and disease in general is far from clear.

What becomes of the nascent fatty acids in the liver? Owing to the layout of the cellular machinery, newly synthesized fatty acids don't just roll off the factory line and straight into the metabolic furnace. Instead, the insulin promoting DNL simultaneously reduces the activity of the fat-burning machinery in the liver and suppresses fatty acid mobiliza-tion from adipose tissue, thereby co-ordinating a body-wide shift from fat burning to fat storage. Once synthesized, the new fatty acids join the TAG droplet within the liver cells, but only temporarily, as the vast majority get packaged up and shipped out. Similar to the generation of chylomicrons by the gut, liver cells package TAG with a different type of apolipoprotein to make very low-density lipoproteins (VLDL) which are released into the bloodstream. These VLDL particles then deliver their cargo to muscle and adipose tissue in the same way that chylomicrons do after a fat-containing meal (via the enzyme LPL). Shrinking with each delivery, eventually the VLDLs become low-density lipoproteins (LDL) particles (which con-tain less fat and are less buoyant/more dense) before being taken out of circulation upon binding to the LDL receptor on the surface of various cell types; either the liver recycles them or other organs cannibalize them for parts.

The liver clearly sits in a precarious position at the heart of the meta-bolic marketplace, acting as a central distributor and processing plant that keeps our warehouse stocked (i.e., fat) and factories operational (e.g., brain, muscle, kidneys etc.). The liver evidently has a large quantity of fat flowing through it every day, although the amount can fluctuate dynamically in accordance to meal-times and physical activity. This unrelenting fat flux means that the liver has to work around the clock to ensure the inflow (e.g., fat from the diet in chylomicrons, free fatty acids from adipose tissue, and fatty acids made by the liver) matches the outflow (e.g., fatty acids shipped out as VLDL or burned by the liver as fuel) to prevent an accumulation of fat which could turn the liver into *foie gras* (Figure 3.6).

While the liver handles its role expertly most of the time, fat can accumulate if inflow exceeds outflow. Losing the precise and integrated regulation of fat storage, synthesis, and usage due to insulin resistance can mean small errors creep in which are magnified over time and can result in liver dysfunction. Fat accumulation in the liver occurs on a sliding scale in which lesser amounts are known as 'steatosis' whereas larger amounts are designated 'non-alcoholic fatty liver disease' (NAFLD).[69] Fatty livers can then become inflamed and fibrotic, a state known as 'steatohepatitis,' with this inflammation potentially causing irreversible damage in the form of scarring or cirrhosis. The development of fatty liver disease is highly complex; increased DNL by the liver[70] has been implicated, with obesity and insulin resistance representing key risk factors.[71]

Amidst the colossal global burden of obesity and metabolic disease, it should perhaps be unsurprising that there is a silent fatty liver pandemic.[72] Fatty livers are associated with poor metabolic and cardiovascular health outcomes,[73] as well as liver cancer; it's no coincidence that liver cancer is one of the fastest growing types of cancer in the US.[74] While the million-dollar question of whether liver-fat accumulation represents a cause or

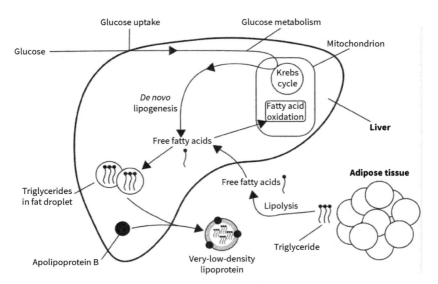

Figure 3.6 Fatty acid flux in the liver.

consequence of metabolic disease remains unanswered (it's probably both[75]), the current approach to treating fatty liver is largely the same as that for obesity and type 2 diabetes. The same litany of diet, exercise, drugs, and/or bariatric surgery (see Chapter 7) tend to benefit NAFLD patients and alleviate its associated complications,[76] thus highlighting the close relationship between obesity, diabetes, and fatty liver disease, as well as the deep integration of the associated organs.

The Essentials of Fatty Acids

The liver's DNL toolkit enables the synthesis of various fatty acids from carbohydrates and amino acids, although it can't make everything that the body needs. The *non-essential* fatty acids that our bodies can make mainly comprise fatty acids with relatively simple structures. For instance, saturated (i.e., no double bonds between carbon atoms) fats like palmitic acid (also found in butter and meat) have a regular structure that mean they are solid at room temperature (Figure 3.3). Conversely, non-essential unsaturated (i.e., contain more than one double bond between carbon atoms) fatty acids like oleic acid (also found in sunflower oil) have irregular structures that render these fatty acids liquid at room temperature. The human body is unable to synthesize more complex polyunsaturated fatty acids like alpha-linolenic acid (an omega-3 fatty acid) or linoleic acid (an omega-6 fatty acid), meaning these fatty acids are *essential* and must be obtained through the diet.[77] These 'good' fats are found in olive oil, eggs, fish, and green leafy vegetables like broccoli and spinach. While many fatty acids are used as metabolic fuel, these molecules also play important roles in the structure of cell membranes as well as signalling in the brain and immune system.[3,78]

One of the highest profile stories concerning dietary fat and health pertains to *trans-fats*. Trans-fats are made through the industrial process of hydrogenation which removes double bonds in unsaturated fatty acids, thereby causing an atomic rearrangement to the *trans* (rather than *cis*) configuration. Human consumption of trans-fats has skyrocketed since the 1950s with the industrialization of the world's diet and the booming popularity of fried fast food, snack food, packaged baked goods, and margarine. A compelling body of evidence indicates that the consumption of trans-fatty acids causes metabolic dysfunction[79] and is associated with an increased risk of cardiovascular disease and premature death.[80] There has been a multi-pronged public health intervention led by various governments in response to this stark message which has achieved its aim of reducing trans-fat consumption to varying degrees of success.[81] Removing trans-fats and other saturated fatty acids is not entirely straightforward, however, as the globalized economy and world's eating habits necessitate their replacement, but with what?

Current data suggest replacing saturated and trans-fats with carbohydrate would *not* reduce the death rate from cardiovascular disease, whereas substitution with mono- or polyunsaturated fatty acids would.[80] Indeed, increased consumption of unsaturated fatty acids (as exemplified by the Mediterranean diet) is associated with a favourable metabolic health profile[82] and reduced incidence of type 2 diabetes.[83] Whether improving the quality of fat in the world's diet could be sustainably achieved and what, if any, impact this might have on cardiovascular health remains to be seen. While the association between saturated/trans-fats and cardiovascular health was clear enough to prompt decisive (and hopefully effective) action, numerous lurching decisions by governments and the food industry have mired other aspects of nutrition in confusion and controversy,[84] with cholesterol being the most notable victim.

Part 4—Cholesterol: Dr Jekyll or Mr Hyde?

Cholesterol may be as feared as much as fat is despised. Most people have heard of 'good' and 'bad' cholesterol, but what does it actually do? In its unmodified form, cholesterol is inserted or removed from cell membranes to regulate their fluidity and permeability.[85] If a cell membrane were a piece of leather, cholesterol would be a salve that can be rubbed in to change the balance between flexibility and rigidity. As the cell membrane is the interface between the internal and external world for billions of cells, this structure—and therefore cholesterol—is involved in roles as diverse as maintaining a cell's structural integrity, co-ordinating signalling within cells,[86] and even nerve impulse conduction.[87]

Bile acids made by the liver and released by the gall bladder to aid fat digestion are modified cholesterol molecules. Cholesterol is also the chemical foundation of all steroid hormones, namely the glucocorticoids (i.e., stress hormones like cortisol) and mineralocorticoids (i.e., salt-regulating hormones like aldosterone) made by the adrenal gland, as well as the sex steroids (e.g., testosterone and oestrogen made by ovaries and testes, respectively). Even vitamin D synthesized in our skin which regulates calcium absorption and bone health has a cholesterol base. Despite its villainous reputation, cholesterol does a lot of good work. Cholesterol metabolism is multi-faceted, complex, and important, so much so, the Nobel Prize in Physiology or Medicine in 1985 was awarded jointly to Michael S. Brown and Joseph L. Goldstein 'for their discoveries concerning the regulation of cholesterol metabolism.'[88]

Cholesterol, Lipoproteins, and Atherosclerosis

How can cholesterol be both good and bad? Understanding this seemingly paradoxical situation requires considering where cholesterol comes from and how it is transported around the body. We obtain some cholesterol from food such as eggs, cheese, and meat; a recent meta-analysis concluded that increased consumption of cholesterol does increase total and LDL cholesterol levels, but that this is *not* associated with an increased risk of cardiovascular disease.[89] Once absorbed by the gut, dietary cholesterol is packaged up with fatty acids into chylomicrons. These chylomicrons deliver TAG and cholesterol around the body until the empty chylomicron remnants are removed from the bloodstream by the liver which cannibalizes these particles for parts. The liver can also synthesize cholesterol, which it packages along with TAG into VLDL for delivery to organs around the body. As the VLDL particles circulate and deliver TAG and cholesterol, they shrink and become LDL particles, which are what doctors often refer to as 'bad' cholesterol.

Low-density lipoprotein levels can be increased in insulin-resistant states which enable greater fatty acid mobilization from adipose tissue and result in the liver generating more VLDL particles.[90] These particles participate in a complex transfer of TAG and cholesterol between lipoprotein types that culminates in increased circulating numbers of small dense LDL (and high-density lipoprotein (HDL)) particles; this insidious shift in the lipoprotein population often precedes the raised glucose levels for which type 2 diabetes is famous.[91] After undergoing a structural change promoted by the metabolic stress induced by insulin-resistant states (e.g., obesity), the LDL apolipoprotein becomes a target for the 'scavenger receptors' present on the surface of immune cells known as macrophages which remove cellular debris generated by immunological warfare waged against foreign invaders.[92] As these cells cannot turn their scavenger receptors off, persistently high LDL levels run the risk of overloading macrophages with cholesterol and turning them into 'foam cells.'

These foam cells can get trapped in blood vessel walls, particularly arteries, and form 'fatty streaks'[93] which serve as the foundation for atherosclerotic plaque development.[94] These unsightly, dangerous structures restrict blood flow and force the heart to work harder, while their rough surface disrupts blood flow and makes it more likely to clot.[93] When the coronary arteries are affected by atherosclerosis, it can be difficult for the heart's consistently high oxygen and nutrient demand to be adequately met; this typically manifests as chest pains (i.e., angina pectoris), particularly during exercise.[95] If the narrowed blood vessel gets completely blocked by a piece of plaque breaking off or a blood clot, the heart muscle's blood supply is cut off; this myocardial infarction (i.e., heart attack) often results in irreversible damage to the heart muscle that can be fatal if not treated rapidly.

What about 'good' cholesterol? HDL are another type of circulating apolipoprotein made by the liver that facilitate the removal of cholesterol from various cell types (i.e., reverse cholesterol transport) to ultimately return it to the liver for recycling or disposal. HDL particles also swipe some cargo from other circulating lipoproteins (i.e., VLDL, LDL, and chylomicrons) as it is delivered around the body, just like passengers swapping between different bus services. Excess cholesterol captured within HDL particles is returned to the liver via several ways, with one pathway involving a specific type of scavenger receptor on the liver cell surface.[96] Bound HDL particles are then relieved of their cholesterol cargo and released back into the circulation to pick up more cholesterol.[97] Alternatively, cholesterol can move from loaded HDL particles back to VLDL, LDL, or chylomicrons before the cholesterol-rich lipoprotein remnants are taken up by the liver, just like someone riding different buses until eventually returning to the terminal. Once back in the liver, getting rid of cholesterol can be tricky, which is perhaps unsurprising given that molecular hoarding played an essential role in our evolution. The liver can dispose of some cholesterol by releasing it directly into the gut to be lost in the faeces, although some is converted into bile acids which facilitate fat digestion; most bile acids are re-absorbed and recycled between the gut and liver, although some are lost in the faeces.

There is a clear message that reducing elevated cholesterol levels brings great health benefits. Analysis of data from 19 different industrialized countries during the 1980s highlighted that the rate at which men died from cardiovascular disease increased in proportion to total cholesterol levels (i.e., HDL, VLDL, and LDL combined).[98] A recent meta-analysis (in which pre-existing data from different studies was pooled and re-analyzed) of nearly 900,000 people[99] has since reported that reducing total cholesterol levels was associated with protection against heart attack deaths in people aged between 40 and 89 years old, although this beneficial effect diminished with increasing age. The role of HDL cholesterol in cardiovascular health is more complicated. Although previous studies have reported that lower levels of HDL are associated with higher rates of cardiovascular death,[99] very high HDL levels have also been found to predict increased risk of premature death in men and women.[100,101] Evidently achieving optimal cardiovascular health involves HDL levels occupying a happy middle ground in conjunction with low total and LDL cholesterol levels.

The relationship between circulating cholesterol levels and cardiovascular disease is most clearly demonstrated in patients with familial hypercholesterolaemia (FH).[102] Although there are several different types of this condition, many patients possess a genetic mutation that renders their LDL receptor non-functional, meaning cholesterol-laden LDL particles cannot be cleared from the bloodstream. The resultant accumulation of circulating LDL greatly increases the risk of developing cardiovascular disease, particularly atherosclerosis, and dying prematurely of a heart attack (usually between their 30s and 40s). Treatment typically involves intensive, life-long treatment with statins, the world's premier cholesterol-lowering drugs. Several clinical trial meta-analyses provide compelling evidence that these cholesterol-lowering drugs not only lower total and LDL cholesterol, but also reduce the rates of fatal and non-fatal heart attacks and strokes, as well as all-cause mortality, with minimal adverse effects in men and women.[103–105] In other words, statins save lives, and lots of them. But how do they work?

Statins inhibit HMG-CoA reductase, a liver enzyme that regulates a critical step in cholesterol synthesis. The modern statin originated from work performed by the Japanese biochemist Akira Endo who proposed that HMG-CoA reductase inhibitors may occur naturally because this enzyme's product maintains the integrity of cell walls in various micro-organisms. His proposal was vindicated in 1976 with the discovery of mevastatin,[106] a naturally occurring HMG-CoA reductase inhibitor produced by the fungus *Penicillium citrinum*. Although mevastatin never made it to market due to adverse effects, a similar molecule was isolated from the fungus *Aspergillus terreus* and reached the market as lovastatin in 1987.[107] Several other statins have been developed since, with this class of drug being among the world's most widely prescribed medications. It seems that cholesterol is neither Dr Jekyll nor Mr Hyde, but is instead misunderstood like fat, having acquired a bad reputation for the disastrous consequences which result from having too much of the 'wrong kind.'

Part 5—Additional Roles that Fat Can Play

Shelter

Fat plays a central role (with the liver) in ensuring our body's dynamic energy demands are consistently met—but that's not all it does. Fat keeps us warm. Maintaining our core temperature is vital for survival so humans have evolved a variety of mechanisms that protect our bodies against extreme temperatures.[108] Our subcutaneous white fat acts as an insulating layer that keeps the cold at bay.[109] But when chilly becomes frigid and a static layer of insulation is insufficient, our body employs more sophisticated strategies that involve activating brown fat (see Chapter 4) and responses such as shivering, seeking shelter, and wearing warmer clothes.

Appetite Regulation

Fat is the body's largest endocrine organ and it releases various hormones ('adipokines'[110]) into the bloodstream which regulate glucose and fat metabolism, appetite, and sexual development, as well as our immune system. The archetypal adipokine is leptin, a proteinaceous hormone that achieved worldwide fame upon its discovery in the mid-1990s.[111] Deriving its name from the Greek term for thin (*leptos*), leptin was identified as a circulating factor that exerts potent appetite-suppressing effects in a series of grotesque yet elegant parabiosis experiments performed during the late 1960s/early 1970s in which the circulatory systems of normal and genetically engineered mice were surgically joined.[112,113] It has since been determined that leptin is secreted by adipocytes and circulates in the plasma at levels directly proportional to the degree of overall fatness,[114] and that it crosses the blood–brain barrier to act on neurons in the hypothalamus to dampen our appetite.[115] It follows that leptin probably signals the size of our fat stores to the brain to influence the complex process of appetite regulation.

The sheer power of leptin to control our feeding behaviour is exemplified in the handful of individuals who possess rare genetic mutations that render their leptin non-functional. The absence of functional leptin leaves such individuals with an insatiable appetite that invariably leads to extreme obesity during childhood.[116] Parents of such children have been known to experience their child's violent temper tantrums at the slightest hint that food might be denied, as well as the need to install padlocks on cupboards and fridges! However, this emotionally draining, unsustainable, and increasingly dangerous situation can be resolved by administering leptin to the patient.[117] After merely days of treatment, a dramatic reduction in appetite is usually observed. Over time, patients shed their excess weight and often return to a normal, healthy weight. Just like insulin injections for type 1 diabetes patients, leptin injections really do give leptin-deficient patients and their families their lives back.

Sexual Development and Function

Leptin doesn't just provide a signal from fat to the brain to regulate feeding behaviour though, as mounting evidence suggests that it plays a key role in co-ordinating puberty and fertility too. Before leptin had been discovered as the key molecule underpinning the obesity displayed by a specific strain of transgenic mice, it was already well-established by the 1970s that these same mice were typically infertile and had perturbed levels of hormones that regulate sexual development and function.[118] Once identified, however, it was soon found that leptin treatment could restore proper sexual development and fertility in both male[119] and female[120] mice. Such discoveries laid the groundwork for investigations into the dizzyingly complex yet impressively precise actions of leptin on the brain, particularly the hypothalamus, to co-ordinate the pituitary gland secretions that choreograph puberty and regulate fertility throughout adulthood.[121]

A picture is emerging which suggests that leptin represents a critical component of a highly complex molecular network that co-ordinates body composition to reproductive biology, a connection that runs remarkably deep. Following early observations in the 1960s that puberty onset in rats correlates more strongly with body size than chronological age,[122] the results of several seminal epidemiological studies prompted the proposal that (female) sexual development requires a minimal amount of body fat (~17%[123,124]). In the modern developed world where food is abundant, however, this ancient connection (see Chapter 2) can be disrupted in women who drastically reduce their body fat content through exercise (particularly professional ballet dancers or gymnasts[125]) or diet (e.g., individuals with anorexia nervosa[126]). Women with low fat mass have correspondingly low levels of leptin as well as low levels of circulating reproductive hormones, a situation which can result in their menstrual cycle ceasing (i.e., amenorrhoea).[127] However, this situation is reversible as women's menstrual cycles (and therefore fertility) return if and when their body fat mass increases above the necessary threshold[128] (~22% body fat is required for regular menstruation[123]); leptin treatment may also represent a viable treatment option in such cases.[129]

It is notable that the average age of puberty onset in girls[130] and boys[131] from around the world has gotten progressively younger over the past decades. Although difficult to pinpoint, it has been proposed that widespread childhood obesity may be playing a major role in this phenomenon.[132] Consistent with animal data, puberty in humans deficient for functional leptin is usually very delayed or doesn't happen at all, with many individuals not developing secondary sexual characteristics such as pubic hair, enlarged breasts, and widened hips in females or facial hair and an Adam's apple in males.[133] However, leptin treatment often corrects many of these abnormalities in addition to reversing the individual's massive appetite and alleviating their obesity.[134] The inter-relation between fat, leptin, and reproductive health is exemplified in the case of a woman with congenital generalized lipodystrophy (i.e., a rare genetic condition defined by little-to-no adipose tissue—see Chapter 7) who displayed an almost complete absence of leptin. Initially infertile, leptin injections not only brought about a significant improvement in this woman's metabolic health and obesity, but also restored her reproductive health such that she was able to naturally conceive and later give birth to a healthy baby boy[135]; leptin injections not only give leptin-deficient individuals their life back, but can also enable its creation.

Although leptin represents an important molecular link between energy metabolism and fertility, it is not alone nor the most important factor. Body fat has a potent influence over fertility in men and women because adipose tissue is home to an arsenal of enzymes that catalyze the activation, interconversion, and inactivation of various steroid hormones which define our reproductive (and metabolic) health.[136] Knowledge of this highly complex aspect of fat biology pre-dates the identification of any biologically active protein hormones like leptin.[137] However, mapping the network of interactions between (gonadal and adipose-derived) sex steroids with the likes of insulin and cortisol which manifest as sex-specific regional fat distribution patterns during puberty and influence fertility remains a daunting investigative challenge.[138]

Obesity puts men at increased risk of infertility because the larger adipose mass can result in greater conversion of testosterone to oestrogen, which then suppresses sperm generation.[139] The severe metabolic stress that obesity imposes also perturbs the levels of other hormones (e.g., insulin and leptin) in ways that can disrupt sperm generation and damage pre-existing sperm.[140] With evidence suggesting that the negative effects of obesity and metabolic disease on male fertility may not be entirely reversible,[141] it follows that keeping fit and not gaining weight in the first place represents the best approach for any prospective father.

Stress

Fat tissue also metabolizes glucocorticoids, the steroid hormones involved in co-ordinating our stress response. Cortisol is the key glucocorticoid in humans and it has wide-ranging, evolutionarily honed effects that promote our chances of survival in situations of acute danger. Primarily acting to promote the mobilization of energy stores to combat danger or retreat from it in the short-term, long-term exposure to elevated levels of glucocorticoids has been implicated in the development of numerous ailments, particularly metabolic and cardiovascular disease.[142] Although their useful immunosuppressive properties are routinely exploited to treat inflammatory conditions and prevent post-transplantation organ rejection, their negative metabolic effects are well-established in the medical community. The complex effects of glucocorticoids on metabolic and cardiovascular health are inextricably linked to their potent influence over body fat distribution[142] (see Chapters 6 and 7).

Immunity

Adipose tissue, energy metabolism, and the immune system share a deep link forged during evolution due to the life-or-death interplay in which metabolic resources are allocated to support host defence and survival.[143] Depending on the abundance of resources and nature of the threat, energy metabolism and immunity co-operate to protect the host by invoking dormancy and/or defence protocols. In the case of surviving an infection, a defensive immune response to fight the infection is mounted, which requires nutrients to build the necessary molecular and cellular tools.[144] This is complemented by the engagement of energy-conserving dormancy behaviours which limit non-essential activities (i.e., growth and reproduction) that typically manifest as malaise, social withdrawal, and loss of libido.[145] Additionally, there is activation of mechanisms that protect tissues from immunological collateral damage (e.g., oxidative stress[146]). Fighting an infection is like fighting a war in which some participants gear up for the frontline while others take shelter to wait the conflict out.

Adipose tissue is resident to a dynamic population of immune cells[147]; white blood cell aggregates were first reported as 'milky spots' residing within human omental fat as early as 1874.[148] Since these initial observations, it has become widely appreciated that the activity of adipose immune cells plays an important role in determining local and whole-body insulin sensitivity and metabolic health.[149] Depending on the type of signal and status of the immune cells, inflammatory signals can exert positive[150] and negative[151] effects on adipocyte (as well as liver and muscle cell) function to influence metabolic health accordingly. Conversely, adipose-derived signals can directly modulate immune cell function,[152] with this complex relationship contributing to the low-grade inflammation in obesity that promotes metabolic and cardiovascular disease,[153] in addition to obesity-related cancers[154] and osteoarthritis.[155] Moreover, obesity impairs our immune system's function[156] in a way that not only reduces our ability to fight off infections, but also decreases the efficacy of vaccines,[157] meaning many individuals remain susceptible to infection by vaccine-preventable diseases.[158] This issue has the potential to severely undermine the efforts to rein in the global COVID-19 pandemic; obesity is already associated with much worse prognoses,[159] most likely due to underlying immune dysfunction.[160] This situation means the weight of the world's population is exacerbating the pandemic as well as protracting the global recovery efforts following vaccine availability.[161]

The vast and growing literature exploring the interplay between energy metabolism and immune function is too large to do justice in a brief overview. Moreover, the biology is so complex and context-specific it is impossible to state whether fat is the 'good guy' or the 'bad guy.' For instance, fat cells within our skin protect us from injury and infection by co-ordinating wound repair and releasing anti-microbial molecules.[162] On the other hand, however, adipose tissue can stand in the way of a complete cure for HIV/AIDS as infected immune cells can hide within fat, out of reach of the immune system and anti-retroviral drugs.[163] Fat can also host various parasitic helminths whose presence might actually enhance adipose function and improve metabolic health.[164] But don't entertain the idea that purposely getting a worm infestation is an easy way to get 'beach body ready'; helminths pose a serious threat to life by inducing life-threatening immune responses[165] as well as malnutrition, anaemia, and reduced cognitive function. The far-reaching relationship between immunity, energy metabolism, and adipose tissue has the ability to touch anybody's life at any stage, often manifesting in a way that reflects its ancient origins and the primal struggle for existence.

Having considered the wide-ranging biology of white fat and its key role (along with the liver) in keeping our metabolic furnace burning, whether we're vegetating on the sofa, trying to run a marathon, or survive a famine, the next chapter considers the other, more esoteric types of fat residing within our bodies.

References

1. Frayn, K. Adipose tissue as a buffer for daily lipid flux. *Diabetologia* **45**, 1201–10 (2002).
2. Frayn, K. N. *Metabolic Regulation: A Human Perspective*. Wiley–Blackwell 2010.
3. Kremmyda, L. S., Tvrzicka, E., Stankova, B., & Zak, A. Fatty acids as biocompounds: their role in human metabolism, health and disease: a review. Part 2: fatty acid physiological roles and applications in human health and disease. *Biomed. Pap. Med. Fac. Univ. Palacky. Olomouc. Czech. Repub.* **155**, 195–218 (2011).
4. Varki, A. Biological roles of glycans. *Glycobiology* **27**, 3–49 (2017).
5. Aghazadeh, Y. & Nostro, M. C. Cell therapy for type 1 diabetes: current and future strategies. *Curr. Diab. Rep.* **17**, 37 (2017).
6. Barrett, E. J. *et al.* Diabetic microvascular disease: an endocrine society scientific statement. *J. Clin. Endocrinol. Metab.* **102**, 4343–410 (2017).
7. Yaribeygi, H., Farrokhi, F. R., Butler, A. E., & Sahebkar, A. Insulin resistance: review of the underlying molecular mechanisms. *J. Cell. Physiol.* **234**, 8152–61 (2019).
8. Walther, T. C. & Farese, R. V. Lipid droplets and cellular lipid metabolism. *Annu. Rev. Biochem.* **81**, 687–714 (2012).
9. Fraser, J. K., Zhu, M., Wulur, I., & Alfonso, Z. Adipose-derived stem cells. *Methods Mol. Biol.* **449**, 59–67 (2008).
10. Nguyen, A. *et al.* Stromal vascular fraction: a regenerative reality? Part 1: current concepts and review of the literature. *J. Plast. Reconstr. Aesthet. Surg.* **69**, 170–9 (2016).

11. Divoux, A. & Clément, K. Architecture and the extracellular matrix: the still unappreciated components of the adipose tissue. *Obes. Rev.* **12**, e494–503 (2011).

12. Gesta, S., Tseng, Y.-H., & Kahn, C. R. Developmental origin of fat: tracking obesity to its source. *Cell* **131**, 242–56 (2007).

13. Frayn, K. N. & Karpe, F. Regulation of human subcutaneous adipose tissue blood flow. *Int. J. Obes. (Lond).* **38**, 1019–26 (2014).

14. Scholten, E. Composite foods: from structure to sensory perception. *Food Funct.* **8**, 481–97 (2017).

15. Gordon, E. L., Ariel-Donges, A. H., Bauman, V., & Merlo, L. J. What is the evidence for 'food addiction?' A systematic review. *Nutrients* **10**, (2018).

16. Coccurello, R. & Maccarrone, M. Hedonic eating and the 'delicious circle': from lipid-derived mediators to brain dopamine and back. *Front. Neurosci.* **12**, 271 (2018).

17. Beauchamp, G. K. Why do we like sweet taste: a bitter tale? *Physiol. Behav.* **164**, 432–7 (2016).

18. Lammert, F. *et al.* Gallstones. *Nat. Rev. Dis. Prim.* **2**, 16024 (2016).

19. Guerciolini, R. Mode of action of orlistat. *Int. J. Obes. Relat. Metab. Disord.* **21 Suppl. 3**, S12–23 (1997).

20. Sahebkar, A. *et al.* Effect of orlistat on plasma lipids and body weight: a systematic review and meta-analysis of 33 randomized controlled trials. *Pharmacol. Res.* **122**, 53–65 (2017).

21. Kersten, S. Physiological regulation of lipoprotein lipase. *Biochim. Biophys. Acta* **1841**, 919–33 (2014).

22. Frayn, K. N. *et al.* Regulation of fatty acid movement in human adipose tissue in the postabsorptive-to-postprandial transition. *Am. J. Physiol.* **266**, E308–17 (1994).

23. Evans, K., Burdge, G. C., Wootton, S. A., Clark, M. L., & Frayn, K. N. Regulation of dietary fatty acid entrapment in subcutaneous adipose tissue and skeletal muscle. *Diabetes* **51**, 2684–90 (2002).

24. Coleman, R. A. & Lee, D. P. Enzymes of triacylglycerol synthesis and their regulation. *Prog. Lipid Res.* **43**, 134–76 (2004).

25. Rahalkar, A. R. *et al.* Novel LPL mutations associated with lipoprotein lipase deficiency: two case reports and a literature review. *Can. J. Physiol. Pharmacol.* **87**, 151–60 (2009).

26. Whalen, J. Gene-therapy approval marks major milestone. *The Wall Street Journal* Nov 2 (2012). Available at: www.wsj.com/articles/SB10001424052970 2037076045780950919940871524.

27. Scott, L. J. Alipogene tiparvovec: a review of its use in adults with familial lipoprotein lipase deficiency. *Drugs* **75**, 175–82 (2015).

28. Sagonowsky, E. With its launch fizzling out, UniQure gives up on $1M+ gene therapy Glybera. *FiercePharma* Apr 20 (2017). Available at: www.fiercepharma. com/pharma/uniqure-gives-up-1m-gene-therapy-glybera.

29. Bryant, L. M. *et al.* Lessons learned from the clinical development and market authorization of Glybera. *Hum. Gene Ther. Clin. Dev.* **24**, 55–64 (2013).

30. Wang, D., Tai, P. W. L., & Gao, G. Adeno-associated virus vector as a platform for gene therapy delivery. *Nat. Rev. Drug Discov.* **18**, 358–78 (2019).

31. Herbison, G. J., Jaweed, M. M., & Ditunno, J. F. Muscle fiber types. *Arch. Phys. Med. Rehabil.* **63**, 227–30 (1982).

32. Scott, W., Stevens, J., & Binder–Macleod, S. A. Human skeletal muscle fiber type classifications. *Phys. Ther.* **81**, 1810–16 (2001).

33. Wasserman, D. H. Four grams of glucose. *Am. J. Physiol. Endocrinol. Metab.* **296**, E11–21 (2009).

34. Poggiogalle, E., Jamshed, H., & Peterson, C. M. Circadian regulation of glucose, lipid, and energy metabolism in humans. *Metabolism* (2018). doi:10.1016/j.metabol.2017.11.017

35. Goodpaster, B. H. & Sparks, L. M. Metabolic flexibility in health and disease. *Cell Metab.* **25**, 1027–36 (2017).

36. Dimitriadis, G., Mitrou, P., Lambadiari, V., Maratou, E., & Raptis, S. A. Insulin effects in muscle and adipose tissue. *Diabetes Res. Clin. Pract.* **93 Suppl. 1**, S52–9 (2011).

37. Nielsen, T. S., Jessen, N., Jørgensen, J. O. L., Møller, N., & Lund, S. Dissecting adipose tissue lipolysis: molecular regulation and implications for metabolic disease. *J. Mol. Endocrinol.* **52**, R199–222 (2014).

38. Sztalryd, C. & Brasaemle, D. L. The perilipin family of lipid droplet proteins: gatekeepers of intracellular lipolysis. *Biochim. Biophys. Acta* **1862**, 1221–32 (2017).

39. Zimmermann, R. *et al.* Fat mobilization in adipose tissue is promoted by adipose triglyceride lipase. *Science* **306**, 1383–6 (2004).

40. Rizack, M. A. Activation of an epinephrine-sensitive lipolytic activity from adipose. *J. Biol. Chem.* **239**, 392–5 (1964).

41. Vaughan, M., Berger, J. E., & Steinberg, D. Hormone-sensitive lipase and monoglyceride lipase activities in adipose tissue. *J. Biol. Chem.* **239**, 401–9 (1964).

42. Trefts, E., Williams, A. S., & Wasserman, D. H. Exercise and the regulation of hepatic metabolism. *Prog. Mol. Biol. Transl. Sci.* **135**, 203–25 (2015).

43. Bartness, T. J., Liu, Y., Shrestha, Y. B., & Ryu, V. Neural innervation of white adipose tissue and the control of lipolysis. *Front. Neuroendocrinol.* **35**, 473–93 (2014).

44. Greenberg, A. S. *et al.* Perilipin, a major hormonally regulated adipocyte-specific phosphoprotein associated with the periphery of lipid storage droplets. *J. Biol. Chem.* **266**, 11341–6 (1991).

45. Barbe, P., Millet, L., Galitzky, J., Lafontan, M., & Berlan, M. In situ assessment of the role of the beta 1-, beta 2- and beta 3-adrenoceptors in the control of lipolysis and nutritive blood flow in human subcutaneous adipose tissue. *Br. J. Pharmacol.* **117**, 907–13 (1996).

46. Clerico, A., Giannoni, A., Vittorini, S., & Passino, C. Thirty years of the heart as an endocrine organ: physiological role and clinical utility of cardiac natriuretic hormones. *Am. J. Physiol. Heart Circ. Physiol.* **301**, H12–20 (2011).

47. Sengenes, C. *et al.* Involvement of a cGMP-dependent pathway in the natriuretic peptide-mediated hormone-sensitive lipase phosphorylation in human adipocytes. *J. Biol. Chem.* **278**, 48617–26 (2003).

48. Rivera-Brown, A. M. & Frontera, W. R. Principles of exercise physiology: responses to acute exercise and long-term adaptations to training. *PM R* **4**, 797–804 (2012).

49. Gremeaux, V. *et al.* Exercise and longevity. *Maturitas* **73**, 312–17 (2012).

50. Kujala, U. M. Evidence on the effects of exercise therapy in the treatment of chronic disease. *Br. J. Sports Med.* **43**, 550–5 (2009).

51. Carroll, A. Closest thing to a wonder drug? Try exercise. *The New York Times* (2016). Available at: www.nytimes.com/2016/06/21/upshot/why-you-should-exercise-no-not-to-lose-weight.html.

52. Cahill, G. F. Fuel metabolism in starvation. *Annu. Rev. Nutr.* **26**, 1–22 (2006).

53. Speakman, J. R. The evolution of body fatness: trading off disease and predation risk. *J. Exp. Biol.* **221**, (2018). doi:10.1242/jeb.167254

54. Ghimire, P. & Dhamoon, A. S. *Ketoacidosis.* StatPearls, 2020.

55. Katz, D. L. Competing dietary claims for weight loss: finding the forest through truculent trees. *Annu. Rev. Public Health* **26**, 61–88 (2005).

56. Gibson, A. A. *et al.* Do ketogenic diets really suppress appetite? A systematic review and meta-analysis. *Obes. Rev.* **16**, 64–76 (2015).

57. Gudzune, K. A. *et al.* Efficacy of commercial weight-loss programs: an updated systematic review. *Ann. Intern. Med.* **162**, 501–12 (2015).

58. Freedman, M. R., King, J., & Kennedy, E. Popular diets: a scientific review. *Obes. Res.* **9 Suppl. 1**, 1S–40S (2001).

59. Lagiou, P. *et al.* Low carbohydrate-high protein diet and incidence of cardiovascular diseases in Swedish women: prospective cohort study. *BMJ* **344**, e4026 (2012).

60. Seidelmann, S. B. *et al.* Dietary carbohydrate intake and mortality: a prospective cohort study and meta-analysis. *Lancet. Public Heal.* **3**, e419–e428 (2018).

61. Halton, T. L. *et al.* Low-carbohydrate-diet score and the risk of coronary heart disease in women. *N. Engl. J. Med.* **355**, 1991–2002 (2006).

62. Koppel, S. J. & Swerdlow, R. H. Neuroketotherapeutics: a modern review of a century-old therapy. *Neurochem. Int.* (2017). doi:10.1016/j.neuint.2017.05.019

63. Puchalska, P. & Crawford, P. A. Multi-dimensional roles of ketone bodies in fuel metabolism, signaling, and therapeutics. *Cell Metab.* **25**, 262–84 (2017).

64. Ameer, F., Scandiuzzi, L., Hasnain, S., Kalbacher, H., & Zaidi, N. De novo lipogenesis in health and disease. *Metabolism* **63**, 895–902 (2014).

65. Acheson, K. J. *et al.* Nutritional influences on lipogenesis and thermogenesis after a carbohydrate meal. *Am. J. Physiol.* **246**, E62–70 (1984).

66. Aarsland, A. & Wolfe, R. R. Hepatic secretion of VLDL fatty acids during stimulated lipogenesis in men. *J. Lipid Res.* **39**, 1280–6 (1998).

67. Strawford, A., Antelo, F., Christiansen, M., & Hellerstein, M. K. Adipose tissue triglyceride turnover, de novo lipogenesis, and cell proliferation in humans measured with 2H2O. *Am. J. Physiol. Endocrinol. Metab.* **286**, E577–88 (2004).

68. Diraison, F. *et al.* Differences in the regulation of adipose tissue and liver lipogenesis by carbohydrates in humans. *J. Lipid Res.* **44**, 846–53 (2003).

69. Vizuete, J., Camero, A., Malakouti, M., Garapati, K., & Gutierrez, J. Perspectives on nonalcoholic fatty liver disease: an overview of present and future therapies. *J. Clin. Transl. Hepatol.* **5**, 67–75 (2017).

70. Lambert, J. E., Ramos-Roman, M. A., Browning, J. D., & Parks, E. J. Increased de novo lipogenesis is a distinct characteristic of individuals with nonalcoholic fatty liver disease. *Gastroenterology* **146**, 726–35 (2014).
71. Qureshi, K. & Abrams, G. A. Prevalence of biopsy-proven non-alcoholic fatty liver disease in severely obese subjects without metabolic syndrome. *Clin. Obes.* **6**, 117–23 (2016).
72. Loomba, R. & Sanyal, A. J. The global NAFLD epidemic. *Nat. Rev. Gastroenterol. Hepatol.* **10**, 686–90 (2013).
73. Lallukka, S. & Yki-Järvinen, H. Non-alcoholic fatty liver disease and risk of type 2 diabetes. *Best Pract. Res. Clin. Endocrinol. Metab.* **30**, 385–95 (2016).
74. Bugianesi, E. *et al.* Expanding the natural history of nonalcoholic steatohepatitis: from cryptogenic cirrhosis to hepatocellular carcinoma. *Gastroenterology* **123**, 134–40 (2002).
75. Yki-Järvinen, H. Non-alcoholic fatty liver disease as a cause and a consequence of metabolic syndrome. *Lancet Diabetes Endocrinol.* **2**, 901–10 (2014).
76. Oseini, A. M. & Sanyal, A. J. Therapies in non-alcoholic steatohepatitis (NASH). *Liver Int.* **37 Suppl. 1**, 97–103 (2017).
77. Di Pasquale, M. G. The essentials of essential fatty acids. *J. Diet. Suppl.* **6**, 143–61 (2009).
78. Tvrzicka, E., Kremmyda, L.-S., Stankova, B., & Zak, A. Fatty acids as biocompounds: their role in human metabolism, health and disease: a review. Part 1: classification, dietary sources and biological functions. *Biomed. Pap. Med. Fac. Univ. Palacky. Olomouc. Czech. Repub.* **155**, 117–30 (2011).
79. Micha, R. & Mozaffarian, D. Trans fatty acids: effects on metabolic syndrome, heart disease and diabetes. *Nat. Rev. Endocrinol.* **5**, 335–44 (2009).
80. Clifton, P. M. & Keogh, J. B. A systematic review of the effect of dietary saturated and polyunsaturated fat on heart disease. *Nutr. Metab. Cardiovasc. Dis.* **27**, 1060–80 (2017).
81. Hyseni, L. *et al.* Systematic review of dietary trans-fat reduction interventions. *Bull. World Health Organ.* **95**, 821–30G (2017).
82. Imamura, F. *et al.* Effects of saturated fat, polyunsaturated fat, monounsaturated fat, and carbohydrate on glucose-insulin homeostasis: a systematic review and meta-analysis of randomised controlled feeding trials. *PLoS Med.* **13**, e1002087 (2016).
83. Koloverou, E., Esposito, K., Giugliano, D., & Panagiotakos, D. The effect of Mediterranean diet on the development of type 2 diabetes mellitus: a meta-analysis of 10 prospective studies and 136,846 participants. *Metabolism* **63**, 903–11 (2014).
84. Bowen, K. J., Sullivan, V. K., Kris-Etherton, P. M., & Petersen, K. S. Nutrition and cardiovascular disease: an update. *Curr. Atheroscler. Rep.* **20**, 8 (2018).
85. Subczynski, W. K., Pasenkiewicz-Gierula, M., Widomska, J., Mainali, L., & Raguz, M. High cholesterol/low cholesterol: effects in biological membranes: a review. *Cell Biochem. Biophys.* **75**, 369–85 (2017).
86. Sezgin, E., Levental, I., Mayor, S., & Eggeling, C. The mystery of membrane organization: composition, regulation and roles of lipid rafts. *Nat. Rev. Mol. Cell Biol.* **18**, 361–74 (2017).

87. Saher, G. & Stumpf, S. K. Cholesterol in myelin biogenesis and hypomyelinating disorders. *Biochim. Biophys. Acta* **1851**, 1083–94 (2015).
88. Brown, M. S. & Goldstein, J. L. A receptor-mediated pathway for cholesterol homeostasis. *Science* **232**, 34–47 (1986).
89. Berger, S., Raman, G., Vishwanathan, R., Jacques, P. F., & Johnson, E. J. Dietary cholesterol and cardiovascular disease: a systematic review and meta-analysis. *Am. J. Clin. Nutr.* **102**, 276–94 (2015).
90. Schofield, J. D., Liu, Y., Rao-Balakrishna, P., Malik, R. A., & Soran, H. Diabetes dyslipidemia. *Diabetes Ther.* **7**, 203–19 (2016).
91. Krauss, R. M. Lipids and lipoproteins in patients with type 2 diabetes. *Diabetes Care* **27**, 1496–504 (2004).
92. Ginhoux, F. & Jung, S. Monocytes and macrophages: developmental pathways and tissue homeostasis. *Nat. Rev. Immunol.* **14**, 392–404 (2014).
93. Badimon, L., Padró, T., & Vilahur, G. Atherosclerosis, platelets and thrombosis in acute ischaemic heart disease. *Eur. Hear. J. Acute Cardiovasc. Care* **1**, 60–74 (2012).
94. Pirillo, A., Bonacina, F., Norata, G. D., & Catapano, A. L. The interplay of lipids, lipoproteins, and immunity in atherosclerosis. *Curr. Atheroscler. Rep.* **20**, 12 (2018).
95. Ford, T. J., Corcoran, D., & Berry, C. Stable coronary syndromes: pathophysiology, diagnostic advances and therapeutic need. *Heart* **104**, 284–92 (2018).
96. Valacchi, G., Sticozzi, C., Lim, Y., & Pecorelli, A. Scavenger receptor class B type I: a multifunctional receptor. *Ann. N. Y. Acad. Sci.* **1229**, E1–7 (2011).
97. Linton, M. F., Tao, H., Linton, E. F., & Yancey, P. G. SR-BI: a multifunctional receptor in cholesterol homeostasis and atherosclerosis. *Trends Endocrinol. Metab.* **28**, 461–72 (2017).
98. Simons, L. A. Interrelations of lipids and lipoproteins with coronary artery disease mortality in 19 countries. *Am. J. Cardiol.* **57**, 5G–10G (1986).
99. Prospective Studies Collaboration *et al.* Blood cholesterol and vascular mortality by age, sex, and blood pressure: a meta-analysis of individual data from 61 prospective studies with 55,000 vascular deaths. *Lancet* **370**, 1829–39 (2007).
100. Madsen, C. M., Varbo, A., & Nordestgaard, B. G. Extreme high high-density lipoprotein cholesterol is paradoxically associated with high mortality in men and women: two prospective cohort studies. *Eur. Heart J.* **38**, 2478–86 (2017).
101. Bowe, B. *et al.* High density lipoprotein cholesterol and the risk of all-cause mortality among U.S. veterans. *Clin. J. Am. Soc. Nephrol.* **11**, 1784–93 (2016).
102. Defesche, J. C. *et al.* Familial hypercholesterolaemia. *Nat. Rev. Dis. Prim.* **3**, 17093 (2017).
103. Cholesterol Treatment Trialists' (CTT) Collaboration *et al.* Efficacy and safety of LDL-lowering therapy among men and women: meta-analysis of individual data from 174,000 participants in 27 randomised trials. *Lancet* **385**, 1397–405 (2015).
104. Chou, R., Dana, T., Blazina, I., Daeges, M., & Jeanne, T. L. Statins for prevention of cardiovascular disease in adults: evidence report and systematic review for the US Preventive Services Task Force. *JAMA* **316**, 2008–24 (2016).

105. Taylor, F. *et al.* Statins for the primary prevention of cardiovascular disease. *Cochrane Database Syst. Rev.* CD004816 (2013). doi:10.1002/14651858. CD004816.pub5

106. Endo, A., Kuroda, M., & Tsujita, Y. ML-236A, ML-236B, and ML-236C, new inhibitors of cholesterogenesis produced by Penicillium citrinium. *J. Antibiot. (Tokyo).* **29**, 1346–8 (1976).

107. Endo, A. The discovery and development of HMG-CoA reductase inhibitors. *J. Lipid Res.* **33**, 1569–82 (1992).

108. Daanen, H. A. M. & Van Marken Lichtenbelt, W. D. Human whole body cold adaptation. *Temp. (Austin, Tex.)* **3**, 104–18 (2016).

109. Stephens, J. M., Halson, S. L., Miller, J., Slater, G. J., & Askew, C. D. Influence of body composition on physiological responses to post-exercise hydrotherapy. *J. Sports Sci.* **36**, 1044–53 (2018).

110. Fasshauer, M. & Blüher, M. Adipokines in health and disease. *Trends Pharmacol. Sci.* **36**, 461–70 (2015).

111. Zhang, Y. *et al.* Positional cloning of the mouse obese gene and its human homologue. *Nature* **372**, 425–32 (1994).

112. Coleman, D. L. & Hummel, K. P. Effects of parabiosis of normal with genetically diabetic mice. *Am. J. Physiol.* **217**, 1298–304 (1969).

113. Coleman, D. L. Effects of parabiosis of obese with diabetes and normal mice. *Diabetologia* **9**, 294–8 (1973).

114. Schwartz, M. W. *et al.* Evidence that plasma leptin and insulin levels are associated with body adiposity via different mechanisms. *Diabetes Care* **20**, 1476–81 (1997).

115. Diéguez, C., Vazquez, M. J., Romero, A., López, M., & Nogueiras, R. Hypothalamic control of lipid metabolism: focus on leptin, ghrelin and melanocortins. *Neuroendocrinology* **94**, 1–11 (2011).

116. Montague, C. T. *et al.* Congenital leptin deficiency is associated with severe early-onset obesity in humans. *Nature* **387**, 903–8 (1997).

117. Farooqi, I. S. *et al.* Effects of recombinant leptin therapy in a child with congenital leptin deficiency. *N. Engl. J. Med.* **341**, 879–84 (1999).

118. Swerdloff, R. S., Batt, R. A., & Bray, G. A. Reproductive hormonal function in the genetically obese (ob/ob) mouse. *Endocrinology* **98**, 1359–64 (1976).

119. Mounzih, K., Lu, R., & Chehab, F. F. Leptin treatment rescues the sterility of genetically obese ob/ob males. *Endocrinology* **138**, 1190–3 (1997).

120. Chehab, F. F., Lim, M. E., & Lu, R. Correction of the sterility defect in homozygous obese female mice by treatment with the human recombinant leptin. *Nat. Genet.* **12**, 318–20 (1996).

121. Elias, C. F. & Purohit, D. Leptin signaling and circuits in puberty and fertility. *Cell. Mol. Life Sci.* **70**, 841–62 (2013).

122. Kennedy, G. C. & Mitra, J. Body weight and food intake as initiating factors for puberty in the rat. *J. Physiol.* **166**, 408–18 (1963).

123. Frisch, R. E. Fatness, menarche, and female fertility. *Perspect. Biol. Med.* **28**, 611–33 (1985).

124. Frisch, R. E. The right weight: body fat, menarche and fertility. *Proc. Nutr. Soc.* **53**, 113–29 (1994).

125. Matejek, N. *et al.* Hypoleptinaemia in patients with anorexia nervosa and in elite gymnasts with anorexia athletica. *Int. J. Sports Med.* **20**, 451–6 (1999).

126. Eckert, E. D. *et al.* Leptin in anorexia nervosa. *J. Clin. Endocrinol. Metab.* **83**, 791–5 (1998).

127. Köpp, W. *et al.* Low leptin levels predict amenorrhea in underweight and eating disordered females. *Mol. Psychiatry* **2**, 335–40 (1997).

128. El Ghoch, M., Calugi, S., Chignola, E., Bazzani, P. V., & Dalle Grave, R. Body fat and menstrual resumption in adult females with anorexia nervosa: a 1-year longitudinal study. *J. Hum. Nutr. Diet.* **29**, 662–6 (2016).

129. Kyriakidis, M., Caetano, L., Anastasiadou, N., Karasu, T., & Lashen, H. Functional hypothalamic amenorrhoea: leptin treatment, dietary intervention and counselling as alternatives to traditional practice – systematic review. *Eur. J. Obstet. Gynecol. Reprod. Biol.* **198**, 131–7 (2016).

130. Kaplowitz, P. B., Slora, E. J., Wasserman, R. C., Pedlow, S. E., & Herman-Giddens, M. E. Earlier onset of puberty in girls: relation to increased body mass index and race. *Pediatrics* **108**, 347–53 (2001).

131. Herman-Giddens, M. E. *et al.* Secondary sexual characteristics in boys: data from the Pediatric Research in Office Settings Network. *Pediatrics* **130**, e1058–68 (2012).

132. NCD Risk Factor Collaboration (NCD-RisC). Worldwide trends in body-mass index, underweight, overweight, and obesity from 1975 to 2016: a pooled analysis of 2416 population-based measurement studies in 128.9 million children, adolescents, and adults. *Lancet* **390**, 2627–42 (2017).

133. Farooqi, I. S. Leptin and the onset of puberty: insights from rodent and human genetics. *Semin. Reprod. Med.* **20**, 139–44 (2002).

134. Farooqi, S. & O'Rahilly, S. Genetics of obesity in humans. *Endocr. Rev.* **27**, 710–18 (2006).

135. Maguire, M., Lungu, A., Gorden, P., Cochran, E., & Stratton, P. Pregnancy in a woman with congenital generalized lipodystrophy: leptin's vital role in reproduction. *Obstet. Gynecol.* **119**, 452–5 (2012).

136. Li, J., Papadopoulos, V., & Vihma, V. Steroid biosynthesis in adipose tissue. *Steroids* **103**, 89–104 (2015).

137. Siiteri, P. K. Adipose tissue as a source of hormones. *Am. J. Clin. Nutr.* **45**, 277–82 (1987).

138. Veldhuis, J. D. *et al.* Endocrine control of body composition in infancy, childhood, and puberty. *Endocr. Rev.* **26**, 114–46 (2005).

139. Davidson, L. M., Millar, K., Jones, C., Fatum, M., & Coward, K. Deleterious effects of obesity upon the hormonal and molecular mechanisms controlling spermatogenesis and male fertility. *Hum. Fertil. (Camb).* **18**, 184–93 (2015).

140. Michalakis, K., Mintziori, G., Kaprara, A., Tarlatzis, B. C., & Goulis, D. G. The complex interaction between obesity, metabolic syndrome and reproductive axis: a narrative review. *Metabolism* **62**, 457–78 (2013).

141. Kahn, B. E. & Brannigan, R. E. Obesity and male infertility. *Curr. Opin. Urol.* **27**, 441–5 (2017).

142. Lee, M.-J., Pramyothin, P., Karastergiou, K., & Fried, S. K. Deconstructing the roles of glucocorticoids in adipose tissue biology and the development of central obesity. *Biochim. Biophys. Acta* **1842**, 473–81 (2014).

143. Wang, A., Luan, H. H., & Medzhitov, R. An evolutionary perspective on immunometabolism. *Science* **363**, (2019). doi:10.1126/science.aar3932

144. Pearce, E. L., Poffenberger, M. C., Chang, C.-H., & Jones, R. G. Fueling immunity: insights into metabolism and lymphocyte function. *Science* **342**, 1242454 (2013).

145. Dantzer, R. & Kelley, K. W. Twenty years of research on cytokine-induced sickness behavior. *Brain. Behav. Immun.* **21**, 153–60 (2007).

146. Du, W., Amarachintha, S., Wilson, A. F., & Pang, Q. SCO2 mediates oxidative stress-induced glycolysis to oxidative phosphorylation switch in hematopoietic stem cells. *Stem Cells* **34**, 960–71 (2016).

147. Ferrante, A. W. The immune cells in adipose tissue. *Diabetes, Obes. Metab.* **15**, 34–8 (2013).

148. Ranvier, L. Du développement et de l'accroissement des vaisseaux sanguins. *Arch Physiol Norm Path* **6**, 429–49 (1874).

149. Kohlgruber, A. C., LaMarche, N. M., & Lynch, L. Adipose tissue at the nexus of systemic and cellular immunometabolism. *Semin. Immunol.* **28**, 431–40 (2016).

150. Brestoff, J. R. & Artis, D. Immune regulation of metabolic homeostasis in health and disease. *Cell* **161**, 146–60 (2015).

151. DiSpirito, J. R. & Mathis, D. Immunological contributions to adipose tissue homeostasis. *Semin. Immunol.* **27**, 315–21 (2015).

152. Iikuni, N., Lam, Q. L. K., Lu, L., Matarese, G., & La Cava, A. Leptin and inflammation. *Curr. Immunol. Rev.* **4**, 70–9 (2008).

153. Jaganathan, R., Ravindran, R., & Dhanasekaran, S. Emerging role of adipocytokines in type 2 diabetes as mediators of insulin resistance and cardiovascular disease. *Can. J. diabetes* (2017). doi:10.1016/j.jcjd.2017.10.040

154. Ackerman, S. E., Blackburn, O. A., Marchildon, F., & Cohen, P. Insights into the link between obesity and cancer. *Curr. Obes. Rep.* **6**, 195–203 (2017).

155. Thijssen, E., van Caam, A., & van der Kraan, P. M. Obesity and osteoarthritis, more than just wear and tear: pivotal roles for inflamed adipose tissue and dyslipidaemia in obesity-induced osteoarthritis. *Rheumatology* **54**, 588–600 (2015).

156. Andersen, C. J., Murphy, K. E., & Fernandez, M. L. Impact of obesity and metabolic syndrome on immunity. *Adv. Nutr.* **7**, 66–75 (2016).

157. Neidich, S. D. *et al.* Increased risk of influenza among vaccinated adults who are obese. *Int. J. Obes.* **41**, 1324–30 (2017).

158. Painter, S. D., Ovsyannikova, I. G., & Poland, G. A. The weight of obesity on the human immune response to vaccination. *Vaccine* **33**, 4422–9 (2015).

159. Simonnet, A. *et al.* High prevalence of obesity in severe acute respiratory syndrome Coronavirus-2 (SARS-CoV-2) requiring invasive mechanical ventilation. *Obesity* **28**, 1195–9 (2020).

160. Sattar, N., McInnes, I. B., & McMurray, J. J. V. Obesity is a risk factor for severe COVID-19 infection. *Circulation* **142**, 4–6 (2020).

161. Ryan, D. H., Ravussin, E., & Heymsfield, S. COVID-19 and the patient with obesity: the editors speak out. *Obesity (Silver Spring)* **28**, 847 (2020).

162. Guerrero-Juarez, C. F. & Plikus, M. V. Emerging nonmetabolic functions of skin fat. *Nat. Rev. Endocrinol.* **14**, 163–73 (2018).

163. Couturier, J. & Lewis, D. E. HIV persistence in adipose tissue reservoirs. *Curr. HIV/AIDS Rep.* (2018). doi:10.1007/s11904-018-0378-z

164. Guigas, B. & Molofsky, A. B. A worm of one's own: how helminths modulate host adipose tissue function and metabolism. *Trends Parasitol.* **31**, 435–41 (2015).

165. Minciullo, P. L. *et al.* Anaphylaxis caused by helminths: review of the literature. *Eur. Rev. Med. Pharmacol. Sci.* **16**, 1513–18 (2012).

4
I Can Get Fat Where? The Other Types of Fat

Brown Adipose Tissue

There has been great interest in brown adipose tissue in recent years, with reports from scientific studies about this particular type of fat even invading the mainstream media on occasion.[1] Rather than playing a role in energy storage, however, the function of brown fat is to produce heat (specifically via non-shivering thermogenesis), which it achieves by burning fatty acids and glucose. After the landmark discovery that this tissue is present in adult humans,[2–4] brown fat has morphed from an academic curiosity into a tantalizing potential treatment, or even cure according to some, for the current global obesity crisis.[5] Should the hype be believed? In order to answer such a question, one must first dive into the biology of brown fat.

Hiding in Plain Sight

In humans, brown fat is most abundant in newborns, accounting for up to 5% of total body weight. It is located primarily in the upper half of the back between the shoulder blades as well as around the heart, kidneys, and pancreas[6] (Figure 4.1). This tissue plays a crucial role in producing heat in newborns who are particularly vulnerable to the potentially fatal effects of heat loss (i.e., hypothermia) owing to their small physical size. Additionally, their developing body lacks sufficient thermal insulation (i.e., subcutaneous fat and body hair), is incapable of shivering, and is essentially reliant on others to retain heat (e.g., via clothing). Brown fat mass typically recedes as the newborn grows, to the point where it was presumed to be largely absent in adults due to the emergence of other biological and

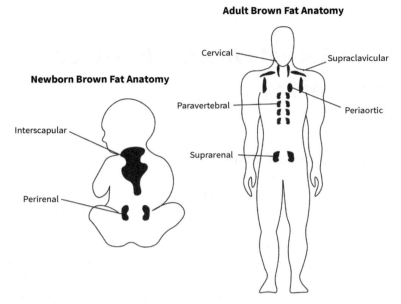

Figure 4.1 Anatomy of brown adipose tissue in humans.

behavioural mechanisms that preserve heat. However, this widespread belief was strongly challenged when new data came to light.

Positron emission tomography (PET) is a scanning technology in which radioactive tracers (such as derivatives of glucose) can be used to locate and visualize anatomical locations that are particularly metabolically active *in vivo* in real-time. This technique is commonly used to diagnose and monitor various types of cancer because the high metabolic rate displayed by tumours to support their unrestrained growth often manifests as distinctive regions of elevated tracer uptake.[7] During the early 2000s, it was noted that highly metabolically active, but otherwise benign, areas were present in adults near the neck and chest region, particularly around the collarbone, with such regions being flagged as potential causes of false positives in cancer diagnoses.[8,9] Further studies revealed that these distinctive hotspots detected during PET scanning were actually functional brown fat depots in adults[2–4] that became increasingly metabolically active upon cold exposure.[10] PET scanning continues to be the gold standard technique for detecting and measuring brown fat mass and activity, although other methods (such as magnetic resonance imaging (see Chapter 5), contrast ultrasound, and near-infrared spectroscopy[11]) have since been developed which are more practical and don't involve exposing study participants to radiation. By the end of the 2000s, the academic community had widely accepted that brown fat exists in adult humans, and their rekindled interest in this previously niche tissue has burned merrily since.

Left Out in the Cold

Brown fat's primary function is thought to be heat production in the context of temperature regulation.[12] Mounting evidence suggests that the advent of the ability to generate heat played an important role in facilitating the evolutionary transition and emergence of endothermic organisms (i.e., those capable of, and dependent on, the internal generation of heat) from their ancient ectothermic ancestors (i.e., those which depend on external heat sources),[13,14] a process which thereby contributed to the evolution of modern humanity.[15] But while brown fat appears to play an important role in newborns, its importance to temperature regulation in adult humans remains somewhat unclear.

This controversy seems to stem mainly from the paucity of data that enables the explicit definition of brown fat to protect adult humans against cold exposure. Concerns have been raised previously that the importance of biological mechanisms (like the activation of brown fat) to humanity's ability to survive in cold environments has been over-emphasized and over-represented in the literature, while highly effective behavioural adaptations pertaining to clothing, shelter, and the timing of physical activity have been overlooked.[16] It follows that there have been numerous calls to re-evaluate how best to study the phenomena that enable humans to survive and thrive in inhospitable environments.[17,18] Little data exist that provide clear comparisons between distinct groups of people who reside in diametrically opposed environments (e.g., Inuits versus indigenous North Africans). Consistent with cold acclimation-inducing brown fat mass expansion, a North-to-South gradient has been observed in which the reported prevalence of spontaneously active brown fat in Boston, US[3] (latitude: 42°21′30″ North) is 4% whereas it is 6.8% in Sherbrooke, Canada[19] (latitude: 45°24′30″ North). Comparisons between Europeans and South-East Asians have yielded equivocal results; one study found no difference between these ethnic groups[20] whereas another reported that brown fat mass and activity was higher in Europeans[21]—it remains unclear whether such differences would even be biologically meaningful. Obtaining a clear picture of this intriguing tissue could provide important insights into our evolutionary history though, specifically our migration from the scorching plains of Africa to cooler climes, as well as indicate whether brown fat represents a viable anti-obesity treatment option in certain ethnicities (who may be heat- or cold-acclimated and have less or more brown fat accordingly).[22]

Cooling Yourself to Live

Despite its ambiguous role, there have been numerous investigations exploring what determines an individual's brown fat mass. Early studies suggested that brown fat is *not* present in a substantial proportion of adults.[23] However, it seems that brown fat actually *is* present in the vast majority of adults, but that it only becomes detectable upon exposure to cold,[10,24] although brown fat mass and its ability to respond to cold exposure declines considerably with increasing age.[25] The most well-developed avenue of brown fat research concerns its relationship with white fat mass and metabolic health. The *least* amount of functional brown fat is typically found in individuals with the highest body mass index (BMI),[26] total fat mass,[27] and visceral fat mass,[24] as well as those with type 2 diabetes.[19] Furthermore, the responsiveness of brown fat to cold exposure is often blunted in obese people,[28] potentially due to inflammation.[29]

Given that brown fat acts as a metabolic furnace that can dispose of (excess) calories to generate heat, it has been proposed that brown fat, or a lack thereof, contributes to the development and/or maintenance of obesity and metabolic disease. The mass of functional brown fat tends to be greatest in lean, metabolically healthy individuals and lowest in those affected by the metabolic complications of obesity.[30] But what comes first—shrinkage and failure of our in-built heater or excessive accumulation of metabolic fuel that doubles as thermal insulation and prompts brown fat to shrink into obsolescence? Reports that brown fat mass and function/activity reportedly increase after bariatric surgery-induced weight loss[31] (see Chapter 7) are interesting, but don't help us determine where brown fat sits on the causal chain or whether it simply reflects overall metabolic health. Despite this ambiguity, scientific and clinical research efforts have grown to investigate the effect of brown fat activation on metabolic health and white adipose mass.[5]

Activating brown fat in humans typically involves exposing individuals to cold. Researchers have pursued two main types of study; one type involves analyzing the acute metabolic effect of activating brown fat, while the other involves looking longer term at the effect of repeated cold stimulation/brown fat activation on metabolic health. Stoking the optimism of those who believe in brown fat's therapeutic potential, several studies have reported that cold exposure (during which time participants were exposed to approximately 18°C/64°F for five to eight hours) is associated with improvements in glucose and fatty acid metabolism as well as overall insulin sensitivity.[32,33] Over the longer-term, brown fat can reportedly be 'trained' such that its mass and responsiveness increase following repeated exposure to cold.[5,34] While this only indicates that humans invoke biological adaptations to compensate for altered environmental conditions, there is the suggestion that such changes impact favourably on body composition and metabolic health. For instance, one study reported that exposing healthy Japanese men to mild cold (17°C/63°F) for two hours every day for six weeks resulted in the emergence and expansion of brown fat coupled with a small but significant decrease in white fat mass.[35]

While the cold-induced reduction in body mass has been difficult to replicate, other studies have reported that cold exposure for several hours each day for weeks or months improves insulin sensitivity.[36,37] Such results are an encouraging proof of principle, but the time, effort, and resources required to achieve these rather modest beneficial effects are a big drawback. Imagine the health benefits that could be attained by using the same hour or so each day to undertake physical activity or cook a nutritious meal compared to simply sitting and getting cold. Reducing indoor temperatures could contribute to the prevention and/or alleviation of obesity, but persistent cold exposure doesn't seem to represent a particularly practical or comfortable method for achieving what would likely amount to a mere beneficial tweak to one's metabolic health for the vast majority of people.[38] Moreover, such measures would likely be stymied by compensatory strategies to protect against the unpleasant sensation of being persistently cold (e.g., wearing extra layers). Faced with this untenable situation, the direction of investigation has shifted to identify chemicals which regulate the development and activity of brown fat.

Start the Fire

Thyroid hormone has a well-established role in the regulation of our overall metabolic rate and may activate brown fat.[39,40] However, it is not clear whether this occurs via direct hormone action or via the sympathetic nervous system. Brown fat mass and activity are higher in women throughout life,[41] suggesting this tissue may contribute to the more favourable metabolic and cardiovascular health risk profile that pre-menopausal women tend to enjoy.[42] As oestrogens can also activate brown fat,[43] brown fat may also be involved in the hot flushes that some women experience during the menopausal transition.[44] Given the complex and broad-acting nature of these types of hormones, however, they don't represent particularly attractive candidates on which to base brown fat-activating drugs.

Brown fat is innervated by the sympathetic nervous system and is readily activated by catecholamines like noradrenaline.[45] However, this neurotransmitter potently increases blood pressure and heart rate—consistent with its key role in co-ordinating the fight-or-flight autonomic response—thus making it inappropriate for therapeutic brown fat activation, especially in the context of obesity. That said, these effects that make the cardiovascular system pump and squeeze harder primarily involve beta-1 adrenoceptors activation; as brown fat activation involves biologically distinct beta-3 adrenoceptors,[46] these different biological effects can be independently modulated with appropriately structured chemicals. Several studies have demonstrated that beta-3 adrenoceptor activators potently increase brown fat activity in rodents, with such treatment reversing obesity and alleviating insulin resistance induced by a fast-food diet.[47,48] These drugs also stimulate the 'browning' of white fat, a phenomenon in which (subcutaneous) adipose tissue acquires some of the heat-producing abilities of brown fat to become so-called 'beige' fat.[49] Surely brown fat activation represents a trail-blazing approach for obesity and metabolic disease treatment that is poised to set the world on fire?

Not quite. An initial human study involving the treatment of lean men with a beta-3 adrenoceptor activator for two months provided somewhat promising results, as after one month the men displayed enhanced glucose tolerance and an increased rate of fat burning.[50] Unfortunately, these effects disappeared by the end of the trial, meaning there was no sustained significant effect (beneficial or otherwise) on insulin sensitivity, energy expenditure, or body composition.[50] Another disappointment followed a few years later when, after a promising early report indicated that a single dose of a different beta-3 adrenoceptor activator significantly increased resting energy expenditure in obese but metabolically normal men,[51] it was subsequently found that treatment for 28 days with the same drug had no lasting overall effect on energy expenditure, body composition, or metabolic health.[52] There have also been numerous other cases in which beta-3 adrenoceptor activators which had proven effective in rodents were found to have no effect in humans.[53] It has been proposed that the transient nature of a therapeutic effect may be due to the 'de-sensitization' of the beta-3 adrenoceptors, a process in which the receptors turn themselves off after a period of sustained activation in a pre-programmed act of self-preservation,[54] a bit like a circuit breaker flipping when the electrical current is too high.

A notable event in this particular story pertains to the report that a single dose of mirabegron, a beta-3 adrenoceptor activator approved for the treatment of overactive bladder in the US, was able to increase energy expenditure in healthy adult men specifically via increased brown fat activity.[55] In an exciting new development, it has since been reported that women treated with mirabegron for four weeks showed increased brown adipose metabolic activity and improved insulin sensitivity, lipid profile, and adiponectin levels (but no change in body composition).[56] It remains to be seen whether these effects persist over the long-term and if they translate to clinically meaningful outcomes. Overall, the beta-3 adrenoceptor story highlights the many difficulties associated with translating science from the laboratory bench to the clinic, many of which are associated with the limitations of animal models. Indeed, notable species differences between mice and humans have been reported with respect to the 'browning' of white adipose tissue.[57] Molecular intricacies aside, mice are far smaller organisms than humans so they lose heat much more easily than we do. This means that brown fat likely plays a far greater role in their biology and that manipulating this tissue will likely produce profound effects that are ultimately limited to mice. Maybe identifying clinically relevant aspects of brown fat biology would require studying human-sized mice ...

It is also possible that drug administration alone is not sufficient to attain health benefits, however small. For example, chemically inducing brown fat expansion might be all well and good, but if the tissue is not active because the environment is sufficiently warm, the burning of (excess) calories will not occur to induce an insulin-sensitizing or weight-loss effect. This was illustrated clearly in a study where a growth factor that promoted the expansion and innervation of brown fat only protected mice from diet-induced obesity when they were kept in a cold environment.[58] Additionally, even though brown fat can be active in relatively warm environmental conditions,[59] if an overweight or obese individual's overall energy expenditure is not greater than their energy consumption, they won't experience any weight loss.[60] Evidently brown fat is proving difficult to harness and it likely doesn't represent the panacea everyone wishes it could be.[38] But what is the actual biological mechanism that brown fat utilizes to link energy metabolism with heat production? Could a deeper understanding of that provide any broader lessons that we can utilize in the fight against the global obesity crisis?

Hot Dam

Brown fat is evolutionarily distinct from white adipose tissue and derives from muscle.[14] Skeletal muscle contributes to temperature regulation as it acts as an effective thermal insulator and can also perform shivering for heat production. Brown fat's distinct heritage manifests as particularly striking morphological features when observed down the microscope.[61] The dense bed of capillaries that run through brown fat enable it to heat large volumes of blood as it passes through. Brown fat also arranges the fatty acids it accumulates in multiple small droplets, rather than the single large droplet present in each white adipocyte. Upon activation, these fatty acids are utilized by the abundant mitochondria present within the brown fat itself; the iron-containing compounds within mitochondria give this tissue its distinctive brown colour.

Recall that mitochondria are the metabolic powerhouses of essentially all cells in the body (barring certain types like red blood cells). These structures utilize the chemical energy contained within nutrients like fatty acids and carbohydrates to generate adenosine triphosphate (ATP), the universal energy currency used to drive essentially all biological processes in the body, from muscle contraction and nerve impulse conduction to hormone secretion and protein synthesis. The mitochondria housed within brown fat are unique though, as they contain a special type of protein called *uncoupling protein 1* (UCP-1; also known as thermogenin) which was originally discovered in 1978.[62] The evolution of UCP-1 represents an important moment in evolutionary history that enabled, or at least facilitated, the emergence of endothermic organisms, which obviously includes humans.[63] To understand how UCP-1 works, however, one must first understand the process of ATP generation in mitochondria.

Adenosine triphosphate generation in mitochondria occurs via 'oxidative phosphorylation', a complex process which operates much the same way as a hydroelectric dam (Figure 4.2). Imagine a mitochondrion acts as a dam receiving water flowing from an elevated pool whose 'potential energy' is harnessed as it turns a turbine which generates electricity. The elevated pool is then refilled by water being pumped up-hill using electricity generated by the dam. In a mitochondrion, the 'elevated pool' comprises acidic particles (i.e., hydrogen ions/protons) trapped between two membranes that flow through a proteinaceous turbine known as *ATP synthase* which generates ATP as it turns. The elevated pool is replenished by the action of the 'electron transport chain', a series of proteins embedded in the inner mitochondrial membrane. These proteins utilize the chemical energy from fatty acids and carbohydrates, converting the energy released from electrons as they move along the protein chain into proton pumping.

This evolutionarily honed biological 'hydroelectric dam' has proven highly effective for the generation of ATP. But where does uncoupling

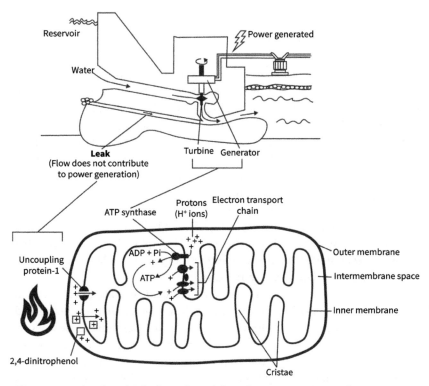

Figure 4.2 Mitochondrial adenosine triphosphate generation and thermogenesis (depicted as a hydroelectric dam).

protein-1 fit in? As its name suggests, UCP-1 'uncouples' the flow of protons from ATP generation, meaning it acts as the biological equivalent of a by-pass that enables water to flow from the elevated pool to the reservoir below *without* engaging the water turbine. In mitochondria, the flow of protons through uncoupling protein-1 results in the dissipation of their potential energy as heat.[12,64] As brown fat has a substantial blood supply, the heat generated by its abundant mitochondria can be quickly transferred to the copious volumes of blood flowing through it to warm the rest of the body. This metabolic 'short circuit' enables brown fat to burn excess calories to generate heat and is the primary reason that has made this tissue such an attractive target for drug development. But with brown fat proving diffi-cult to harness for therapeutic gain, could the broader concept of metabolic uncoupling represent a potentially viable approach for the treatment of obesity?

Conscious Uncoupling

Chemicals which mimic the action of UCP-1 exist and can be used to an-swer such a burning question. Coming from a rather unlikely background, the most famous metabolic uncoupling agent is 2,4-dinitrophenol (DNP),[65] a compound which has enjoyed a storied and controversial existence since its discovery approximately 100 years ago. DNP was originally used on an industrial scale to make explosives in French munitions factories during World War I. During this time, a number of factory workers experienced DNP poisoning with reports highlighting conspicuous symptoms such as high temperatures, excessive sweating, and—most intriguingly—substantial reductions in body weight.[66] Capitalizing on these findings, scientists from Stanford University in the US explored the possibility that DNP might represent a uniquely effective diet pill and undertook a series of studies accordingly during the 1920s and 1930s.[67,68]

On the back of some impressive results in clinical trials, DNP was soon being touted as an effective weight-loss aid in the US that was being sold in over-the-counter medicines to the public. It soon became clear, how-ever, that DNP was (and continues to be) a very dangerous chemical. As the number of adverse events piled up (including an outbreak of individuals developing cataracts[69]), the US Food and Drug Administration were forced to act, eventually deeming DNP 'extremely dangerous and not fit for human consumption' in 1938[70]; DNP was withdrawn from the market shortly thereafter. Such horrible effects are perhaps unsurprising for a chemical that is not only highly explosive, but also acts as a pesticide and fungicide.

2,4-Dinitrophenol achieves its 'therapeutic' effects by chemically dissipating the proton gradient across the inner mitochondrial membrane, thus uncoupling ATP generation from the flow of protons; the extent of uncoupling directly reflects the dose of DNP. This metabolic uncoupling makes ATP production more inefficient, meaning more calories are required to generate the same amount of ATP. With this metabolic uncoupling underpinning both weight loss and heat production, it is easy to believe the anecdotes that DNP was supposedly given to Russian troops to help them stay warm on the frigid battlefields during World War II, at least until they lost too much weight to survive the freezing conditions or fight properly.[71] Unlike uncoupling protein-1, however, DNP's action is not limited to brown fat as it can permeate tissues throughout the body. This makes DNP very dangerous, with its toxicity arising not because of compromised ATP production (in which vital biological processes simply cease), but from the excessive generation of heat that can manifest as fatal hyperthermia (body temperature can rise as high as 44°C/111°F[65]), an agonizing situation in which the body essentially cooks itself.

Individual responses to DNP vary considerably,[72] meaning taking DNP can be like playing Russian roulette. There have been numerous reports of DNP overdoses causing death as a result of accidental[73] or intentional exposure.[74,75] Despite the dangers associated with its use and legislation banning its sale for human consumption, DNP is readily available on the Internet under a variety of names and is often marketed as a 'safe weight-loss aid.' Indeed, DNP continues to be used by some bodybuilders and athletes who wish to rapidly reduce (white) fat mass, while others use it as a diet aid despite a number of deaths in the UK.[76] One notable case concerns the unfortunate death of Eloise Aimee Parry, a young student who died after taking eight DNP capsules (rather than the recommended one, in a bid to get faster results) that had been sold to her as a safe slimming aid.[77]

2,4-Dinitrophenol is a dangerous industrial chemical not fit for human consumption. However, it has been reported that long-term treatment of rats with a *very* low dose of DNP safely alleviated diet-induced type 2 diabetes and liver fat accumulation.[78] There is some lingering academic interest in harnessing the power of mitochondrial uncoupling as a method for treating obesity,[79] but it remains unclear whether this would be well-received by the public and/or clinical community. Stranger things have happened though. For instance, there is a vast and growing market for

SGLT2 inhibitors used to treat metabolic disease, particularly type 2 diabetes; somewhat ironically, these drugs precipitate weight loss and improve insulin sensitivity by promoting glucose excretion in the urine.[80] With the colossal scale of the obesity crisis meaning all options warrant consideration, DNP deserves at least revisiting, albeit in a way that would avoid repeating historical mistakes. It would certainly make for an explosive story if a century-old industrial chemical turned out to be the cure for the global obesity crisis.

Burning the Midnight Oil—Or Not

There is a growing appreciation of the importance of circadian phenomena (i.e., how biological processes vary over time) in essentially all aspects of human biology, with brown fat being no exception. Reactive spikes of brown adipose tissue activity upon cold exposure are actually overlaid on a recurring pattern of fluctuating daily activity in humans. Indeed, brown fat is typically most active around waking, with its activity declining throughout the remainder of the day.[81] This pattern of activity has been associated with increased glucose[82] and fat[83] metabolism in the morning compared to the afternoon or evening.

As brown fat is often thought to act as a metabolic furnace that can dispose of (excess) calories, the greater clearance of ingested fat and carbohydrate early in the day has prompted speculation that an individual's eating pattern may affect their risk of developing obesity and metabolic disease. Consistent with this, an observational study that examined the correlation between an individual's BMI and their daily pattern of food consumption in a variety of countries highlighted that those who ate more in the evening compared to the morning were more likely to have an increased BMI.[84] In the context of weight loss, study results have highlighted that a larger calorie intake at breakfast than dinner is associated with better weight loss in obese women,[85] with late eaters showing an impaired ability to shed the pounds.[86] Such data suggest that there might be substance to the adage that we should eat 'breakfast like a king, lunch like a prince, and dinner like a pauper.'[87] But before deciding to never eat an evening meal again, or acting as though breakfast calories 'don't count', there is a great deal we do not understand about the biological effects of nutritional timing.[88] Moreover, the total amount of calories consumed during the day is far more important than the timing of eating in determining body mass and composition.[60] Indeed, individuals who miss breakfast and then compensate by eating more during the rest of the day reportedly have a larger BMI,[89] just like those who snack between meals.[90]

With modern society increasingly operating on a 24-hour schedule, it is important to understand how the timing of dietary patterns may contribute to society's worsening health. Bearing the brunt of a topsy-turvy, or even absent, daily routine, it is well-established that shift workers have a significantly increased risk of developing all manner of health problems, particularly (central) obesity[91] and metabolic disease[92]; disrupted circadian biology may play an important role in this context.[93] While our ability to handle meals varies throughout the day, human studies have shown that misalignment between meal times and one's biological rhythm can cause desynchronization between the central clock in the brain's hypothalamus and the peripheral clocks within metabolically important tissues such as adipose tissue.[94] Moreover, these internal misalignments can manifest as perturbations in insulin sensitivity and glucose metabolism that may underpin the increased metabolic disease risk shown by shift workers.[95] Could brown fat be involved in this phenomenon? While there is a paucity of human data, one study of mice found that those housed in a persistently lit environment (which obliterates their normal sleep-wake cycle) not only developed obesity and metabolic disease, but also showed substantially reduced brown fat activity[96]; it remains unclear whether this effect is causative or correlative. Either way, understanding how time, diet, and work patterns interact to influence our health will be crucial to devising effective solutions which minimize the harm done by the entrenched 24-hour nature of modern society.

The scientific and clinical communities are at a crossroads with this curious organ. There is fairly good evidence which suggests brown fat plays a role in everyday energy expenditure in many humans, contributing to their basal metabolic rate and performing diet-induced thermogenesis[97,98] (in which a portion of recently ingested food is burned for heat). However, it remains unclear whether disrupted brown fat biology plays a significant causal role in the development of obesity and its associated metabolic complications. While some people are optimistic about the promise of brown fat (or metabolic uncoupling) as a possible treatment for obesity and metabolic disease, not everyone shares it, and ultimately a great many obstacles remain to be overcome to turn its potential into reality.

Bone Marrow Adipose Tissue

In contrast to brown fat's almost celebrity-like status, bone marrow adipose tissue has remained relatively obscure since its discovery. Originally discovered by anatomists in the late 1800s who found it to be particularly abundant in individuals who had died from arsenic poisoning,[99] bone marrow fat sits at the interface between the skeleton, blood cell production, and energy metabolism. These anatomists also noted that amidst the extensively fat-infiltrated bone of these unfortunate individuals, few red or white blood cells were present in their bone marrow, consistent with the modern appreciation that arsenic is toxic to blood cell-producing bone marrow stem cells.[100] This observation prompted the suggestion that haematopoiesis (i.e., the generation of new blood cells) and bone marrow fat mass were inversely related (i.e., when one goes up, the other goes down).

These intriguing observations laid dormant for many decades until the advent of chemotherapy in the middle of the twentieth century (which enabled the effective treatment of cancer) prompted a re-examination of early findings.[101] Echoing prior reports, bone marrow from individuals who had undergone chemotherapy (which involves using chemicals that are toxic to haematopoietic stem cells) tended to contain lots of fat but few blood cells.[102] While haematologists were well aware of the relationship between blood cell production and bone marrow fat, bone biologists were relatively late to the show, but have since provided some crucial insights into bone marrow fat.

Research performed during the 1960s highlighted that bone marrow fat accumulation occurs normally during early development,[103] with fat filling many of the gaps in bones that make up the appendicular skeleton (i.e., the bones which support our limbs), thus suggesting that bone marrow fat is not simply a vestigial interloper within our skeleton. Bone marrow fat mass increases throughout life, although the pattern of accrual varies between the sexes. For instance, bone marrow fat mass increases slowly throughout life in men whereas it increases sharply in women between the ages of 55 to 65,[104] suggesting it may be associated with menopause[105]; this relationship is apparent in various ethnicities.[106,107] Research in the 1960s and 1970s also highlighted a reciprocal relationship between bone mineral density and bone marrow fat; the bones of individuals with osteoporosis are defined not only by reduced bone mineral content, but also by increased bone marrow fat mass.[108] This pattern is so robust that bone marrow fat mass can be reliably used to identify individuals at increased risk of bone fracture, particularly older members of society,[109,110] as well as younger individuals who have not yet started to experience bone mass loss.[111–113]

Fat and Thin Bones

What influences bone marrow fat mass? And is there more to this story than our bones simply turning to jelly as we age? Mounting evidence suggests that bone marrow fat actually represents the crucial interface between our metabolic and bone health. Large-scale studies have provided compelling data that obesity is associated with poor bone health[114,115] and increased fracture risk[116] in men and women. Recent meta-analyses have also reported that the risk of hip fracture is particularly pronounced in individuals with central/abdominal obesity[117,118]; it currently remains unclear whether this relationship holds for other bones. Additionally, women with larger amounts of visceral fat mass tend to have higher bone marrow fat content[119] and may be at a greater risk of bone fracture[120] accordingly.

This relationship is also present in individuals with metabolic disease and is often related to central obesity. Indeed, bone marrow fat mass is increased in men[121] and women[122] with type 2 diabetes and is reportedly positively correlated with visceral fat mass in the latter. This interplay between metabolic health, bone mineral density, and bone marrow fat mass might explain why individuals who are (centrally) obese[116,117] and/or diabetic[123] tend to have impaired bone health and are at increased risk of having a fracture. These data also highlight how subcutaneous fat plays a protective role in bone health[115] as well as metabolic and cardiovascular health[124] (see Chapters 5 and 6). The literature examining the relationship between regional, rather than overall, fat mass and bone health is still developing, with age, sex, and ethnicity-specific nuances remaining to be elucidated,[125] with some inconsistencies between visceral fat and bone health having been reported.[126] As it stands though, the current evidence suggests that (central) obesity and/or metabolic disease are not good for your bones. And although an overweight BMI might be associated with a lower fracture risk,[118,127,128] that does not mean putting on weight and moving up to the overweight BMI bracket is a wise move for your bones (or general health for that matter).

(Central) obesity and metabolic disease are associated with bones becoming fatter, but this seemingly simple statement is underpinned by an array of complex mechanisms including hormonal perturbations. For example, the increased bone marrow fat mass observed in women with ex-panded visceral fat mass is accompanied by reduced levels of circulating IGF-1, a growth factor which promotes bone growth and mineralization.[119] Perturbations to testosterone and oestrogen levels arising from dysfunc-tional, obese adipose tissue may also affect bone health.[114,129] Data from current experimental animal models suggest that various circulating mo-lecular signals act on the (finite) pool of universal progenitor cells present in bone marrow, directing them to become adipocytes at the expense of bone cells,[130] thus providing a mechanism to explain the reciprocal rela-tionship between bone marrow fat and bone mineral content. Indeed, the expanded bone marrow fat mass observed in diet-induced obese mice[131] tends to impair the animal's ability to regenerate bone and generate new blood cells.[132,133]

On a more positive note, bone marrow fat accumulation driven by high-fat diet feeding can be suppressed by exercise, at least in mice[134]; as this effect was achieved via wheel running, it remains unclear what specific ex-ercise type (e.g., aerobic or weight-bearing) is most effective. In addition to preventing its accumulation, exercise also limits the expansion of bone marrow fat mass in obese mice.[135] Bone marrow fat mass in mice can also be reduced by dietary restriction,[136] with this finding aligning with data from human studies indicating that bone marrow fat mass decreases during weight loss induced by bariatric surgery[137] (see Chapter 7). Much of the molecular minutiae currently charted in animal models requires validation in humans, but an abundance of clinical evidence suggests there are signifi-cant similarities between species.[101]

Within the reciprocal relationship between bone fat and mineral con-tent, losing bone marrow fat does not necessarily mean that bone regener-ates or miraculously becomes stronger; the mechanical integrity of obese mice's bones did not recover after dietary restriction-induced weight loss and bone marrow fat mass retraction.[136] It is not currently unclear whether obesity permanently damages bone health, which is a scary proposition given its global prevalence. It is possible, however, that performing (weight-bearing) exercise protects bone structure and integrity during weight loss; such knowledge may be crucial for all manner of patient groups, particu-larly elderly people and post-operative bariatric surgery patients who have a greatly increased risk of bone fractures.[138]

Another important factor that can influence bone health in the context of obesity and diabetes is the medication used to treat these conditions. For instance, the thiazolidinediones (TZDs) are insulin-sensitizing agents that exert their beneficial effects on metabolic health primarily through actions on subcutaneous adipose tissue (see Chapters 6 and 7). However, these drugs are controversial due to the number of side effects associated with their use, particularly the increased risk of bone fracture.[139] Bone health is already diminished in obesity and metabolic disease,[140] so exacerbating this issue is not exactly ideal. Data from mouse studies suggest a curious scenario in which some beneficial and deleterious effects of the TZDs actually arise from bone. These drugs increase bone marrow fat mass,[141] an effect which may simultaneously weaken bone strength while increasing circulating levels of the insulin-sensitizing adiponectin. This TZD-induced expansion of bone marrow fat may be somewhat attenuated by exercise though, at least in mice.[142,143]

Having explored the relationship between bone marrow fat, skeletal integrity, and metabolic health, it's time to pose the killer question. *What exactly does bone marrow fat do?* Despite the accumulation of knowledge about its biology over the past 100 years, the specific biological role of bone marrow fat remains enigmatic. Many fundamental issues pertaining to the biology of bone marrow fat in health and disease will likely remain unanswered due to the technical difficulties that accompany the study of a physically tough, often inaccessible tissue like bone both *in vitro* and *in vivo*. Based on current data, however, there is growing consensus that bone marrow fat is a source of circulating adiponectin.[144] This would be consistent with it simply acting as an extension of white adipose tissue, but it is the circumstances under which bone marrow fat secretes more adiponectin into the circulation that make this observation so intriguing. Indeed, circulating adiponectin levels tend to increase during calorie restriction, with this apparently being underpinned by an expansion of bone marrow fat mass.[145] Yes, you read that correctly; bone marrow fat *expands* during prolonged calorie restriction. Initial observations of bone marrow fat expansion during calorie restriction in humans and rabbits date back to the 1970s.[146] Evidently bone marrow fat is part of a larger, much more complex biological network linking bone health and energy metabolism than is currently appreciated.

There has been a concerted effort to elucidate the specific molecular signals which control the expansion of bone marrow fat during calorie restriction. The glucocorticoids are a prime candidate as their levels typically increase during starvation to ensure the body's energy demands are met. Persistent exposure to high levels of glucocorticoids can induce bone thinning in people to the extent that they can cause osteoporosis.[147]

The observation that bone marrow fat expansion in starved rodents (but not rabbits[148]) is accompanied by a parallel increase in circulating glucocorticoid levels raises the possibility that these hormones contribute to this curious interplay between bone and energy metabolism. Other evidence implicates the adipokine leptin[149] whose levels typically decline during starvation.[150] In this case, it may be significant that leptin-sensitive progenitor cells residing in the bone marrow are the main source of bone cells and adipocytes in adult mice.[151] As starvation is such a complex metabolic state involving many moving parts, the expansion of bone marrow fat may be driven by several coincident changes acting in isolation or tandem, directly or indirectly. Faced with making sense of such a dizzyingly complex scene, scientists and clinicians have turned to a distinct set of patients, specifically those with anorexia nervosa, whose condition could provide some important, clinically relevant insights into the interplay between bone health and metabolic status.

Thin Body, Fat Bones

The self-induced starvation which defines the physical manifestation of anorexia nervosa (which primarily affects young women) has widespread consequences on an individual's health. One such effect is an increased risk of developing osteoporosis[152] that renders individuals prone to bone fracture.[153] What is less well-appreciated, however, is that the weakening of bones in anorexia nervosa patients is accompanied by a substantial expansion of bone marrow fat mass.[154–156] The extent of bone marrow fat expansion appears to be directly proportional to the amount of weight loss,[157] thus reinforcing the notion that bone marrow fat is exquisitely sensitive to an individual's nutritional and metabolic status. This expansion of bone marrow fat is particularly concerning, as the diversion of the finite number of progenitor cells in the bone marrow towards the fat lineage reduces one's capacity for haematopoiesis and may have serious health consequences, such as increased infection risk, that may not be immediately obvious from standard clinical tests.[157]

It has been proposed that the elevated circulating cortisol levels observed in anorexia nervosa patients represents the crucial link between the metabolic response to their self-induced starvation and the simultaneous loss of bone mineral and expansion of bone marrow fat mass, as well as psychological distress.[158] However, anorexia nervosa is defined by numerous other hormonal changes in addition to elevated cortisol levels, any of which may contribute to the impaired bone health that patients typically experience. For instance, sex hormone deficiency, growth hormone resistance, or even perturbations to gut hormones such as peptide-YY and ghrelin all represent potential molecular culprits that warrant further investigation.[159]

Bone marrow adipose tissue has peculiar biological properties that play a hitherto unclear role in mammalian and human biology.[160] Indeed, bone marrow fat expands not only when subcutaneous and visceral fat mass expand, but also when they retract.[161] What is clear, however, is that bone marrow fat represents an important link between energy metabolism,[162] bone health,[163] and blood cell production.[164] As it sits at this crucial interface, perturbations to this tissue likely contribute to complications related to skeletal integrity and immunity (via impaired haematopoiesis) at opposite ends of the nutritional spectrum. Hopefully a greater understanding of this curious type of fat will translate to better management of patients particularly affected by altered bone marrow fat mass, such as those with anorexia nervosa, cancer patients undergoing chemotherapy, and the vast number of obese people with impaired bone health.

Other Types of Fat

This chapter focused specifically on the more prominent 'other' types of fat that reside in the body, but it will become apparent in the remaining chapters that white (subcutaneous and visceral) adipose tissue is remarkably heterogeneous too. Before moving ahead though, it is worth briefly acknowledging that other white fat depots exist which display unique biological properties that contribute to our body's functioning in myriad ways. For instance, the fat surrounding the heart (i.e., epicardial fat) which resides between the myocardium (i.e., heart muscle) and the visceral pericardium (i.e., inner lining of the abdominal cavity) secretes a variety of adipokines and cytokines that modulate vascular health and function.[165] As epicardial fat mass is positively correlated with BMI and waist circumference[166] and apparently shares many biological features with visceral fat,[167] this fat depot may link overall and regional fat mass with the vascular complications of obesity and metabolic disease.

(White) fat pads give our bodies their distinctive shape and appearance, with these physical attributes often exerting a strong influence over our self-esteem. While the motive for cosmetic surgery might be principally aesthetic, the underlying reason might range from a simple attempt to delay or reverse the aging process to a desire to conceal the physical manifestation of a vanishingly rare type of lipodystrophy[168] (see Chapter 7). The fat pads in the face[169] and pubic area (i.e., mons pubis[170]) are notable deposits of aesthetically important subcutaneous fat that can be highly distressing if shaped 'abnormally' (according to dynamic social interpretations). Fat also protects the body's soft tissues from mechanical forces, with the fat pads on the soles and balls of our feet[171] and in our joints[172] providing the internal cushioning that makes walking a comfortable and effective method of locomotion. Not only does fat represent the internal fuel source that enabled evolution to kick into high gear, it probably also contributed to the migration and evolution of the (bipedal) human race.[173] Understanding the biology of these and other fat deposits that each contribute to our everyday lives might provide important insights not only into the pathogenesis of obesity, diabetes, or lipodystrophy, but also our evolutionary history. And with that, it's time to refocus our attention on subcutaneous and visceral fat to examine the relationship between overall and regional (white) fat mass with metabolic and cardiovascular health.

References

1. Harding, A. 'Brown fat' burns calories -- may lead to new obesity treatments. *CNN* (2009). Available at: www.cnn.com/2009/HEALTH/04/10/brown.fat. obesity/.
2. Nedergaard, J., Bengtsson, T., & Cannon, B. Unexpected evidence for active brown adipose tissue in adult humans. *Am. J. Physiol. Endocrinol. Metab.* **293**, E444–52 (2007).
3. Cypess, A. M. *et al.* Identification and importance of brown adipose tissue in adult humans. *N. Engl. J. Med.* **360**, 1509–17 (2009).
4. Virtanen, K. A. *et al.* Functional brown adipose tissue in healthy adults. *N. Engl. J. Med.* **360**, 1518–25 (2009).
5. Ruiz, J. R. *et al.* Role of human brown fat in obesity, metabolism and cardiovascular disease: strategies to turn up the heat. *Prog. Cardiovasc. Dis.* (2018). doi:10.1016/j.pcad.2018.07.002
6. Heaton, J. M. The distribution of brown adipose tissue in the human. *J. Anat.* **112**, 35–9 (1972).
7. Sheikhbahaei, S. *et al.* Molecular imaging and precision medicine: PET/computed tomography and therapy response assessment in oncology. *PET Clin.* **12**, 105–18 (2017).
8. Yeung, H. W. D., Grewal, R. K., Gonen, M., Schöder, H., & Larson, S. M. Patterns of (18)F-FDG uptake in adipose tissue and muscle: a potential source of false-positives for PET. *J. Nucl. Med.* **44**, 1789–96 (2003).

9. Cohade, C., Osman, M., Pannu, H. K., & Wahl, R. L. Uptake in supraclavicular area fat ('USA-Fat'): description on 18F-FDG PET/CT. *J. Nucl. Med.* **44**, 170–6 (2003).

10. van Marken Lichtenbelt, W. D. *et al.* Cold-activated brown adipose tissue in healthy men. *N. Engl. J. Med.* **360**, 1500–8 (2009).

11. Ong, F. J. *et al.* Recent advances in the detection of brown adipose tissue in adult humans: a review. *Clin. Sci.* **132**, 1039–54 (2018).

12. Fenzl, A. & Kiefer, F. W. Brown adipose tissue and thermogenesis. *Horm. Mol. Biol. Clin. Investig.* **19**, 25–37 (2014).

13. Oelkrug, R. *et al.* Brown fat in a protoendothermic mammal fuels eutherian evolution. *Nat. Commun.* **4**, 2140 (2013).

14. Oelkrug, R., Polymeropoulos, E. T., & Jastroch, M. Brown adipose tissue: physiological function and evolutionary significance. *J. Comp. Physiol. B.* **185**, 587–606 (2015).

15. Steegmann, A. T., Cerny, F. J., & Holliday, T. W. Neandertal cold adaptation: physiological and energetic factors. *Am. J. Hum. Biol.* **14**, 566–83 (2002).

16. Daanen, H. A. M. & Van Marken Lichtenbelt, W. D. Human whole body cold adaptation. *Temp. (Austin, Tex.)* **3**, 104–18 (2016).

17. Steegmann, A. T. Human cold adaptation: an unfinished agenda. *Am. J. Hum. Biol.* **19**, 218–27 (2007).

18. Bahler, L., Holleman, F., Booij, J., Hoekstra, J. B., & Verberne, H. J. Hot heads & cool bodies: the conundrums of human brown adipose tissue (BAT) activity research. *Eur. J. Intern. Med.* **40**, 26–9 (2017).

19. Ouellet, V. *et al.* Outdoor temperature, age, sex, body mass index, and diabetic status determine the prevalence, mass, and glucose-uptake activity of 18F-FDG-detected BAT in humans. *J. Clin. Endocrinol. Metab.* **96**, 192–9 (2011).

20. Admiraal, W. M. *et al.* Cold-induced activity of brown adipose tissue in young lean men of South-Asian and European origin. *Diabetologia* **56**, 2231–7 (2013).

21. Bakker, L. E. H. *et al.* Brown adipose tissue volume in healthy lean south Asian adults compared with white Caucasians: a prospective, case-controlled observational study. *Lancet Diabetes Endocrinol.* **2**, 210–17 (2014).

22. Sellayah, D. The impact of early human migration on brown adipose tissue evolution and its relevance to the modern obesity pandemic. *J. Endocr. Soc.* **3**, 372–86 (2019).

23. Cronin, C. G. *et al.* Brown fat at PET/CT: correlation with patient characteristics. *Radiology* **263**, 836–42 (2012).

24. Saito, M. *et al.* High incidence of metabolically active brown adipose tissue in healthy adult humans: effects of cold exposure and adiposity. *Diabetes* **58**, 1526–31 (2009).

25. Yoneshiro, T. *et al.* Age-related decrease in cold-activated brown adipose tissue and accumulation of body fat in healthy humans. *Obesity (Silver Spring)* **19**, 1755–60 (2011).

26. Pace, L. *et al.* Determinants of physiologic 18F-FDG uptake in brown adipose tissue in sequential PET/CT examinations. *Mol. Imaging Biol.* **13**, 1029–35 (2011).

27. Vijgen, G. H. E. J. *et al.* Brown adipose tissue in morbidly obese subjects. *PLoS One* **6**, e17247 (2011).

28. Orava, J. *et al.* Blunted metabolic responses to cold and insulin stimulation in brown adipose tissue of obese humans. *Obesity (Silver Spring)* 21, 2279–87 (2013).

29. Villarroya, F., Cereijo, R., Gavaldà-Navarro, A., Villarroya, J., & Giralt, M. Inflammation of brown/beige adipose tissues in obesity and metabolic disease. *J. Intern. Med.* (2018). doi:10.1111/joim.12803

30. Matsushita, M. *et al.* Impact of brown adipose tissue on body fatness and glucose metabolism in healthy humans. *Int. J. Obes.* 38, 812–17 (2014).

31. Vijgen, G. H. E. J. *et al.* Increase in brown adipose tissue activity after weight loss in morbidly obese subjects. *J. Clin. Endocrinol. Metab.* 97, E1229–33 (2012).

32. Chondronikola, M. *et al.* Brown adipose tissue improves whole-body glucose homeostasis and insulin sensitivity in humans. *Diabetes* 63, 4089–99 (2014).

33. Iwen, K. A. *et al.* Cold-induced brown adipose tissue activity alters plasma fatty acids and improves glucose metabolism in men. *J. Clin. Endocrinol. Metab.* 102, 4226–34 (2017).

34. Chen, K. Y. *et al.* Brown fat activation mediates cold-induced thermogenesis in adult humans in response to a mild decrease in ambient temperature. *J. Clin. Endocrinol. Metab.* 98, E1218–23 (2013).

35. Yoneshiro, T. *et al.* Recruited brown adipose tissue as an antiobesity agent in humans. *J. Clin. Invest.* 123, 3404–8 (2013).

36. Blondin, D. P. *et al.* Increased brown adipose tissue oxidative capacity in cold-acclimated humans. *J. Clin. Endocrinol. Metab.* 99, E438–46 (2014).

37. Lee, P. *et al.* Temperature-acclimated brown adipose tissue modulates insulin sensitivity in humans. *Diabetes* 63, 3686–98 (2014).

38. Marlatt, K. L., Chen, K. Y., & Ravussin, E. Is activation of human brown adipose tissue a viable target for weight management? *Am. J. Physiol. Regul. Integr. Comp. Physiol.* (2018). doi:10.1152/ajpregu.00443.2017

39. Lahesmaa, M. *et al.* Hyperthyroidism increases brown fat metabolism in humans. *J. Clin. Endocrinol. Metab.* 99, E28–35 (2014).

40. Cioffi, F., Gentile, A., Silvestri, E., Goglia, F., & Lombardi, A. Effect of iodothyronines on thermogenesis: focus on brown adipose tissue. *Front. Endocrinol.* 9, 254 (2018).

41. Pfannenberg, C. *et al.* Impact of age on the relationships of brown adipose tissue with sex and adiposity in humans. *Diabetes* 59, 1789–93 (2010).

42. Colafella, K. M. M. & Denton, K. M. Sex-specific differences in hypertension and associated cardiovascular disease. *Nat. Rev. Nephrol.* (2018). doi:10.1038/nrneph.2017.189

43. González-García, I., Tena-Sempere, M., & López, M. Estradiol regulation of brown adipose tissue thermogenesis. *Adv. Exp. Med. Biol.* 1043, 315–35 (2017).

44. Aldiss, P., Budge, H., & Symonds, M. E. Is a reduction in brown adipose thermogenesis responsible for the change in core body temperature at menopause? *Cardiovasc. Endocrinol.* 5, 155–6 (2016).

45. Muzik, O., Mangner, T. J., Leonard, W. R., Kumar, A., & Granneman, J. G. Sympathetic innervation of cold-activated brown and white fat in lean young adults. *J. Nucl. Med.* 58, 799–806 (2017).

46. Lowell, B. B. & Flier, J. S. Brown adipose tissue, beta 3-adrenergic receptors, and obesity. *Annu. Rev. Med.* **48**, 307–16 (1997).

47. Umekawa, T. *et al.* Anti-obesity and anti-diabetic effects of CL316,243, a highly specific beta 3-adrenoceptor agonist, in Otsuka Long-Evans Tokushima Fatty rats: induction of uncoupling protein and activation of glucose transporter 4 in white fat. *Eur. J. Endocrinol.* **136**, 429–37 (1997).

48. Ghorbani, M. & Himms-Hagen, J. Appearance of brown adipocytes in white adipose tissue during CL 316,243-induced reversal of obesity and diabetes in Zucker fa/fa rats. *Int. J. Obes. Relat. Metab. Disord.* **21**, 465–75 (1997).

49. Marlatt, K. L. & Ravussin, E. Brown adipose tissue: an update on recent findings. *Curr. Obes. Rep.* **6**, 389–96 (2017).

50. Weyer, C., Tataranni, P. A., Snitker, S., Danforth, E., & Ravussin, E. Increase in insulin action and fat oxidation after treatment with CL 316,243, a highly selective beta3-adrenoceptor agonist in humans. *Diabetes* **47**, 1555–61 (1998).

51. van Baak, M. A. *et al.* Acute effect of L-796568, a novel beta 3-adrenergic receptor agonist, on energy expenditure in obese men. *Clin. Pharmacol. Ther.* **71**, 272–9 (2002).

52. Larsen, T. M. *et al.* Effect of a 28-d treatment with L-796568, a novel beta(3)-adrenergic receptor agonist, on energy expenditure and body composition in obese men. *Am. J. Clin. Nutr.* **76**, 780–8 (2002).

53. Buemann, B., Toubro, S., & Astrup, A. Effects of the two beta3-agonists, ZD7114 and ZD2079 on 24-hour energy expenditure and respiratory quotient in obese subjects. *Int. J. Obes. Relat. Metab. Disord.* **24**, 1553–60 (2000).

54. Summers, R. J., Kompa, A., & Roberts, S. J. β-Adrenoceptor subtypes and their desensitization mechanisms. *J. Auton. Pharmacol.* **17**, 331–43 (1997).

55. Cypess, A. M. *et al.* Activation of human brown adipose tissue by a β3-adrenergic receptor agonist. *Cell Metab.* **21**, 33–8 (2015).

56. O'Mara, A. E. *et al.* Chronic mirabegron treatment increases human brown fat, HDL cholesterol, and insulin sensitivity. *J. Clin. Invest.* **130**, 2209–19 (2020).

57. Zuriaga, M. A., Fuster, J. J., Gokce, N., & Walsh, K. Humans and mice display opposing patterns of 'browning' gene expression in visceral and subcutaneous white adipose tissue depots. *Front. Cardiovasc. Med.* **4**, 27 (2017).

58. Boon, M. R. *et al.* BMP7 activates brown adipose tissue and reduces diet-induced obesity only at subthermoneutrality. *PLoS One* **8**, e74083 (2013).

59. Weir, G. *et al.* Substantial metabolic activity of human brown adipose tissue during warm conditions and cold-induced lipolysis of local triglycerides. *Cell Metab.* **27**, 1348–55.e4 (2018).

60. Katz, D. L. Competing dietary claims for weight loss: finding the forest through truculent trees. *Annu. Rev. Public Health* **26**, 61–88 (2005).

61. Townsend, K. & Tseng, Y.-H. Brown adipose tissue: recent insights into development, metabolic function and therapeutic potential. *Adipocyte* **1**, 13–24 (2012).

62. Nicholls, D. G., Bernson, V. S., & Heaton, G. M. The identification of the component in the inner membrane of brown adipose tissue mitochondria responsible for regulating energy dissipation. *Experientia. Suppl.* **32**, 89–93 (1978).

63. Gaudry, M. J., Campbell, K. L., & Jastroch, M. Evolution of UCP1. *Handb. Exp. Pharmacol.* (2018). doi:10.1007/164_2018_116

64. Christiansen, E. N., Pedersen, J. I., & Grav, H. J. Uncoupling and recoupling of oxidative phosphorylation in brown adipose tissue mitochondria. *Nature* **222**, 857–60 (1969).

65. Grundlingh, J., Dargan, P. I., El-Zanfaly, M., & Wood, D. M. 2,4-dinitrophenol (DNP): a weight loss agent with significant acute toxicity and risk of death. *J. Med. Toxicol.* **7**, 205–12 (2011).

66. Perkins, R. G. A study of the munitions intoxications in France. *Public Health Rep.* **24**, 2335–74 (1919).

67. Tainter, M. L., Stockton, A. B., & Cutting, W. C. Use of dinitrophenol in obesity and related conditions. *J. Am. Med. Assoc.* **101**, 1472 (1933).

68. Cutting, W. C., Mehrtens, H. G., & Tainter, M. L. Actions and uses of dinitrophenol. *J. Am. Med. Assoc.* **101**, 193 (1933).

69. Margo, C. E. & Harman, L. E. Diet pills and the cataract outbreak of 1935: reflections on the evolution of consumer protection legislation. *Surv. Ophthalmol.* **59**, 568–73 (2014).

70. Colman, E. Dinitrophenol and obesity: an early twentieth-century regulatory dilemma. *Regul. Toxicol. Pharmacol.* **48**, 115–17 (2007).

71. Kurt, T. L. *et al.* Dinitrophenol in weight loss: the poison center and public health safety. *Vet. Hum. Toxicol.* **28**, 574–5 (1986).

72. Simkins, S. Dinitrophenol and desiccated thyroid in the treatment of obesity. *J. Am. Med. Assoc.* **108**, 2110 (1937).

73. Leftwich, R. B., Floro, J. F., Neal, R. A., & Wood, A. J. Dinitrophenol poisoning: a diagnosis to consider in undiagnosed fever. *South. Med. J.* **75**, 182–4 (1982).

74. Miranda, E. J., McIntyre, I. M., Parker, D. R., Gary, R. D., & Logan, B. K. Two deaths attributed to the use of 2–4-dinitrophenol. *J. Anal. Toxicol.* **30**, 219–22 (2006).

75. McFee, R. B., Caraccio, T. R., McGuigan, M. A., Reynolds, S. A., & Bellanger, P. Dying to be thin: a dinitrophenol related fatality. *Vet. Hum. Toxicol.* **46**, 251–4 (2004).

76. Office for National Statistics. Number of deaths where dinitrophenol (DNP) was mentioned on the death certificate, England and Wales, 2007 to 2016. (2017). Available at: www.ons.gov.uk/peoplepopulationandcommunity/birthsdeathsandmarriages/deaths/adhocs/007648numberofdeathswheredinitrophenoldnpwasmentionedonthedeathcertificateenglandandwales2007to2016.

77. Food Standards Authority. FSA welcomes guilty verdict in DNP trial. (2018). Availabe at: www.food.gov.uk/news-alerts/news/fsa-welcomes-guilty-verdict-in-dnp-trial

78. Perry, R. J., Zhang, D., Zhang, X.-M., Boyer, J. L., & Shulman, G. I. Controlled-release mitochondrial protonophore reverses diabetes and steatohepatitis in rats. *Science* **347**, 1253–6 (2015).

79. Harper, J. A., Dickinson, K., & Brand, M. D. Mitochondrial uncoupling as a target for drug development for the treatment of obesity. *Obes. Rev.* **2**, 255–65 (2001).

80. Sizar, O., Podder, V., & Talati, R. *Empagliflozin*. StatPearls, 2020. doi:30422520

81. Froy, O. & Garaulet, M. The circadian clock in white and brown adipose tissue: mechanistic, endocrine, and clinical aspects. *Endocr. Rev.* **39**, 261–73 (2018).

82. Lee, P. *et al.* Brown adipose tissue exhibits a glucose-responsive thermogenic biorhythm in humans. *Cell Metab.* **23**, 602–9 (2016).

83. van den Berg, R. *et al.* A diurnal rhythm in brown adipose tissue causes rapid clearance and combustion of plasma lipids at wakening. *Cell Rep.* **22**, 3521–33 (2018).

84. Summerbell, C. D., Moody, R. C., Shanks, J., Stock, M. J., & Geissler, C. Relationship between feeding pattern and body mass index in 220 free-living people in four age groups. *Eur. J. Clin. Nutr.* **50**, 513–19 (1996).

85. Jakubowicz, D., Barnea, M., Wainstein, J., & Froy, O. High caloric intake at breakfast vs. dinner differentially influences weight loss of overweight and obese women. *Obesity (Silver Spring)* **21**, 2504–12 (2013).

86. Garaulet, M. *et al.* Timing of food intake predicts weight loss effectiveness. *Int. J. Obes.* **37**, 604–11 (2013).

87. Knapton, S. Breakfast like a king, lunch like a prince and dine like a pauper to stay healthy, say scientists. *The Telegraph* (2016). Available at: www.telegraph. co.uk/science/2016/06/22/breakfast-like-a-king-lunch-like-a-prince-and-dine-like-a-pauper/.

88. Almoosawi, S., Vingeliene, S., Karagounis, L. G., & Pot, G. K. Chrono-nutrition: a review of current evidence from observational studies on global trends in time-of-day of energy intake and its association with obesity. In *Proceedings of the Nutrition Society* (2016). doi:10.1017/S0029665116000306

89. Dubois, L., Girard, M., Potvin Kent, M., Farmer, A., & Tatone-Tokuda, F. Breakfast skipping is associated with differences in meal patterns, macronutrient intakes and overweight among pre-school children. *Public Health Nutr.* **12**, 19–28 (2009).

90. Howarth, N. C., Huang, T. T.-K., Roberts, S. B., Lin, B.-H., & McCrory, M. A. Eating patterns and dietary composition in relation to BMI in younger and older adults. *Int. J. Obes.* **31**, 675–84 (2007).

91. Sun, M. *et al.* Meta-analysis on shift work and risks of specific obesity types. *Obes. Rev.* **19**, 28–40 (2018).

92. Knutsson, A. & Kempe, A. Shift work and diabetes--a systematic review. *Chronobiol. Int.* **31**, 1146–51 (2014).

93. Froy, O. & Garaulet, M. The circadian clock in white and brown adipose tissue: mechanistic, endocrine, and clinical aspects. *Endocr. Rev.* **39**, 261–73 (2018).

94. Wehrens, S. M. T. *et al.* Meal timing regulates the human circadian system. *Curr. Biol.* **27**, 1768–75.e3 (2017).

95. Morris, C. J., Purvis, T. E., Mistretta, J., & Scheer, F. A. J. L. Effects of the internal circadian system and circadian misalignment on glucose tolerance in chronic shift workers. *J. Clin. Endocrinol. Metab.* **101**, 1066–74 (2016).

96. Kooijman, S. *et al.* Prolonged daily light exposure increases body fat mass through attenuation of brown adipose tissue activity. *Proc. Natl. Acad. Sci. U. S. A.* **112**, 6748–53 (2015).

97. Hibi, M. *et al.* Brown adipose tissue is involved in diet-induced thermogenesis and whole-body fat utilization in healthy humans. *Int. J. Obes.* **40**, 1655–61 (2016).

98. Trayhurn, P. Origins and early development of the concept that brown adipose tissue thermogenesis is linked to energy balance and obesity. *Biochimie* **134**, 62–70 (2017).

99. Stockman, R. The action of arsenic on the bone-marrow and blood. *J. Physiol.* **23**, 376–82.2 (1898).

100. Pereira, J. A. *et al.* Effects of inorganic arsenic on bone marrow hematopoietic cells: an emphasis on apoptosis and Sca-1/c-Kit positive population. *J. Stem Cells* **5**, 117–27 (2010).

101. Lanske, B. & Rosen, C. Bone marrow adipose tissue: the first 40 years. *J. Bone Miner. Res.* **32**, 1153–6 (2017).

102. Gordon, M. Y., King, J. A., & Gordon-Smith, E. C. Bone marrow fibroblasts, fat cells and colony-stimulating activity. *Br. J. Haematol.* **46**, 151–2 (1980).

103. Emery, J. L. & Follett, G. F. Regression of bone-marrow haemopoiesis from the terminal digits in the foetus and infant. *Br. J. Haematol.* **10**, 485–9 (1964).

104. Griffith, J. F. *et al.* Bone marrow fat content in the elderly: a reversal of sex difference seen in younger subjects. *J. Magn. Reson. Imaging* **36**, 225–30 (2012).

105. Baum, T. *et al.* Anatomical variation of age-related changes in vertebral bone marrow composition using chemical shift encoding-based water-fat magnetic resonance imaging. *Front. Endocrinol.* **9**, 141 (2018).

106. Shen, W. *et al.* Ethnic and sex differences in bone marrow adipose tissue and bone mineral density relationship. *Osteoporos. Int.* **23**, 2293–301 (2012).

107. Shen, W. *et al.* Relationship between MRI-measured bone marrow adipose tissue and hip and spine bone mineral density in African-American and Caucasian participants: the CARDIA study. *J. Clin. Endocrinol. Metab.* **97**, 1337–46 (2012).

108. Meunier, P., Aaron, J., Edouard, C., & Vignon, G. Osteoporosis and the replacement of cell populations of the marrow by adipose tissue. A quantitative study of 84 iliac bone biopsies. *Clin. Orthop. Relat. Res.* **80**, 147–54 (1971).

109. Patsch, J. M. *et al.* Bone marrow fat composition as a novel imaging biomarker in postmenopausal women with prevalent fragility fractures. *J. Bone Miner. Res.* **28**, 1721–8 (2013).

110. Schwartz, A. V *et al.* Vertebral bone marrow fat associated with lower trabecular BMD and prevalent vertebral fracture in older adults. *J. Clin. Endocrinol. Metab.* **98**, 2294–300 (2013).

111. Di Iorgi, N. *et al.* Bone acquisition in healthy young females is reciprocally related to marrow adiposity. *J. Clin. Endocrinol. Metab.* **95**, 2977–82 (2010).

112. Shen, W. *et al.* MRI-measured bone marrow adipose tissue is inversely related to DXA-measured bone mineral in Caucasian women. *Osteoporos. Int.* **18**, 641–7 (2007).

113. Di Iorgi, N., Rosol, M., Mittelman, S. D., & Gilsanz, V. Reciprocal relation between marrow adiposity and the amount of bone in the axial and appendicular skeleton of young adults. *J. Clin. Endocrinol. Metab.* **93**, 2281–6 (2008).

114. Bredella, M. A. *et al.* Determinants of bone microarchitecture and mechanical properties in obese men. *J. Clin. Endocrinol. Metab.* **97**, 4115–22 (2012).

115. Gilsanz, V. *et al.* Reciprocal relations of subcutaneous and visceral fat to bone structure and strength. *J. Clin. Endocrinol. Metab.* **94**, 3387–93 (2009).

116. Kim, S. H., Yi, S.-W., Yi, J.-J., Kim, Y. M., & Won, Y. J. Association between body mass index and the risk of hip fracture by sex and age: a prospective cohort study. *J. Bone Miner. Res.* (2018). doi:10.1002/jbmr.3464

117. Sadeghi, O., Saneei, P., Nasiri, M., Larijani, B., & Esmaillzadeh, A. Abdominal obesity and risk of hip fracture: a systematic review and meta-analysis of prospective studies. *Adv. Nutr.* **8**, 728–38 (2017).

118. Li, X., Gong, X., & Jiang, W. Abdominal obesity and risk of hip fracture: a meta-analysis of prospective studies. *Osteoporos. Int.* **28**, 2747–57 (2017).

119. Bredella, M. A. *et al.* Vertebral bone marrow fat is positively associated with visceral fat and inversely associated with IGF-1 in obese women. *Obesity (Silver Spring)* **19**, 49–53 (2011).

120. Machado, L. G. *et al.* Visceral fat measured by DXA is associated with increased risk of non-spine fractures in nonobese elderly women: a population-based prospective cohort analysis from the São Paulo Ageing & Health (SPAH) Study. *Osteoporos. Int.* **27**, 3525–33 (2016).

121. Sheu, Y. *et al.* Vertebral bone marrow fat, bone mineral density and diabetes: The Osteoporotic Fractures in Men (MrOS) study. *Bone* **97**, 299–305 (2017).

122. Baum, T. *et al.* Does vertebral bone marrow fat content correlate with abdominal adipose tissue, lumbar spine bone mineral density, and blood biomarkers in women with type 2 diabetes mellitus? *J. Magn. Reson. Imaging* **35**, 117–24 (2012).

123. Kim, T. Y. & Schafer, A. L. Diabetes and bone marrow adiposity. *Curr. Osteoporos. Rep.* **14**, 337–44 (2016).

124. Karpe, F. & Pinnick, K. E. Biology of upper-body and lower-body adipose tissue--link to whole-body phenotypes. *Nat. Rev. Endocrinol.* **11**, 90–100 (2015).

125. Hind, K., Pearce, M., & Birrell, F. Total and visceral adiposity are associated with prevalent vertebral fracture in women but not men at age 62 years: The Newcastle Thousand Families Study. *J. Bone Miner. Res.* **32**, 1109–15 (2017).

126. Liu, C.-T. *et al.* Visceral adipose tissue is associated with bone microarchitecture in the Framingham Osteoporosis Study. *J. Bone Miner. Res.* **32**, 143–50 (2017).

127. Xiang, B.-Y. *et al.* Body mass index and the risk of low bone mass-related fractures in women compared with men: a PRISMA-compliant meta-analysis of prospective cohort studies. *Medicine* **96**, e5290 (2017).

128. Søgaard, A. J. *et al.* Age and sex differences in body mass index as a predictor of hip fracture: A NOREPOS Study. *Am. J. Epidemiol.* **184**, 510–19 (2016).

129. Lecka-Czernik, B. *et al.* Marrow adipose tissue: skeletal location, sexual dimorphism, and response to sex steroid deficiency. *Front. Endocrinol.* **8**, 188 (2017).

130. da Silva, S. V., Renovato-Martins, M., Ribeiro-Pereira, C., Citelli, M., & Barja-Fidalgo, C. Obesity modifies bone marrow microenvironment and directs bone marrow mesenchymal cells to adipogenesis. *Obesity (Silver Spring)* **24**, 2522–32 (2016).

131. Doucette, C. R. *et al.* A high fat diet increases bone marrow adipose tissue (MAT) but does not alter trabecular or cortical bone mass in C57BL/6J mice. *J. Cell. Physiol.* **230**, 2032–7 (2015).

132. Ambrosi, T. H. *et al.* Adipocyte accumulation in the bone marrow during obesity and aging impairs stem cell-based hematopoietic and bone regeneration. *Cell Stem Cell* **20**, 771–84.e6 (2017).

133. Tencerova, M. *et al.* High-fat diet-induced obesity promotes expansion of bone marrow adipose tissue and impairs skeletal stem cell functions in mice. *J. Bone Miner. Res.* **33**, 1154–65 (2018).

134. Styner, M. *et al.* Bone marrow fat accumulation accelerated by high fat diet is suppressed by exercise. *Bone* **64**, 39–46 (2014).

135. Styner, M. *et al.* Exercise decreases marrow adipose tissue through ß-oxidation in obese running mice. *J. Bone Miner. Res.* **32**, 1692–702 (2017).

136. Scheller, E. L. *et al.* Changes in skeletal integrity and marrow adiposity during high-fat diet and after weight loss. *Front. Endocrinol.* **7**, 102 (2016).

137. Kim, T. Y. *et al.* Bone marrow fat changes after gastric bypass surgery are associated with loss of bone mass. *J. Bone Miner. Res.* **32**, 2239–47 (2017).

138. Lu, C.-W. *et al.* Fracture risk after bariatric surgery: a 12-year nationwide cohort study. *Medicine* **94**, e2087 (2015).

139. Schwartz, A. V *et al.* Effects of TZD use and discontinuation on fracture rates in ACCORD bone study. *J. Clin. Endocrinol. Metab.* **100**, 4059–66 (2015).

140. Napoli, N. *et al.* Mechanisms of diabetes mellitus-induced bone fragility. *Nat. Rev. Endocrinol.* **13**, 208–19 (2017).

141. Sulston, R. J. *et al.* Increased circulating adiponectin in response to thiazolidinediones: investigating the role of bone marrow adipose tissue. *Front. Endocrinol.* **7**, 128 (2016).

142. Pagnotti, G. M. & Styner, M. Exercise regulation of marrow adipose tissue. *Front. Endocrinol.* **7**, 94 (2016).

143. Styner, M. *et al.* Exercise regulation of marrow fat in the setting of PPARγ agonist treatment in female C57BL/6 mice. *Endocrinology* **156**, 2753–61 (2015).

144. Scheller, E. L., Burr, A. A., MacDougald, O. A., & Cawthorn, W. P. Inside out: bone marrow adipose tissue as a source of circulating adiponectin. *Adipocyte* **5**, 251–69

145. Cawthorn, W. P. *et al.* Bone marrow adipose tissue is an endocrine organ that contributes to increased circulating adiponectin during caloric restriction. *Cell Metab.* **20**, 368–75 (2014).

146. Tavassoli, M., Eastlund, D. T., Yam, L. T., Neiman, R. S., & Finkel, H. Gelatinous transformation of bone marrow in prolonged self-induced starvation. *Scand. J. Haematol.* **16**, 311–19 (1976).

147. Henneicke, H., Gasparini, S. J., Brennan-Speranza, T. C., Zhou, H., & Seibel, M. J. Glucocorticoids and bone: local effects and systemic implications. *Trends Endocrinol. Metab.* **25**, 197–211 (2014).

148. Cawthorn, W. P. *et al.* Expansion of bone marrow adipose tissue during caloric restriction is associated with increased circulating glucocorticoids and not with hypoleptinemia. *Endocrinology* **157**, 508–21 (2016).

149. Chen, X. X. & Yang, T. Roles of leptin in bone metabolism and bone diseases. *J. Bone Miner. Metab.* **33**, 474–85 (2015).

150. Müller, M. J. *et al.* Metabolic adaptation to caloric restriction and subsequent refeeding: the Minnesota Starvation Experiment revisited. *Am. J. Clin. Nutr.* **102**, 807–19 (2015).

151. Zhou, B. O., Yue, R., Murphy, M. M., Peyer, J. G., & Morrison, S. J. Leptin-receptor-expressing mesenchymal stromal cells represent the main source of bone formed by adult bone marrow. *Cell Stem Cell* **15**, 154–68 (2014).

152. Rigotti, N. A., Neer, R. M., Skates, S. J., Herzog, D. B., & Nussbaum, S. R. The clinical course of osteoporosis in anorexia nervosa. A longitudinal study of cortical bone mass. *JAMA* **265**, 1133–8 (1991).

153. Faje, A. T. *et al.* Fracture risk and areal bone mineral density in adolescent females with anorexia nervosa. *Int. J. Eat. Disord.* **47**, 458–66 (2014).

154. Ecklund, K. *et al.* Bone marrow fat content in 70 adolescent girls with anorexia nervosa: magnetic resonance imaging and magnetic resonance spectroscopy assessment. *Pediatr. Radiol.* **47**, 952–62 (2017).

155. Ecklund, K. *et al.* Bone marrow changes in adolescent girls with anorexia nervosa. *J. Bone Miner. Res.* **25**, 298–304 (2010).

156. Bredella, M. A. *et al.* Increased bone marrow fat in anorexia nervosa. *J. Clin. Endocrinol. Metab.* **94**, 2129–36 (2009).

157. Abella, E. *et al.* Bone marrow changes in anorexia nervosa are correlated with the amount of weight loss and not with other clinical findings. *Am. J. Clin. Pathol.* **118**, 582–8 (2002).

158. Lawson, E. A. *et al.* Hypercortisolemia is associated with severity of bone loss and depression in hypothalamic amenorrhea and anorexia nervosa. *J. Clin. Endocrinol. Metab.* **94**, 4710–16 (2009).

159. Schorr, M. & Miller, K. K. The endocrine manifestations of anorexia nervosa: mechanisms and management. *Nat. Rev. Endocrinol.* **13**, 174–86 (2017).

160. Craft, C. S. & Scheller, E. L. Evolution of the marrow adipose tissue microenvironment. *Calcif. Tissue Int.* **100**, 461–75 (2017).

161. Fazeli, P. K. & Klibanski, A. The paradox of marrow adipose tissue in anorexia nervosa. *Bone* (2018). doi:10.1016/j.bone.2018.02.013

162. Suchacki, K. J. & Cawthorn, W. P. Molecular interaction of bone marrow adipose tissue with energy metabolism. *Curr. Mol. Biol. reports* **4**, 41–9 (2018).

163. Muruganandan, S., Govindarajan, R., & Sinal, C. J. Bone marrow adipose tissue and skeletal health. *Curr. Osteoporos. Rep.* **16**, 434–42 (2018).

164. Hawkes, C. P. & Mostoufi-Moab, S. Fat-bone interaction within the bone marrow milieu: impact on hematopoiesis and systemic energy metabolism. *Bone* (2018). doi:10.1016/j.bone.2018.03.012

165. Patel, V. B., Shah, S., Verma, S., & Oudit, G. Y. Epicardial adipose tissue as a metabolic transducer: role in heart failure and coronary artery disease. *Heart Fail. Rev.* **22**, 889–902 (2017).

166. Wang, C.-P. *et al.* Increased epicardial adipose tissue (EAT) volume in type 2 diabetes mellitus and association with metabolic syndrome and severity of coronary atherosclerosis. *Clin. Endocrinol.* **70**, 876–82 (2009).

167. Nagy, E., Jermendy, A. L., Merkely, B., & Maurovich-Horvat, P. Clinical importance of epicardial adipose tissue. *Arch. Med. Sci.* **13**, 864–74 (2017).

168. Lightbourne, M. & Brown, R. J. Genetics of lipodystrophy. *Endocrinol. Metab. Clin. North Am.* **46**, 539–54 (2017).

169. Wollina, U., Goldman, A., & Tchernev, G. Fillers and facial fat pads. *Open Access Maced. J. Med. Sci.* **5**, 403–8 (2017).

170. Alter, G. J. Management of the mons pubis and labia majora in the massive weight loss patient. *Aesthetic Surg. J.* **29**, 432–42.

171. Dalal, S., Widgerow, A. D., & Evans, G. R. D. The plantar fat pad and the diabetic foot--a review. *Int. Wound J.* **12**, 636–40 (2015).

172. Zwick, R. K., Guerrero-Juarez, C. F., Horsley, V., & Plikus, M. V. Anatomical, physiological, and functional diversity of adipose tissue. *Cell Metab.* **27**, 68–83 (2018).

173. Holowka, N. B. & Lieberman, D. E. Rethinking the evolution of the human foot: insights from experimental research. *J. Exp. Biol.* **221**, jeb174425 (2018).

5

What Shape Is Healthy? Body Composition, Body Shape, and Health

Part 1 1—Measuring Fat

Body Mass Index

Simple measures of a body's physical properties such as height and weight are rather limited in what they can tell us. The need to obtain more information from simple anthropometric measures led to the development of the body mass index (BMI) as an index of 'relative fatness', that is, fatness relative to height. Far from being a modern stroke of genius, the calculation used to determine BMI was originally described nearly two centuries ago by a Belgian named Adolphe Quetelet (1796–1874). Primarily interested in defining the 'normal' (average) man, Quetelet pioneered the use of mathematical and statistical techniques to study the physical characteristics and social phenomena of humans.[1] In doing so, he kick-started the field of anthropometry (in addition to making several important contributions to mathematics, astronomy, sociology, and statistics throughout his life).

Drawing upon data organized in innovative (at the time) height–weight tables to categorize adult's and children's weight relative to an ideal for their height, Quetelet struggled to fit the data to the normal, bell-shaped (i.e., Gaussian) distribution displayed by many other natural phenomena. This was because a wide range of weights can be associated with a given height in men and women. His solution to this problem manifested as the 'Quetelet index', which was calculated by dividing weight (in kilograms) by the square of height (in metres). This masterstroke was published in a trailblazing article entitled *Recherches sur le poids de l'homme aux différent âges*

('Research on the weight of man at different ages') in 1832 and later in his book in 1835.[1]

Undoubtably a significant development in the academic world, the Quetelet index was a solution to a problem that didn't exist at the time and so entered a prolonged state of obscure dormancy. While people who fell on the extreme end of Quetelet's index in terms of corpulence certainly existed, the vast majority of deaths in the 1800s[2] and 1900s[3] were caused by infectious diseases. This situation would change, however, as the world transformed through the onward march of industrialization and globalization. Responding to cramped, often unhygienic living conditions, particularly amongst the growing working classes, public health officials in Europe (and later North America) instituted sanitation reforms that contributed to the reduction in the burden of disease from many infectious diseases.[4] This paved the way for society to undergo the 'epidemiological transition', in which non-communicable, chronic illnesses became increasingly responsible for a greater burden of morbidity and mortality in industrialized countries.[5]

It was well-established at the time that obesity negatively influenced various aspects of health, but it was only during the twentieth century that the diseases and premature death associated with obesity started to affect a substantial and growing number of people. With this mounting public health problem threatening to prove very costly, it soon caught the attention of a particularly powerful stakeholder who stood to lose a great deal unless something was done: the insurance industry. In the early 1900s, actuaries began to notice that insurance companies were paying out an increased number of death claims held by heavier policyholders.[6] Suddenly being able to define and identify 'normal/healthy' body weight became an issue of paramount importance for the insurance industry to shield themselves from crippling pay-outs driven by the burgeoning obesity crisis. Evidently the prospect of a big medical bill was more effective at prompting action than the fact that a growing proportion of the population was getting sick and dying in a preventable manner; little may have changed on this front.

Leading the charge to tackle this burgeoning problem was Louis I. Dublin (1882–1969), an American statistician and the vice president of the Metropolitan Life Insurance Company. Driven by a sense of urgency, Dublin collected huge amounts of data in a bid to define 'normal' weight. History, however, ultimately repeated itself. Encountering the same frustratingly wide range of weights associated with a given height in men and women as Quetelet, Dublin's solution involved arbitrarily dividing the distribution of weights at a given height into three groups. At the low end of the spectrum, people were deemed to be of 'desirable weight'; in the middle were people of 'undesirable weight' (20–25% above desirable weight); and at the top were the 'morbidly obese' individuals (70–100% above desirable weight). These cut-offs were adopted into practice and, for the first time, people were sold more/less expensive premiums based on weight-related measures, with higher premiums associated with higher weight.[7,8] With obesity representing a major cost borne by health insurers and taxpayers,[9] the question of whether obese people should pay more for their health insurance and care has become an increasingly high-stakes, contentious debate involving issues of health, morality, and economics, with global implications.

It soon became clear, however, that this approach was unsatisfactory in that it didn't fix the underlying mathematical problem. The pressure to devise a reliable and practical measure of relative weight was mounting, especially in the wake of World War II, when the burden of obesity and its related diseases (specifically type 2 diabetes and cardiovascular disease) was starting to grow at an alarming rate as living standards increased. Concerted efforts were made in epidemiological and clinical studies to test various anthropometric indices that combined height and weight in myriad ways. It became clear from the results of these studies in the 1960s that Quetelet's index from over 130 years earlier was the best of the bunch.[10,11]

Eager to put this recently fashioned, or re-discovered, tool to the test, Quetelet's index was employed during the fourth wave of the famous longitudinal 'Framingham Heart Study of Cardiovascular Risk.'[12] The eminent American physiologist Ancel Keys (1904–2004) demonstrated the utility of the index in a subsequent study in which he confirmed the validity of Quetelet's index and renamed it the 'Body Mass Index' in 1972.[13] Although the calculation uses total body weight, Quetelet's Index/BMI has always been intended to provide an estimate of *fat mass*. Used as an expression of 'relative weight' in countless studies since, BMI has played a crucial role in our investigation of the relationship between obesity and human morbidity and mortality. It is a useful index of relative weight, most of the time, for most people. Additionally, it is easy to assess, to the point that anyone can calculate their BMI by using a set of scales, a tape measure, and a calculator (Figure 5.1).

Body mass index is limited, however, in a number of ways. Firstly, the calculation was devised and validated using data from European and North American populations, thus raising concerns regarding its generalizability and applicability. Rather than trying to re-engineer the calculation though, this issue has been partially addressed by devising ethnicity-specific BMI cut-offs[14] (see Table 5.1). As with any (medical) cut-off, social and cultural

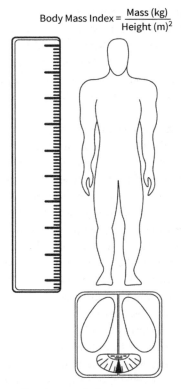

$$\text{Body Mass Index} = \frac{\text{Mass (kg)}}{\text{Height (m)}^2}$$

Figure 5.1 Calculation of body mass index.

Table 5.1 Body mass index categories for European and Asian populations

	Underweight	Normal Weight	Overweight	Obese
European	$<18.5\,\text{kg/m}^2$	$18.5\text{--}24.9\,\text{kg/m}^2$	$25\text{--}29.9\,\text{kg/m}^2$	$>30\,\text{kg/m}^2$
Asian		$18.5\text{--}23\,\text{kg/m}^2$	$23\text{--}27.5\,\text{kg/m}^2$	$27.5\text{--}32.5\,\text{kg/m}^2$

Source data from WHO Expert Consultation. Appropriate body-mass index for Asian populations and its implications for policy and intervention strategies. *Lancet* **363**, 157–63 (2004).

meanings of indexes and their thresholds may vary by place and time, thereby challenging possible standardization.

Additionally, the nature of the calculation limits its ability to determine whether an individual has an appropriate body mass relative to their frame.[15] The BMI calculation typically provides an *over-estimate* of relative body weight/fat mass in tall people but an *under-estimate* in individuals of short stature. In other words, people with small frames who carry relatively greater amounts of fat (e.g., a retired jockey who's put on a few pounds) might have a normal BMI, whereas tall individuals of otherwise healthy proportions (e.g., a sturdy basketball player) may be labelled overweight. Relatedly, BMI doesn't account for differences in body composition. As muscle is denser than fat, a bull-like rugby player could be labelled overweight, even obese, whereas someone with a proportionately low muscle mass in conjunction with a substantial paunch could have a normal BMI. BMI can also change in the absence of weight changes due to age-related loss of height, for instance. While not its primary purpose, the most notable limitation to BMI's utility relates to the fact that it provides no information on body fat *distribution*.

Waist-Hip Ratio

With general obesity casting such a large shadow over perceptions and understandings around fat, the more nuanced observation that body fat distribution plays a more important role in determining health outcomes than overall fat mass has occurred relatively late in the history of medicine. The earliest scientific articles outlining rudimentary techniques to measure specific fat pads to explore the relationship between body fat distribution and health were published during the 1910s (*Die Dicke des Fettpolsters bei gesunden und kranken Kindern*[16] or 'The thickness of the fat pad in healthy and sick children'). This body of literature developed slowly over the following few decades with contributions made by German, French, Italian, Russian, American, and British researchers. It wasn't until the 1940s and 1950s, however, that this fledgling field received a much-needed boost with the publication of two seminal papers by the eminent French physician Dr Jean Vague.

In arguably the clearest account of the time, Dr Vague attempted to formally delineate the different body fat distribution patterns typical of men and women by offering a standardized approach to their measurement using callipers (a pinching device). He also popularized the terms *android* and *gynoid* to describe the distinct patterns of fat distribution exhibited by men and women, respectively.[17] More importantly, he provided compelling evidence that android fat patterning (i.e., preferential upper body fat accumulation) was associated with an increased incidence of type 2 diabetes and atherosclerosis, whereas these diseases were significantly less common in individuals exhibiting lower body fat accumulation (i.e., gynoid).[18]

Early studies used callipers to measure the thickness of skinfolds at specific locations on the body to obtain information on regional fat mass. At their crudest, these simple tools were used to measure the thickness of the 'spare tyre' around one's stomach, the 'bingo wings' hanging from one's arm, and various other anatomical locations. In an ambitious attempt to use these data, Dr Vague proposed a formula that used these skinfold measurements to generate a single numerical value (an 'index of masculine differentiation') which reflected the extent of upper body fat accumulation in an individual.[18] While Dr Vague's work and publications would nonetheless lay the groundwork and direction of health-focused anthropometry, his formula did not catch on due to its unwelcoming complexity and the practical difficulties associated with using callipers to obtain reliable and reproducible data.

Just as the health implications of central obesity were starting to manifest after the end of World War II, it became clear that the techniques available for studying body fat distribution were inadequate, similar to the circumstances that drove the development of BMI for estimating relative fat mass. Pressure was building in the 1950s to develop a simple, accurate, and practical measure of body fat distribution, but the silence wouldn't be broken until the early 1980s with the publication of an article concluding that waist-hip ratio (WHR) represented the most useful measure of body fat distribution[19] out of a number of novel 'body girth ratios.' WHR's utility was solidified in 1983 in a study which reported that men and women with a preponderance of upper body fat accumulation tended to have worse metabolic health.[20] From these promising early studies, WHR not only vindicated the evidence gathered during the first half of the twentieth century, it also established itself as the simple, practical, and effective measure of body fat distribution that the scientific and clinical communities had been looking for. And it didn't take long for WHR to be rolled out in large-scale investigations.[21]

Waist-hip ratio is very simple to obtain. The standardized method for measuring the body circumferences used in the WHR formula outlined by the World Health Organization (WHO)[22] involves wrapping a tape measure around the narrowest part of your waist (just above the navel) and then around the widest part of your buttocks for the hips (Figure 5.2). To calculate WHR, divide the waist circumference (in centimetres) by the hip circumference (in centimetres). The number generated by the WHR calculation is often used to represent the extent of abdominal fat accumulation. As the typical shape of a man and woman is different, the WHO has designated sex-specific WHR cut-offs; men whose WHR >0.9 are defined as centrally obese whereas for women the cut-off is WHR >0.85. Similar to the historical development of the BMI, these cut-offs were devised using data collected from primarily European and North American populations; it should be unsurprising that ethnicity-specific WHR cut-offs have been proposed.[23] Waist circumference can also be used in isolation, with central obesity in Europeans being defined as >102cm/40in in men and >88cm/35in in women.[23]

Compared to BMI, WHR is a far less controversial anthropometric index. Having proven to be highly useful in clinical, epidemiological, and scientific settings, body circumferences and WHR do have limitations, although none as serious as those plaguing BMI. The main issue relates to

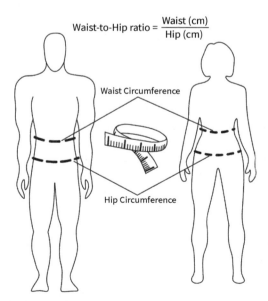

Figure 5.2 Calculation of waist-to-hip ratio.

the fact that body circumferences not only reflect fat mass, but also the underlying bone structures and lean mass (i.e., muscle and visceral organs). However, this might not be such a big issue, as studies involving waist and hip circumferences have provided such compelling evidence that body shape (underpinned by fat distribution) is a strong indicator of health outcomes that different, more sensitive ways of measuring regional fat mass are now required to advance our understanding. While the tape measure and scales will undoubtedly always have their place, technological advances have provided several powerful methods that can measure body composition precisely and capture the spatial distribution of adipose, lean, and bone tissue.[24] These include dual-energy X-ray absorptiometry, computed tomography, magnetic resonance imaging, and bioelectrical impedance analysis.

Dual-Energy X-Ray Absorptiometry

Dual-energy X-ray absorptiometry (DXA) is a prime example of a technology that was developed and refined for one purpose which later proved to be useful for something completely different as well. Originally designed to measure bone mineral density (BMD), DXA is primarily used in the clinical diagnosis and monitoring of osteoporosis, the disease in which bones become weaker and can break more easily.[25] John Cameron and James Sorenson originally invented single-photon absorptiometry and refined the method during the 1960s.[26] The more advanced second incarnation of this technique, which utilized a different radioactive material that emitted X-rays at two energy levels (hence *dual*-photon/energy X-ray absorptiometry) was developed during the 1970s[27] and became available for clinical use in the following decade.

The first report of DXA being used to measure body composition involving the quantification of fat and fat-free mass was published in 1981.[28] Great strides have since been made to optimize the capturing and processing of images to enhance the accuracy, precision, and clinical utility of this imaging technique.[29,30] DXA has proven to be a very convenient, relatively cheap, and versatile research tool that is safe for almost anyone, with pregnant women being the most notable exception. The dose of radiation involved in a DXA scan is almost negligible, with one scan involving exposure equivalent to approximately three hours of natural background radiation.[31]

Having a DXA scan is a lot like being photocopied; the patient lies still on the scanner bed for about 10–15 minutes while a mechanical arm beaming X-rays moves across their body (Figure 5.3). DXA utilizes the basic principle that different types of body tissue absorb X-ray energy at different rates. Imagine a beam of X-rays as a jet of water that would blow straight through a sandcastle (e.g., soft tissue), but reflect away from the pole of a sun umbrella (e.g., hard tissue) that the sandcastle was built around. Upon determining the absorption of X-rays at each scanning position, it is possible to discriminate between bone, fat, and lean tissue, as well as determine their regional masses.[32] Once all of these data are crunched, a detailed three-dimensional image of a person's body and its composition is obtained.

Dual-energy X-ray absorptiometry can accurately measure body composition and regional fat mass across a range of body shapes and sizes in a highly reproducible manner.[33] As effective as it is though, DXA isn't perfect. The primary limitation of DXA concerns the fact that, although it can discern fat from other types of tissue (i.e., bone and visceral organs), it is unable to directly discriminate between different types of fat. This means that DXA cannot, for example, directly differentiate subcutaneous from visceral fat in the abdomen, nor can it accurately identify brown fat. Fortunately a work-around (validated against computed tomography (CT) data; see below) exists in the form of sophisticated algorithms that can predict visceral fat mass from standard DXA images,[34,35] thus enhancing the utility of this already valuable technique. The other main issue afflicting DXA, and all imaging techniques, is the capacity of the equipment to accommodate individuals of a larger frame and/or shape. Some individuals can simply be too large (be they tall or corpulent) to fit on the scanning area of the bed. While

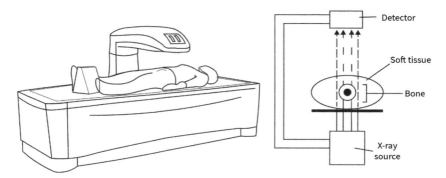

Figure 5.3 Dual X-ray absorptiometry.

it is possible to shepherd such bodies onto the bed and do a half-scan, such data are inherently sub-optimal. Although these practical issues might only affect a small number of study participants, they do have to be considered by scientists and clinicians. In sum, DXA is very useful for measuring body composition and regional fat mass, but it can't directly discern between different types of fat; its bigger brother, CT, however, can.

Computed Tomography

Computed tomography (CT) is a powerful technique that uses similar principles to DXA scanning, albeit with much higher doses of radiation, to accurately measure both body composition and fat distribution. CT scans involve measuring the absorption of X-rays projected from different angles at specific levels on an individual's body (Figure 5.4). Computer software then processes this information to produce high-resolution, two-dimensional cross-sections ('slices') from which different types of tissue can be discerned with exquisite sensitivity[36]; three-dimensional tissue volumes can be calculated from multiple slices. CT has blossomed over time from a primitive technique developed in the 1940s[37] to a technological tour de force used to diagnose and monitor cancer. As this particular use of CT scanning became established, it quickly became clear that unlocking this technology's potential would require maximizing its ability to discriminate between different types of tissue in the healthy and diseased state.

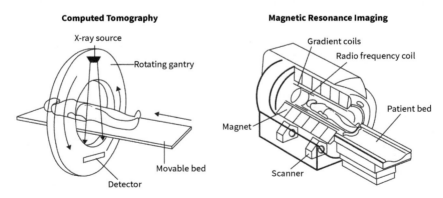

Figure 5.4 Computed tomography and magnetic resonance imaging.

The modern CT scanner was actually invented by two scientists working independently on opposite sides of the Atlantic Ocean.[38] Godfrey Hounsfield, a British engineer working for Electrical and Musical Industries (EMI) laboratories in England, and Allan Cormack, a South African-born physicist based at Tufts University in the US, both separately produced the first CT scanners in 1972. Installation of the first machines, which were originally designed for scanning the head only, occurred between 1974 and 1976, with systems capable of scanning the whole body becoming available in the latter year. Advances in scanning technique and image interpretation meant that CT was achieving its intended goal of reliably discriminating fat from cancerous masses by the late 1970s.[39] Soon after this milestone was reached, it was possible to accurately distinguish fatty tumours (i.e., lipomas) from normal adipose tissue[40]; this is a bit like being able to locate individual pieces of rotten fruit nestled within a pile of fresh produce just by looking at it.

Repurposing the wealth of knowledge and expertise used to identify fat while detecting cancer, CT scanning has been used since the 1980s to accurately distinguish subcutaneous and visceral fat in the abdomen.[41] CT scanning has since established itself as the gold-standard imaging technique for the study of body fat distribution. Commonly used to quantify abdominal subcutaneous and visceral fat,[42] this technique has also proven highly useful in the investigation of the relationship between ectopic fat accumulation (notably in the liver[43] as well as skeletal and cardiac muscle[44]) and health outcomes. The source of CT's strength is, however, also its weakness. The high-resolution images for which it is famed are obtained at the expense of exposing individuals to a significant dose of radiation. Compared to a DXA scan which involves exposure to around three hours of natural background radiation, a single CT scan exposes an individual to approximately three *years* of background radiation.[31] CT scanning is therefore unsuitable for pregnant women and growing children, as well as studies involving a series of measurements. Reports that lower radiation doses can be used to accurately measure abdominal fat from a single slice[45] have helped renew interest in CT scanning, but this technique remains somewhat limited by its very power, especially in the research setting. Stuck between DXA not being powerful enough and CT being too strong, researchers and clinicians with a penchant for studying visceral fat who want to peer inside your body with a high degree of accuracy can do so safely in the realm of magnetic resonance imaging.

Magnetic Resonance Imaging

More commonly associated with the heart and brain, magnetic resonance imaging (MRI) has proven highly useful in the study of body composition and regional fat distribution. MRI uses strong magnetic fields, electric field gradients, and radio waves to generate images in which different tissue types are distinguished based on their unique magnetic resonance properties.[46] Akin to CT scanning, MRI involves the generation of single or multiple two-dimensional slices at specific levels on an individual's body which highly advanced software then processes to determine body composition and regional fat mass (Figure 5.4). As ionizing radiation is not utilized, MRI is safe to use in vulnerable populations and longitudinal studies involving serial measurements.

The groundwork for MRI was laid in 1946 when the Swiss-American physicist Felix Bloch and the American physicist Edward Purcell independently discovered the phenomenon of magnetic resonance; they would later share the Nobel Prize in 1952 for their work. MRI was used solely for chemical and physical analysis of non-living materials until the 1970s, when the American physician Raymond Damadian showed that MRI could be used to study the human body too. Damadian's landmark 1971 study used MRI to illustrate differences in the nuclear resonance properties of healthy and cancerous tissue,[47] thus kick-starting the race to develop MRI and positioning it as a tool that could help unlock the secrets of the human body.

The first MRI scan of living human tissue was performed by Peter Mansfield's team in 1976 on fellow scientist Andrew Maudsley's obliging finger. Meanwhile, Damadian constructed the first full-body MRI machine— optimistically named 'Indomitable'—and performed the first full-body scan the following year, in which it took almost five hours to produce one image of his collaborator Larry Minkoff's thorax.[48] While he may have blazed the trail, however, Damadian's imaging technique never became a practically usable method and does not underpin the MR imaging that is routinely used today.

A significant collective effort involving numerous scientists over the next 20 years transformed these early MRI incarnations into the modern technological tour de force present in many hospitals today. By adapting advances in CT imaging, computer technology to generate images from MRI data was developed in 1973 by Godfrey Hounsfield (who actually went on to share the 1979 Nobel Prize in Physiology or Medicine with Allan McLeod Cormack for developing CT scanning), with a technique to rapidly capture images being reported in 1977 by Peter Mansfield. These revolutionary developments in medical imaging were recognized in 2003 with the conferral of the Nobel

Prize in Physiology or Medicine to the physicist Peter Mansfield and chemist Paul Lauterbur. Despite contributing to MRI's inception, Damadian was controversially overlooked for the Nobel Prize, for reasons yet to be explained.[49]

Magnetic resonance imaging now rivals CT scanning as an imaging technique used to study body composition and fat distribution in various health contexts, including ectopic fat accumulation in the liver, heart, pancreas, and skeletal muscle[50] as well as bone marrow fat[51] (see Chapter 4). Exploiting the unique physics involved, functional MRI (fMRI) is used to visualize and measure not only blood-flow, but also the amount of oxygen-carrying blood at a specific location within the body. Like being able to estimate the internal temperature of a house by monitoring the amount of smoke coming out of the chimney, this technique has proven instrumental in the study of healthy and diseased brains since the landmark study which reported that a reduced amount of oxygenated blood reflects a local increase in neural activity.[52] Functional MRI has played a crucial role in identifying the brain structures involved in appetite regulation and how their activity is affected by the presence or absence of food, obesity, social situations, habits, and personality traits, as well as factors such as stress.[53]

Magnetic resonance imaging is generally a very safe technique, although the very strong magnets involved do pose their own unique set of risks.[54] As one might expect, MRI is not recommended for people who have metallic objects such as cochlear implants, cardiac pacemakers, metal pins, or shrapnel within their bodies. Rigorous safety procedures are also usually enforced to minimize the risk of injury or death by magnetic objects moving at high speeds. Space within an MRI scanner is already at a premium as the wires used to generate the magnetic field required for imaging are tightly coiled, meaning the typical experience of being scanned can be claustrophobia-inducing for some, and it is not uncommon for larger individuals to get slightly stuck in MRI scanners. Evidently there are several powerful imaging technologies used in research and clinical settings to accurately measure body composition and fat distribution. In contrast to these expensive technologies whose use requires special access, however, it is possible to bring a bit of science into the home or gym at little cost.

Bioelectrical Impedance Analysis

If you're using a home body-fat analyser to monitor your slimming progress, imagine a pair of frog legs doing a victory dance when you triumphantly slip into a pair of trousers that used to be too tight. Why? Because this method of measuring body fat mass in the comfort of your own home relies on the principles of 'animal electricity'. This phenomenon was discovered in 1780 by the Italian physician, physicist, biologist, and philosopher Luigi Galvani (1737–1798) when he observed a dead frog's legs jerking around upon being zapped with static electricity from his metal scalpel.[55] The discovery that muscles contract and neurons fire by conducting electricity laid the groundwork for the field of electrophysiology, in addition to inspiring classic literature such as Mary Shelley's *Frankenstein*.

Building on the fact that different body tissues have distinct electrical properties, studies performed during the late 1950s and 1960s highlighted how it was possible to use a small, harmless electrical current to determine the volume of total water in a person's body.[56] Further development of this research culminated in the mid-1980s with the emergence of bioelectrical impedance analysis (BIA), a technique that enables the determination of body composition[57] (but not regional fat distribution). BIA has since become very popular owing to the development of relatively cheap, commercially available, portable, and simple-to-use devices that involve gripping or standing on a metallic pad with bare skin—far more pleasant and user-friendly than sticking electrodes into one's body.

As the name suggests, BIA involves measuring the electrical impedance (i.e., resistance) of a small electrical current running through body tissues to estimate total body water, which is then used to estimate fat-free mass (i.e., lean mass). Fat mass is approximated by subtracting fat-free mass from total body mass.[58] Being able to quickly, easily, and cheaply estimate body composition means that BIA represents a highly accessible way to bring some science into the home or gym. However, this technique is largely unsuitable for many research or clinical purposes[59] because it estimates body composition using a physical characteristic that can vary considerably. Indeed, factors such as dehydration, recent exercise, recent food consumption, and even the posture adopted during analysis can affect the reading.[60] To get the most out of BIA in the home or gym, be sure to standardize the measurement process and perform repeated measurements often.

Weapon of Choice

Magnetic resonance imaging, CT, and DEXA are clearly very powerful tools that can accurately measure body composition and regional fat mass.

They are not, however, interchangeable, meaning researchers need to pick the most appropriate imaging method when designing a study. For instance, examining visceral fat should ideally involve CT or MRI scanning, not DXA. Considering the wide range of shapes and sizes that people come in, it should be unsurprising that the pattern of fat distribution can vary considerably between individuals according to MRI[61] and CT scanning.[62] Our innards often don't look anything near as neat or tidy as the textbooks would have us believe, with our internal anatomy often proving more variable than our external appearance. This variation means that MRI or CT scanning results can change substantially depending on where an image is taken.[63] It's a bit like trying to determine the composition of a cake by looking at a wafer-thin slice through it; if you hit or miss a particularly large cluster of currants or clod of icing, you could get very different results.

There have been claims that single slice imaging protocols are able to accurately quantify visceral fat mass, but there is no clear consensus over which is the best anatomical landmark to use[64] (e.g., which vertebral level or distance from the navel). Such observations highlight how there is no shortcut, and that obtaining the most accurate measurement of regional fat mass or body composition inevitably entails using multi-slice imaging protocols. Thinking of our cake again, we'd get a far more accurate idea of how much icing or currants it contains by looking at multiple slices rather than pinning all our hopes on a single slice (Figure 5.5). While multi-slice protocols are certainly more expensive, they provide better quality data and are preferred for the construction of large datasets like the UK Biobank[65] which will contain detailed data on nearly 500,000 people when complete. The imaging technologies available are providing a mind-boggling amount of detail and information that was almost inconceivable even a handful of years ago. So, what has been found using these imaging and anthropometric techniques?

Part 2—What Are You Made Of? How Body Composition Relates to Health

The Weight of the World

Body mass index has been used in epidemiological studies for many decades and has proven to be a highly effective predictor of health outcomes despite its mathematical shortcomings. The simplicity of BMI means that it has been possible to easily gather huge quantities of data relatively cheaply.

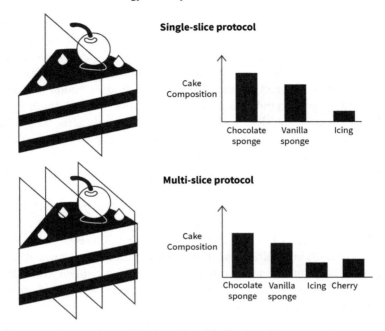

Figure 5.5 Comparison of single and multi-slice imaging protocols.

This is exemplified in a recent meta-analysis of data from 239 studies in which ten million participants from four continents (Asia, Australia and New Zealand, Europe, and North America) were followed for ~13 years. After crunching statistics for this colossal dataset, the results were strikingly clear; overweight (BMI 25–30kg/m^2) and obesity (BMI >30kg/m^2) were strongly associated with an increased risk of all-cause mortality (i.e., premature death).[66]

Breaking things down, increased BMI was associated with higher rates of death due to coronary heart disease, stroke, respiratory disease, and various cancers. It is important to note that this meta-analysis used universal BMI cut-offs which 'should' be lower for certain ethnicities[14] (particularly Asians), meaning the death rates for certain populations may actually be higher, thereby strengthening these already striking associations. Note that the death rates for these aforementioned diseases were also higher for individuals at the very bottom end of the scale (i.e., underweight, BMI <18.5kg/m^2) compared to people of normal weight (BMI 20–25kg/m^2). This finding is likely underpinned by the underweight BMI category capturing people who are predisposed or are already ill due to malnourishment, an eating disorder (e.g., anorexia and bulimia), or wasting syndromes related to cancer or HIV/AIDS, for example.

Other large-scale studies add weight to this already compelling case and indicate that a larger BMI is associated with increased risk of developing type 2 diabetes,[67] cardiovascular disease,[68] or both[69] in men and women alike. Although studies like this can't tell us *why* a greater BMI is associated with an increased risk of developing disease and/or premature death, the results from another type of study suggest that BMI plays a causal role and is not an innocent bystander. *Mendelian randomization studies* use the information generated in genome-wide association studies (GWAS) which have identified specific genetic variants associated with traits such as BMI. Noting that the same trait may be associated with altered disease risk, the GWAS data can be used to examine whether people carrying more of the genetic variants associated with the trait have an altered disease risk. If they do, this suggests that the trait plays a causal role in altering their risk of disease development.[70] Imagine a number of genes are associated with being tall and that being tall is associated with an increased risk of banging one's head. If people are grouped according to how many 'tall genes' they are carrying, we would likely see that those with the most 'tall genes' would bang their head the most; these people would probably also be the tallest too. In this case, it can be inferred that the 'tall genes' *cause* the tallness that is associated with an increased risk of banging one's head.

Mendelian randomization studies have been used to examine the relationship between BMI and metabolic and cardiovascular disease. Current results indicate that the risk of developing type 2 diabetes or coronary heart disease, heart failure, and stroke[71] is highest in individuals carrying the most genetic variants associated with increased BMI.[72] This means that it can be reasonably inferred that increased BMI plays a causal role in promoting the development of these diseases. However, we know that BMI only provides a crude estimate of body composition. So, what is actually driving this association? Is fat or lean mass more important? To obtain an answer, we have to use something more advanced than a set of scales and a tape measure.

Distorted Reflections

Body mass index is principally used as an index of relative fatness, so it is reassuring that BMI correlates strongly with fat mass percentage—as determined by DXA scanning—in children[73] and adults.[74] However, the strength of these correlations varies by sex, age, and ethnicity.[75] This is problematic if we want to use BMI to reliably determine whether an individual is overweight or obese. To determine how good BMI is at identifying obesity, there have been studies that compare whether people get the same classification according to BMI and body fat percentage, the latter being a more detailed measure which takes overall body frame into account. Defining obesity as BMI >30kg/m^2 or >30% body fat for women and >25% body fat for men, it has been reported that only ~50% of adults[76] and ~70% of children[77] were given the same label from each method.

These results tell us that BMI is a rather poor measure of relative weight/fatness that incorrectly classifies ~50% of adults and ~30% of children as healthy when they are actually carrying excess body fat (relative to their frame) and thus are at increased risk of developing metabolic and cardiovascular disease. To use the technical jargon, these data indicate that BMI is *specific* as it correctly identifies people who are a healthy weight as being a healthy weight most of the time (i.e., 'true positive'). However, it is not very *sensitive* as it miscategorizes many people who are overweight or obese as normal (i.e., 'true negative'). As BMI has been used as the world's primary index of fatness, its use may have painted a misleadingly rosier picture of reality, which is a worrying prospect to say the least. But what underpins the relationship between BMI and an increased risk of disease and premature death?

To answer this question, we need to look at how the size of specific body compartments correlate with disease and death. Take the most obvious culprit; fat. DXA-derived body composition data provide a clear message that increased fat mass percentage is strongly associated with a greater risk of developing type 2 diabetes[78] and premature death.[79] While not mind-blowing, these data provide the crystal-clear message that carrying more fat, particularly excessive amounts, is bad for your health. But how much is too much?

Drawing a Line

When attempting to delineate *excessive* from *normal*, it is important to remember that the primary aim of the work which culminated in the (re-) discovery of BMI was to devise a measure of *relative* weight. It is well-appreciated that BMI has serious limitations, but this is far from a wholly negative thing. Indeed, the realization that BMI has poor sensitivity (i.e., it fails to identify many obese people as such) and the fact that there is a wide range of fat mass percentages at any given BMI have been turned to our advantage in the quest to find what constitutes a healthy body composition.

Part of the puzzle that can help define where the 'excessive' boundary rests pertains to the discovery during the 1980s of individuals who are classified as having a normal BMI but are 'metabolically obese.'[80] As the name suggests, these are people with a normal BMI who exhibit the metabolic characteristics akin to an obese person at increased risk of developing metabolic and/or cardiovascular disease (e.g., raised fasting insulin and triglyceride levels coupled with insulin resistance[81]). Detailed examination of these individuals has highlighted that they carry significantly more fat than their metabolically normal counterparts,[82] are more likely to develop type 2 diabetes[83] and heart disease,[84] and are at increased risk of dying prematurely[85] despite falling in the normal BMI category. A meta-analysis of studies using largely similar criteria estimated that the global prevalence of 'metabolically obese, normal weight' stands at a staggering 20%.[86] Evidently the current BMI-centric approach is inadequate and the current definition of obesity needs to be overhauled to emphasize the importance of excess body fat relative to overall body mass in relation to health.[87] However, this approach runs the risk of overlooking the crucial role that *lean mass* plays in determining our health.

Lean on Me

Lean mass refers to everything in your body that isn't fat, which therefore includes muscle, visceral organs, body water, and skin (bone mass is typically excluded). Understanding the relationship between lean mass and health outcomes has been a priority in the field of geriatric medicine due to the phenomenon of age-related wasting, meaning the majority of the literature focuses on older populations. The results from many large-scale studies of body composition using DXA provide the robust and consistent message that increased lean mass is associated with reduced rates of all-cause mortality in elderly Asians,[88] Europeans,[89] and Americans[90], with this association holding throughout adulthood.[91] It follows that lean mass is also negatively associated with the risk of developing type 2 diabetes.[92] Thinking of lean mass as roughly the reciprocal of fat mass and identifying that it has an opposite association with health outcomes is not exactly mind-blowing.

However, such compelling data highlight the need to re-evaluate the definition of obesity and health in terms of overall body composition and move away from focusing on relative fatness in isolation.

A concept that has emerged from this more holistic way of thinking pertains to 'sarcopenic obesity' (sarcopenia is the process of skeletal muscle wastage typically associated with aging). This term primarily concerns individuals who have low amounts of lean mass in conjunction with an excessive amount of fat relative to their frame, a bit like a sausage that looks fine from the outside, but actually contains a surprisingly high amount of fat and gristle on the inside. Individuals who fit this bill have been referred to as 'thin outside, fat inside.'[93] Such individuals tend to have the worst (metabolic) health prospects,[94] with premature death occurring far more frequently in sarcopenic obese individuals[95] amongst the older population, particularly men.[96] This association holds throughout adulthood, with individuals who carry the least amount of fat in conjunction with the highest amounts of lean mass experiencing the lowest risk of all-cause mortality.[97] Being a gristly sausage is not good for one's health!

Although lean mass undoubtedly plays a crucial role in determining our health, having a large amount is not necessarily a ticket to a disease-free life; you have to actually be fit and strong to reap the health benefits conferred by a larger muscle mass.[98] Indeed, the substantial risk of developing type 2 diabetes at high BMI is increased further when it occurs in conjunction with muscle weakness[99] (assessed via hand-grip strength). Strength training confers wide-ranging health benefits, reducing rates of premature death, cancer, and cardiovascular disease.[100] The fact that the current generation of children is weaker and less fit than previous generations[101] is particularly alarming. With a mounting body of compelling evidence indicating that cardiorespiratory fitness is another crucial factor which determines overall health,[102,103] public health may continue to deteriorate due to ever-decreasing levels of physical activity and declining fitness levels, despite stabilizing obesity rates.[104] Sitting still for too long is bad for your health, even if your figure suggests otherwise!

Too Good to Be True

Without diminishing the clear message that the data convey about how body composition relates to health, a significant number of individuals complicate the somewhat neat narrative that a normal weight is necessary to be healthy. That complication comes in the controversial form of 'metabolically healthy obesity' (MHO), a phenomenon characterized by people who carry excessive amounts of fat relative to their frame in the apparent absence of metabolic or cardiovascular disease.[105] Proponents of this phenomenon argue that some people can elude the health-related pitfalls of obesity, but over-emphasizing the frequency of this situation runs the risk of fatally undermining the prevailing public health message that you can't be obese and healthy, that you can't have your cake and eat it too. With the stakes being so high, it's important to tread carefully. So, does MHO actually exist?

There is no easy answer to this question given that over 30 different definitions have been used to identify MHO, resulting in prevalence rates varying widely between 3% and 43%.[106] The US apparently hosts far more MHO individuals than Europe,[86] meaning there are a large number of people whose bodies can carry an excessive amount of fat while somehow retaining apparently good metabolic health (e.g., as assessed by insulin sensitivity[107]). Whether or not insulin-sensitive obese individuals exist is not the major issue, however (they do[108]). Instead, the primary concern is whether MHO is benign and if MHO individuals remain healthy over the long-term.[109] In other words, can you be obese and healthy?

The simple answer is a resounding *no*, with the evidence increasingly suggesting that despite the existence of MHO individuals, obesity and good health are highly unlikely to co-exist. While MHO and its definition (particularly with respect to body composition) require further study, an extensive meta-analysis has clearly demonstrated that although a large proportion of the obese population may be metabolically healthy at the time of examination, MHO people are still at greatly increased risk of developing metabolic and cardiovascular disease over the long-term.[110,111] When and how the various obesity-related diseases manifest likely depends on the duration and extent of prevailing obesity. It would not be inappropriate to think of MHO individuals as smokers who have not developed lung cancer, but whose risk continues to creep up every moment they continue smoking.

While it may be possible to technically identify individuals who have metabolically benign obesity at the time of measurement, there are *no* subgroups of overweight/obese individuals who are *less* at risk of dying from cardiovascular disease compared to their normal weight counterparts over the long-term[112]; all are at increased risk instead. Consistent with this, the risk of carotid atherosclerosis, a key risk factor for having a heart attack, was reported to be highest in obese individuals in a study compared to normal weight people despite *every* participant in the study being deemed meta-bolically healthy at the outset.[113] In similar studies using clearly defined groups of metabolically healthy people, overweight and obesity were ro-bustly associated with an increased risk of developing type 2 diabetes[114] and non-alcoholic fatty liver disease.[115] MHO doesn't protect against the devel-opment of various cancers either.[116] The evidence keeps mounting and it paints a damning picture. It seems extremely unlikely that you can be obese and healthy,[117] and a good doctor is unlikely to tell you otherwise.

As compelling as the data are, the same problem that loomed large at the start of this chapter hangs over this controversial topic area as well. The investigation of MHO has been hampered by the fact that BMI has been used to categorize people as normal weight, overweight, or obese. While a number of people who are obese according to BMI can be metabolically healthy at the time of examination, this state offers no protection against developing various diseases over the long-term. There may be a spectrum of physiological 'resilience' in which certain bodies can apparently handle the immense metabolic strain imposed by obesity better than others for a temporary, ill-defined period. This 'protection' is merely illusory though, because being overweight or obese inevitably catches up with the vast ma-jority of people's health. If anything, MHO is a disingenuous concept that may lull people into a false sense of security about their health.[118] Moving forward from here, data gathered over decades indicates that *where* an indi-vidual carries their fat, rather than *how much* they have, plays the important role in influencing an individual's disease risk.

Part 3—The Shape of Things to Come: How Body Fat Distribution Relates to Health

Waisted

The general message is simple; upper body fat accumulation is associated with a significantly increased risk of disease and premature death in men and women of many different ethnicities. A meta-analysis comprising in-formation on over 650,000 people clearly showed that a larger waist circum-ference was strongly associated with a higher rate of all-cause mortality in Caucasian men and women from America and Europe across the BMI spec-trum[119]; this association has also been observed in African Americans[120] and Asians.[121] So what? Surely waist circumference just reflects general obesity and identifies the same individuals who are already obese and likely to get sick or die early anyway? Not quite. In a number of head-to-head comparisons, measures of upper body fat accumulation (i.e., waist circumference or WHR) have been repeatedly found to be much more strongly associated with the risk of premature death and disease than BMI, as illustrated in another meta-analysis examining data on over 406,000 people from Europe, Asia, and the US. When evaluating the effect of a comparable increase in overall fatness or upper body fat accumulation on the risk of having a fatal heart attack, a five-unit increase in BMI was associated with a 16% increase in risk whereas a 0.1-unit increase in WHR was associated with an 82% increase in risk.[122] In other words, the expansion of one's waist is associated with a far greater risk of having a heart attack than the underlying increase in overall body weight or BMI would otherwise suggest. Watch your waistline!

Upper body fat accumulation is also associated with an increased risk of developing cardiovascular and metabolic disease, specifically type 2 diabetes.[123] A meta-analysis of over 259,200 people of various ethnicities reported that a universal waist circumference cut-off of >102cm for men or >88cm for women was a better predictor of type 2 diabetes risk compared to obesity (defined by BMI >30kg/m^2).[124] Several other hefty reports indicate that abdominal obesity is associated with an increased risk of developing lung[125] and colorectal cancer.[126] A wardrobe full of XL-sized clothes indicates that XL-sized medical problems are likely lurking under the surface, with the extent that one's gut protrudes possibly reflecting the degree of damage.

Just as excessive fatness (according to BMI) is not an innocent bystander in the slow-motion wreckage of one's health that is obesity, Mendelian randomization studies have provided convincing evidence that central obesity plays a causal role in increasing the risk of getting sick or dying prematurely. By using genetic markers associated with body fat distribution, it has been found that individuals who have a greater genetic predisposition to upper body fat accumulation are at increased risk of developing type 2 diabetes and coronary heart disease[127] as well as having a stroke.[128] Perhaps surreptitiously casting a discriminating eye over your relatives' figures may provide some useful information about whether big bellies run in the family and if the biological cards are potentially stacked in your favour, as well as how much work may be required to offset the risk.

Evidently this information has implications that strike deep into our clinical and scientific understanding of the relationship between fat and health. The prevailing message that obesity puts one's health at serious risk absolutely still stands. However, looking at a rough index of fatness in isolation is suboptimal when trying to determine the risk of someone getting sick, sicker, or dying. Possible solutions will likely involve using a combination of anthropometric indices[129] that assess relative fatness and body fat distribution while accounting for sex, age, and ethnicity.[130] Evidently there is plenty of room to hone our ability to reliably and accurately predict the health prospects of anyone that may walk into a doctor's office.

These data also mean that many overweight and obese individuals may find that their health outlook is actually worse than they might have thought. This is because the vast majority may not be 'just' obese, but are actually *centrally* obese, with the attendant risks to their health being greater than previously appreciated. In addition, many non-obese people previously thought to be low risk might now find themselves having to re-evaluate their health situation. For instance, a study including over 170,000 people of normal BMI ($18.5–24.9 kg/m^2$) and waist circumference (<90cm in men or <80 cm in women) found that even in this group of otherwise healthy people, a larger waist circumference was associated with a greater prevalence of metabolic disturbances[131] in men and women, although the increased risk was smaller compared to increased waist circumference in conjunction with an overweight or obese BMI.[123] We should all keep a watchful eye on our waistline (and physical fitness levels), whatever size or shape we may be.

The Hips of Health

It's not all bad news though. Lower body fat accumulation, independent of overall fatness, *protects* against the development of metabolic and cardiovascular disease in men and women. This phenomenon was most clearly demonstrated in the INTERHEART study of over 27,000 individuals from 52 countries representing several major ethnicities. After confirming that abdominal obesity was associated with worse cardiovascular health, the authors made the remarkable discovery that the risk of having a heart attack actually *decreased* with increasing hip circumference, independently of BMI.[132] So, a peachy bum and shapely legs may be more than just easy on the eye to some; they might also be guardians of heart health!

Several other large-scale studies have replicated and confirmed the observation that lower body fat accumulation has a beneficial (or at least neutral) relationship with metabolic and cardiovascular health. Increased hip circumference has been associated with a reduced risk of coronary heart disease in the European Prospective Investigation into Cancer and Nutrition (EPIC) study of over 24,500 people,[133] while the Netherlands-based Hoorn study reported that increased hip and thigh circumference were both associated with a lower incidence of type 2 diabetes.[134] Moreover, a Mendelian randomization study using data from over 164,000 people in the UK Biobank indicated that lower body fat plays a causal role in protecting against the development of coronary heart disease and type 2 diabetes.[135] The quest for the best answer to the eternally vexing 'does my bum look big in this?' just got harder!

Although the associations between waist and hip circumference with health outcomes are convincing and robust, what body compartment is actually driving these relationships? Note that body circumferences are only crude measures of regional fat mass; waist and hip circumference reflect not only fat mass, but also muscle, internal organs, and bone structures. So, what makes abdominal obesity so unhealthy? And what is special about lower body fat that enables it to protect against metabolic and cardiovascular disease? To answer such questions, we need to examine body composition and regional fat mass data collected using the various sophisticated imaging techniques outlined earlier.

Compartmentalizing the Issue

Due to the strong association between upper body fat accumulation and poor health outcomes, abdominal obesity has been subject to intense scrutiny. Recall that there are two main types of fat within the abdomen, namely subcutaneous (under the skin) and visceral (surrounding the organs). Current data indicate that visceral fat is much more strongly correlated to the risk of developing metabolic and cardiovascular disease than its subcutaneous counterpart, although the relationship is complex. Moreover, discerning these types of fat requires imaging technology as waist circumference does not specifically reflect visceral fat mass; waist circumference actually correlates better with overall and subcutaneous fat mass, albeit in an age-, sex-, and ethnicity-specific manner.[136] Analysis of abdominal CT scans from over 32,500 people highlighted that increased *visceral* fat mass area was strongly associated with a *greater* risk of sudden death, whereas a greater *subcutaneous* fat mass area was associated with a *lower* risk of all-cause mortality.[137] Similar results were found upon analysis of DXA data from the Oxford Biobank in which accumulation of subcutaneous fat—particularly in the lower body, but also in the abdomen—was associated with a significantly lower risk of developing metabolic disturbances in men and women.[138]

The latter study also noted that greater visceral fat accumulation, irrespective of total fatness, is strongly associated with a higher incidence of insulin resistance and hypertension. These DXA-derived measures of regional fat mass exhibited substantially stronger associations than the corresponding body circumference. A larger visceral fat mass is associated with a greater incidence of fat accumulation in the liver whereas a larger subcutaneous fat mass protects against this.[139] The different types of abdominal fat are also associated with opposing outcomes in the context of cancer; gastrointestinal, respiratory, and renal cancer patients with proportionally more subcutaneous abdominal fat reportedly survive the longest,[140] while increased visceral fat mass is associated with worse survival rates for colorectal and pancreatic cancer.[141]

The plot therefore thickens—again. While the public message that 'obesity is bad for your health' is certainly not wrong, the relationship between fat and health is far more complicated than previously thought. Moving beyond the messy, potentially futile, affair of trying to clearly discern whether someone is obese or not, it has become increasingly apparent that it is important to know not just *how much* fat someone is carrying, but also *where* it is stored. These features are inextricably linked, and carrying an excessive amount of fat, especially in your upper body, is bad for your health. However, the extent of damage appears to reflect the balance between storage in subcutaneous and visceral fat; expansion of subcutaneous fat, particularly in the lower body, protects against the development of metabolic and cardiovascular disease whereas accumulation of visceral fat predicts disease and premature death.

It can be helpful to think of the relationship between fat mass and distribution with health as though it were a road network. To keep traffic flowing smoothly and safely (i.e., to achieve and maintain good health), the vast majority of cars (i.e., fatty acids) would ideally be driving on a smooth, well-lit multi-lane highway (i.e., subcutaneous fat). Some cars may travel on the dangerous, narrow backroads (i.e., visceral fat), with the risk of collisions or breakdowns increasing if more cars are diverted because of congestion or lane closure on the highway. The risk and frequency of accidents can be reduced primarily by reducing the overall number of cars on the road, followed by keeping as many cars as possible on well-maintained highways and away from the dangerous backroads.

So, how can having a big bum or tum have diametrically opposed relationships with the risk of having a heart attack or getting type 2 diabetes? Answering such a question involves again dispelling the misconception that fat is all the same—a major theme throughout this book. Ignoring the more esoteric types of fat in the body (e.g., brown adipose tissue and bone marrow fat), data gathered over decades indicate that the white fat deposits under our skin surrounding our abdomen, bum, legs, and internal organs exhibit distinct characteristics to perform discrete (evolutionarily defined) biological roles. Within this context, evidence is increasingly laying the blame for the development of metabolic and cardiovascular disease at the door of subcutaneous fat that has stopped working properly. Chapter 6 explores how the biological properties of fat tissue vary around the body so we can make sense of the associations between regional fat mass and health. However, before moving on to the nitty-gritty biology of the different fat depots, let's first consider how body composition and fat distribution vary between different groups of people in a bit more detail.

Part 4—The Cards We're Dealt: Body Composition and Fat Distribution Patterns

Men Are from Mars, Women Are from Venus

There are significant differences in the body composition and fat distribution patterns between men and women. For instance, women have ~10% greater total fat mass percentage compared to men of the same BMI throughout life, whereas men carry proportionally more lean mass[142]; this pattern transcends ethnicity and is applicable to men and women in general. The differences in body composition between men and women are also accompanied by quite obvious differences in body shape. At a comparable level of overall fatness, men and women store their fat in very different ways. Women tend to have a greater proportion of subcutaneous fat than men,[143] with this fat being located in their abdomen and particularly around the thighs[144]; this partitioning pattern gives rise to the rounded legs and buttocks that play a major role in defining the archetypal feminine shape. Women also tend to carry less visceral fat than men.[143]

These differences in body shape and composition emerge as body mass increases during puberty, with this increase being driven mainly by lean mass in boys while adipose tissue makes a larger contribution in girls (these changes also occur in an ethnicity-specific manner[145] to give rise to distinct fat distribution patterns in adults[143]). Given the striking differences in body fat distribution displayed by men and women, it should be unsurprising that some of the genetic variants associated with regional fat accumulation only have an effect in men or women; this contrasts to those associated with overall obesity which often have a comparable effect in both sexes.[146] After eventually emerging from the bubbling pubertal cauldron of hormones and genes as an adult, the conspicuous lumps and bumps that have developed not only define an individual's biological sex, but also influence their health.

According to an analysis of UK Biobank data, the prevalence of type 2 diabetes was found to be substantially higher in Caucasian, Black, South Asian, and Chinese men compared to their female counterparts.[147] While men may be more likely to develop type 2 diabetes, however, women may be particularly vulnerable to the deleterious cardiovascular effects of this disease. For instance, amongst people with type 2 diabetes, heart attacks occur at an earlier age and the survival rate is lower in women compared to men.[148] If life were a boxing match, women seem to be better able to avoid being hit than men, but if (heart) disease manages to land a punch, women's bodies fare much worse than those of men. Cardiovascular disease is amongst the leading causes of death in women, but its incidence lags about ten years behind men,[149] although this gap closes with increasing age.[150] This loss of protection against cardiovascular disease in women may be due to *menopause*, the phenomenon in which women's oestrogen levels naturally decline (see Chapter 7).

Same but Different

Humans clearly come in all shapes and sizes, with certain physical characteristics being more common in distinct ethnic groups. Large-scale ongoing efforts to more accurately quantify the body composition (i.e., fat and lean mass[151,152]) of people according to age, sex, and ethnicity (e.g., the UK Biobank) are providing crucial insights that have far-reaching implications for predicting health risks, improving patient outcomes, and lowering healthcare costs. However, we only need to look at the world of sport to see how natural history has provided members of certain ethnicities with attributes that provide an advantage on the basketball court, running track, or weightlifting arena.[153] It has been reported that Asian Indians tend to carry more fat, both overall and in the abdomen, compared to their European and Polynesian counterparts; they also tend to have less lean mass, skeletal muscle, and bone mineral.[154] Such physical features may be a contributing factor to India's pretty poor track record at the Olympics, despite having a huge population of potential sports stars from which to draw. Indeed, as of 2020, India has won a mere 28 medals in 34 Olympic tournaments, whereas Great Britain has won 883 medals over 51 tournaments and New Zealand has won 120 medals in 39 tournaments.

While much remains to be learned about the specific reasons contributing to ethnicity-specific bodily differences, data from anthropological studies suggest that decreasing annual temperature is associated with increasing BMI, meaning survival in colder environments favours larger energy stores and lean mass.[155] Additionally, ethnicity-specific differences in body fat distribution may be a response to distinct immunological challenges posed by different environments; it has been proposed that intramuscular adipose tissue in African populations reflects an adaptation to malaria which provides local fuel to muscle tissue recruited in the fever defence mechanism, whereas the preponderance for visceral adiposity (noting its inflammation-prone nature) in South Asian populations may be an adaptation to gut-borne infections that often accompany monsoon rainfall.[156] Moreover, ethnicity-specific differences can be neutralized when individuals share the same environment.[157]

Other DXA data suggest that young healthy Hispanic men carry a greater total fat mass than African American, Asian, or non-Hispanic white men, and that they also tend to carry this fat around their abdomen.[158] Compared with Whites, Black ethnic populations have a higher skeletal muscle mass and higher fat mass among women.[151] Non-Hispanic white women also tend to have the lowest total and regional fat mass compared to the increasing amounts carried by their Asian, Hispanic, and African American counterparts,[159] with African women carrying much more subcutaneous but similar amounts of visceral fat to their White counterparts.[160] The next chapter explores the biology of fat located in different parts of the body to put the relationship between overall and regional body fat mass with health outcomes in context.

References

1. Eknoyan, G. Adolphe Quetelet (1796–1874)—the average man and indices of obesity. *Nephrol. Dial. Transplant* 23, 47–51 (2008).
2. Jones, D. S., Podolsky, S. H., & Greene, J. A. The burden of disease and the changing task of medicine. *N. Engl. J. Med.* 366, 2333–8 (2012).
3. Office for National Statistics. Causes of death over 100 years. 2017.
4. Dubos, R. J. *Mirage of Health: Utopias, Progress, and Biological Change.* Rutgers University Press, 1959.
5. Omran, A. R. The epidemiologic transition: a theory of the epidemiology of population change. 1971. *Milbank Q.* 83, 731–57 (2005).
6. Association of Life Insurance Medical Directors and the Actuarial Society of America. *Medico-Actuarial Mortality Investigation. Vol.1.* (1912).
7. Eknoyan, G. A history of obesity, or how what was good became ugly and then bad. *Adv. Chronic Kidney Dis.* 13, 421–7 (2006).
8. Bray, G. A. Life insurance and overweight. *Obes. Res.* 3, 97–9 (1995).
9. Tremmel, M., Gerdtham, U.-G., Nilsson, P. M., & Saha, S. Economic burden of obesity: a systematic literature review. *Int. J. Environ. Res. Public Health* 14, 435 (2017).
10. Billewicz, W. Z., Kemsley, W. F., & Thomson, A. M. Indices of adiposity. *Br. J. Prev. Soc. Med.* 16, 183–8 (1962).
11. Khosla, T. & Lowe, C. R. Indices of obesity derived from body weight and height. *Br. J. Prev. Soc. Med.* 21, 122–8 (1967).
12. Florey, C. du V. The use and interpretation of ponderal index and other weight–height ratios in epidemiological studies. *J. Chronic Dis.* 23, 93–103 (1970).
13. Keys, A., Fidanza, F., Karvonen, M. J., Kimura, N., & Taylor, H. L. Indices of relative weight and obesity. *J. Chronic Dis.* 25, 329–43 (1972).
14. World Health Organization Expert Consultation. Appropriate body-mass index for Asian populations and its implications for policy and intervention strategies. *Lancet* 363, 157–63 (2004).
15. Taylor, R. S. Letter to the editor. *Paediatr. Child Health* 15, 258 (2010).
16. Batkin, S. Die Dicke des Fettpolsters bei gesunden und kranken Kindern. *Jahrb. f. Kinderheilk* 82, 103 (1915).
17. Vague, J. La différenciation sexuelle; facteur déterminant des formes de l'obésité. *Presse Med.* 55, 339 (1947).
18. Vague, J. The degree of masculine differentiation of obesities: a factor determining predisposition to diabetes, atherosclerosis, gout, and uric calculous disease. *Am. J. Clin. Nutr.* 4, 20–34 (1956).
19. Hartz, A. J., Rupley, D. C., Kalkhoff, R. D., & Rimm, A. A. Relationship of obesity to diabetes: influence of obesity level and body fat distribution. *Prev. Med. (Baltim).* 12, 351–7 (1983).
20. Krotkiewski, M., Björntorp, P., Sjöström, L., & Smith, U. Impact of obesity on metabolism in men and women. Importance of regional adipose tissue distribution. *J. Clin. Invest.* 72, 1150–62 (1983).

21. Larsson, B. *et al.* Abdominal adipose tissue distribution, obesity, and risk of cardiovascular disease and death: 13 year follow-up of participants in the study of men born in 1913. *Br. Med. J. (Clin. Res. Ed).* **288**, 1401–4 (1984).

22. World Health Organization. Waist circumference and waist-hip ratio: report of a WHO expert consultation. World Health Organization, 8–11 (2008). doi:10.1038/ejcn.2009.139

23. Qiao, Q. & Nyamdorj, R. The optimal cutoff values and their performance of waist circumference and waist-to-hip ratio for diagnosing type II diabetes. *Eur. J. Clin. Nutr.* **64**, 23–9 (2010).

24. Seabolt, L. A., Welch, E. B., & Silver, H. J. Imaging methods for analyzing body composition in human obesity and cardiometabolic disease. *Ann. N. Y. Acad. Sci.* **1353**, 41–59 (2015).

25. Compston, J. E., McClung, M. R., & Leslie, W. D. Osteoporosis. *Lancet* **393**, 364–76 (2019).

26. Cameron, J. R. & Sorenson, J. Measurement of bone mineral in vivo: an improved method. *Science* **142**, 230–2 (1963).

27. DePuey, E. G., Thompson, W. L., Alagarsamy, V., & Burdine, J. A. Bone mineral content determined by functional imaging. *J. Nucl. Med.* **16**, 891–5 (1975).

28. Peppler, W. W. & Mazess, R. B. Total body bone mineral and lean body mass by dual-photon absorptiometry. I. Theory and measurement procedure. *Calcif. Tissue Int.* **33**, 353–9 (1981).

29. Al-Antari, M. A. *et al.* Non-local means filter denoising for DEXA images. *Conf. Proc.... Annu. Int. Conf. IEEE Eng. Med. Biol. Soc.* **2017**, 572–5 (2017).

30. Martineau, P., Bazarjani, S., & Zuckier, L. S. Artifacts and incidental findings encountered on dual-energy X-ray absorptiometry: atlas and analysis. *Semin. Nucl. Med.* **45**, 458–69 (2015).

31. X-Ray Safety Information. www.radiologyinfo.org/en/info.cfm?pg=safety-xray#part3.

32. Toombs, R. J., Ducher, G., Shepherd, J. A., & De Souza, M. J. The impact of recent technological advances on the trueness and precision of DXA to assess body composition. *Obesity (Silver Spring)* **20**, 30–9 (2012).

33. LaForgia, J., Dollman, J., Dale, M. J., Withers, R. T., & Hill, A. M. Validation of DXA body composition estimates in obese men and women. *Obesity (Silver Spring)* **17**, 821–6 (2009).

34. Kaul, S. *et al.* Dual-energy X-ray absorptiometry for quantification of visceral fat. *Obesity (Silver Spring)* **20**, 1313–18 (2012).

35. Bosch, T. A. *et al.* Visceral adipose tissue measured by DXA correlates with measurement by CT and is associated with cardiometabolic risk factors in children. *Pediatr. Obes.* **10**, 172–9 (2015).

36. Mazonakis, M. & Damilakis, J. Computed tomography: what and how does it measure? *Eur. J. Radiol.* **85**, 1499–504 (2016).

37. Hartley, J. B. Tomography in the diagnosis of lung carcinoma. *Proc. R. Soc. Med.* **39**, 531–4 (1946).

38. Asiado, T. CT scan: computed axial tomography (CAT) scan. *Decoded* (2011).

39. Cohen, W. N., Seidelmann, F. E., & Bryan, P. J. Computed tomography of localized adipose deposits presenting as tumor masses. *Am. J. Roentgenol.* **128**, 1007–11 (1977).

40. Viamonte, M. & Viamonte, M. Radiology and pathology of fat. *Crit. Rev. Diagn. Imaging* **16**, 93–123 (1981).

41. Borkan, G. A. *et al.* Assessment of abdominal fat content by computed tomography. *Am. J. Clin. Nutr.* **36**, 172–7 (1982).

42. Lee, Y.-H., Hsiao, H.-F., Yang, H.-T., Huang, S.-Y., & Chan, W. P. Reproducibility and repeatability of computer tomography-based measurement of abdominal subcutaneous and visceral adipose tissues. *Sci. Rep.* **7**, 40389 (2017).

43. Graffy, P. M. & Pickhardt, P. J. Quantification of hepatic and visceral fat by CT and MR imaging: relevance to the obesity epidemic, metabolic syndrome and NAFLD. *Br. J. Radiol.* **89**, 20151024 (2016).

44. Eastwood, S. V *et al.* Thigh fat and muscle each contribute to excess cardiometabolic risk in South Asians, independent of visceral adipose tissue. *Obesity (Silver Spring)* **22**, 2071–9 (2014).

45. Yoon, D. Y. *et al.* Comparison of low-dose CT and MR for measurement of intra-abdominal adipose tissue: a phantom and human study. *Acad. Radiol.* **15**, 62–70 (2008).

46. Marzola, P., Boschi, F., Moneta, F., Sbarbati, A., & Zancanaro, C. Preclinical in vivo imaging for fat tissue identification, quantification, and functional characterization. *Front. Pharmacol.* **7**, 336 (2016).

47. Damadian, R. Tumor detection by nuclear magnetic resonance. *Science* **171**, 1151–3 (1971).

48. Damadian, R., Goldsmith, M., & Minkoff, L. NMR in cancer: XVI. FONAR image of the live human body. *Physiol. Chem. Phys.* **9**, 97–100, 108 (1977).

49. Macchia, R. J., Termine, J. E., & Buchen, C. D. Raymond V. Damadian, M.D.: magnetic resonance imaging and the controversy of the 2003 Nobel Prize in Physiology or Medicine. *J. Urol.* **178**, 783–5 (2007).

50. Thomas, E. L., Fitzpatrick, J. A., Malik, S. J., Taylor-Robinson, S. D., & Bell, J. D. Whole body fat: content and distribution. *Prog. Nucl. Magn. Reson. Spectrosc.* **73**, 56–80 (2013).

51. Singhal, V. & Bredella, M. A. Marrow adipose tissue imaging in humans. *Bone* (2018). doi:10.1016/j.bone.2018.01.009

52. Kwong, K. K. *et al.* Dynamic magnetic resonance imaging of human brain activity during primary sensory stimulation. *Proc. Natl. Acad. Sci. U. S. A.* **89**, 5675–9 (1992).

53. Neseliler, S., Han, J.-E., & Dagher, A. The use of functional magnetic resonance imaging in the study of appetite and obesity. In *Appetite and Food Intake: Central Control*, 2nd ed. CRC Press/Taylor & Francis, 2017.

54. Watson, R. E. Lessons learned from MRI safety events. *Curr. Radiol. Rep.* **3**, 37 (2015).

55. Piccolino, M. Animal electricity and the birth of electrophysiology: the legacy of Luigi Galvani. *Brain Res. Bull.* **46**, 381–407 (1998).

56. Chumlea, W.C. & Guo, S. S. Bioelectrical impedance: a history, research issues, and recent consensus. In *Emerging Technologies for Nutrition Research: Potential for Assessing Military Performance Capability*. National Academies Press, 1997.
57. Kushner, R. F. & Schoeller, D. A. Estimation of total body water by bioelectrical impedance analysis. *Am. J. Clin. Nutr.* 44, 417–24 (1986).
58. Kyle, U. G. *et al.* Bioelectrical impedance analysis--part I: review of principles and methods. *Clin. Nutr.* 23, 1226–43 (2004).
59. Johnson Stoklossa, C. A., Forhan, M., Padwal, R. S., Gonzalez, M. C., & Prado, C. M. Practical considerations for body composition assessment of adults with class II/III obesity using bioelectrical impedance analysis or dual-energy X-ray absorptiometry. *Curr. Obes. Rep.* 5, 389–96 (2016).
60. Kushner, R. F., Gudivaka, R., & Schoeller, D. A. Clinical characteristics influencing bioelectrical impedance analysis measurements. *Am. J. Clin. Nutr.* 64, 423S–427S (1996).
61. Thomas, E. L. & Bell, J. D. Influence of undersampling on magnetic resonance imaging measurements of intra-abdominal adipose tissue. *Int. J. Obes. Relat. Metab. Disord.* 27, 211–18 (2003).
62. Greenfield, J. R., Samaras, K., Chisholm, D. J., & Campbell, L. V. Regional intra-subject variability in abdominal adiposity limits usefulness of computed tomography. *Obes. Res.* 10, 260–5 (2002).
63. So, R. *et al.* Visceral adipose tissue volume estimated at imaging sites 5–6 cm above L4–L5 is optimal for predicting cardiovascular risk factors in obese Japanese men. *Tohoku J. Exp. Med.* 227, 297–305 (2012).
64. Shen, W. *et al.* A single MRI slice does not accurately predict visceral and subcutaneous adipose tissue changes during weight loss. *Obesity (Silver Spring)* 20, 2458–63 (2012).
65. Sudlow, C. *et al.* UK biobank: an open access resource for identifying the causes of a wide range of complex diseases of middle and old age. *PLoS Med.* 12, e1001779 (2015).
66. Global BMI Mortality Collaboration *et al.* Body-mass index and all-cause mortality: individual-participant-data meta-analysis of 239 prospective studies in four continents. *Lancet* 388, 776–86 (2016).
67. Abdullah, A., Peeters, A., de Courten, M., & Stoelwinder, J. The magnitude of association between overweight and obesity and the risk of diabetes: a meta-analysis of prospective cohort studies. *Diabetes Res. Clin. Pract.* 89, 309–19 (2010).
68. Mongraw-Chaffin, M. L., Peters, S. A. E., Huxley, R. R., & Woodward, M. The sex-specific association between BMI and coronary heart disease: a systematic review and meta-analysis of 95 cohorts with 1.2 million participants. *Lancet Diabetes Endocrinol* 3, 437–49 (2015).
69. Kivimäki, M. *et al.* Overweight, obesity, and risk of cardiometabolic multimorbidity: pooled analysis of individual-level data for 120,813 adults from 16 cohort studies from the USA and Europe. *Lancet Public Heal.* 2, e277–e285 (2017).

70. Bennett, D. A. & Holmes, M. V. Mendelian randomisation in cardiovascular research: an introduction for clinicians. *Heart* **103**, 1400–7 (2017).

71. Hägg, S. *et al.* Adiposity as a cause of cardiovascular disease: a Mendelian randomization study. *Int. J. Epidemiol.* **44**, 578–86 (2015).

72. Corbin, L. J. *et al.* BMI as a modifiable risk factor for type 2 diabetes: refining and understanding causal estimates using Mendelian randomization. *Diabetes* **65**, 3002–7 (2016).

73. Martin-Calvo, N., Moreno-Galarraga, L., & Martinez-Gonzalez, M. A. Association between body mass index, waist-to-height ratio and adiposity in children: a systematic review and meta-analysis. *Nutrients* **8**, (2016).

74. Flegal, K. M. *et al.* Comparisons of percentage body fat, body mass index, waist circumference, and waist-stature ratio in adults. *Am. J. Clin. Nutr.* **89**, 500–8 (2009).

75. Heymsfield, S. B., Peterson, C. M., Thomas, D. M., Heo, M., & Schuna, J. M. Why are there race/ethnic differences in adult body mass index-adiposity relationships? A quantitative critical review. *Obes. Rev.* **17**, 262–75 (2016).

76. Okorodudu, D. O. *et al.* Diagnostic performance of body mass index to identify obesity as defined by body adiposity: a systematic review and meta-analysis. *Int. J. Obes.* **34**, 791–9 (2010).

77. Javed, A. *et al.* Diagnostic performance of body mass index to identify obesity as defined by body adiposity in children and adolescents: a systematic review and meta-analysis. *Pediatr. Obes.* **10**, 234–44 (2015).

78. Bower, J. K., Meadows, R. J., Foster, M. C., Foraker, R. E., & Shoben, A. B. The association of percent body fat and lean mass with HbA1c in US adults. *J. Endocr. Soc.* **1**, 600–8 (2017).

79. Zong, G. *et al.* Total and regional adiposity measured by dual-energy X-ray absorptiometry and mortality in NHANES 1999–2006. *Obesity (Silver Spring)* **24**, 2414–21 (2016).

80. Ruderman, N. B., Schneider, S. H., & Berchtold, P. The 'metabolically-obese,' normal-weight individual. *Am. J. Clin. Nutr.* **34**, 1617–21 (1981).

81. Ruderman, N., Chisholm, D., Pi-Sunyer, X., & Schneider, S. The metabolically obese, normal-weight individual revisited. *Diabetes* **47**, 699–713 (1998).

82. Kim, M. K. *et al.* Normal weight obesity in Korean adults. *Clin. Endocrinol.* **80**, 214–20 (2014).

83. Meigs, J. B. *et al.* Body mass index, metabolic syndrome, and risk of type 2 diabetes or cardiovascular disease. *J. Clin. Endocrinol. Metab.* **91**, 2906–12 (2006).

84. Shea, J. L., King, M. T. C., Yi, Y., Gulliver, W., & Sun, G. Body fat percentage is associated with cardiometabolic dysregulation in BMI-defined normal weight subjects. *Nutr. Metab. Cardiovasc. Dis.* **22**, 741–7 (2012).

85. Batsis, J. A. *et al.* Normal weight obesity and mortality in United States subjects ≥60 years of age (from the Third National Health and Nutrition Examination Survey). *Am. J. Cardiol.* **112**, 1592–8 (2013).

86. Wang, B. *et al.* Prevalence of metabolically healthy obese and metabolically obese but normal weight in adults worldwide: a meta-analysis. *Horm. Metab. Res.* **47**, 839–45 (2015).

87. Oliveros, E., Somers, V. K., Sochor, O., Goel, K., & Lopez-Jimenez, F. The concept of normal weight obesity. *Prog. Cardiovasc. Dis.* **56**, 426–33 (2014).

88. Han, S. S. *et al.* Lean mass index: a better predictor of mortality than body mass index in elderly Asians. *J. Am. Geriatr. Soc.* **58**, 312–17 (2010).

89. Spahillari, A. *et al.* The association of lean and fat mass with all-cause mortality in older adults: the cardiovascular health study. *Nutr. Metab. Cardiovasc. Dis.* **26**, 1039–47 (2016).

90. Brown, J. C., Harhay, M. O., & Harhay, M. N. Appendicular lean mass and mortality among prefrail and frail older adults. *J. Nutr. Health Aging* **21**, 342–5 (2017).

91. Navaneethan, S. D., Kirwan, J. P., Arrigain, S., & Schold, J. D. Adiposity measures, lean body mass, physical activity and mortality: NHANES 1999–2004. *BMC Nephrol.* **15**, 108 (2014).

92. Son, J. W. *et al.* Low muscle mass and risk of type 2 diabetes in middle-aged and older adults: findings from the KoGES. *Diabetologia* **60**, 865–72 (2017).

93. Thomas, E. L. *et al.* The missing risk: MRI and MRS phenotyping of abdominal adiposity and ectopic fat. *Obesity (Silver Spring)* **20**, 76–87 (2012).

94. Srikanthan, P. & Karlamangla, A. S. Relative muscle mass is inversely associated with insulin resistance and prediabetes. Findings from the third National Health and Nutrition Examination Survey. *J. Clin. Endocrinol. Metab.* **96**, 2898–903 (2011).

95. Batsis, J. A., Mackenzie, T. A., Emeny, R. T., Lopez-Jimenez, F., & Bartels, S. J. Low lean mass with and without obesity, and mortality: results from the 1999–2004 National Health and Nutrition Examination Survey. *J. Gerontol. A. Biol. Sci. Med. Sci.* **72**, 1445–51 (2017).

96. Tian, S. & Xu, Y. Association of sarcopenic obesity with the risk of all-cause mortality: a meta-analysis of prospective cohort studies. *Geriatr. Gerontol. Int.* **16**, 155–66 (2016).

97. Sørensen, T. I. A., Frederiksen, P., & Heitmann, B. L. Levels and changes in body mass index decomposed into fat and fat-free mass index: relation to long-term all-cause mortality in the general population. *Int. J. Obes.* (2020). doi:10.1038/s41366-020-0613-8

98. Li, R. *et al.* Associations of muscle mass and strength with all-cause mortality among US older adults. *Med. Sci. Sports Exerc.* (2017). doi:10.1249/MSS.0000000000001448

99. Cuthbertson, D. J. *et al.* Dynapenic obesity and the risk of incident type 2 diabetes: the English Longitudinal Study of Ageing. *Diabet. Med.* **33**, 1052–9 (2016).

100. Stamatakis, E. *et al.* Does strength-promoting exercise confer unique health benefits? A pooled analysis of data on 11 population cohorts with all-cause, cancer, and cardiovascular mortality endpoints. *Am. J. Epidemiol.* **187**, 1102–12 (2018).

101. Sandercock, G. R. H. & Cohen, D. D. Temporal trends in muscular fitness of English 10-year-olds 1998–2014: an allometric approach. *J. Sci. Med. Sport* (2018). doi:10.1016/j.jsams.2018.07.020

102. Kodama, S. *et al.* Cardiorespiratory fitness as a quantitative predictor of all-cause mortality and cardiovascular events in healthy men and women: a meta-analysis. *JAMA* **301**, 2024–35 (2009).

103. Zaccardi, F. *et al.* Cardiorespiratory fitness and risk of type 2 diabetes mellitus: a 23-year cohort study and a meta-analysis of prospective studies. *Atherosclerosis* **243**, 131–7 (2015).

104. Sandercock, G. R. H., Ogunleye, A., & Voss, C. Six-year changes in body mass index and cardiorespiratory fitness of English schoolchildren from an affluent area. *Int. J. Obes.* **39**, 1504–7 (2015).

105. Karelis, A. D. Metabolically healthy but obese individuals. *Lancet* **372**, 1281–3 (2008).

106. Velho, S., Paccaud, F., Waeber, G., Vollenweider, P., & Marques-Vidal, P. Metabolically healthy obesity: different prevalences using different criteria. *Eur. J. Clin. Nutr.* **64**, 1043–51 (2010).

107. Stefan, N. *et al.* Identification and characterization of metabolically benign obesity in humans. *Arch. Intern. Med.* **168**, 1609–16 (2008).

108. Chen, D. L. *et al.* Phenotypic characterization of insulin-resistant and insulin-sensitive obesity. *J. Clin. Endocrinol. Metab.* **100**, 4082–91 (2015).

109. Phillips, C. M. Metabolically healthy obesity across the life course: epidemiology, determinants, and implications. *Ann. N. Y. Acad. Sci.* **1391**, 85–100 (2017).

110. Lin, H., Zhang, L., Zheng, R., & Zheng, Y. The prevalence, metabolic risk and effects of lifestyle intervention for metabolically healthy obesity: a systematic review and meta-analysis: A PRISMA-compliant article. *Medicine* **96**, e8838 (2017).

111. Mongraw-Chaffin, M. *et al.* Metabolically healthy obesity, transition to metabolic syndrome, and cardiovascular risk. *J. Am. Coll. Cardiol.* **71**, 1857–65 (2018).

112. Eckel, N., Meidtner, K., Kalle-Uhlmann, T., Stefan, N., & Schulze, M. B. Metabolically healthy obesity and cardiovascular events: a systematic review and meta-analysis. *Eur. J. Prev. Cardiol.* **23**, 956–66 (2016).

113. Kim, T. J. *et al.* Metabolically healthy obesity and the risk for subclinical atherosclerosis. *Atherosclerosis* **262**, 191–7 (2017).

114. Chang, Y. *et al.* Metabolically healthy obesity is associated with an increased risk of diabetes independently of nonalcoholic fatty liver disease. *Obesity (Silver Spring)* **24**, 1996–2003 (2016).

115. Chang, Y. *et al.* Metabolically healthy obesity and the development of nonalcoholic fatty liver disease. *Am. J. Gastroenterol.* **111**, 1133–40 (2016).

116. Sinn, D. H. *et al.* Metabolically-healthy obesity is associated with higher prevalence of colorectal adenoma. *PLoS One* **12**, e0179480 (2017).

117. Kramer, C. K., Zinman, B., & Retnakaran, R. Are metabolically healthy overweight and obesity benign conditions?: a systematic review and meta-analysis. *Ann. Intern. Med.* **159**, 758–69 (2013).

118. Magkos, F. Metabolically healthy obesity: what's in a name? *Am. J. Clin. Nutr.* **110**, 533–9 (2019).

119. Cerhan, J. R. *et al.* A pooled analysis of waist circumference and mortality in 650,000 adults. *Mayo Clin. Proc.* **89**, 335–45 (2014).

120. Katzmarzyk, P. T. *et al.* Anthropometric markers of obesity and mortality in white and African American adults: the Pennington Center Longitudinal Study. *Obesity (Silver Spring)* **21**, 1070–5 (2013).

121. Lim, R. B. T. *et al.* Anthropometrics indices of obesity, and all-cause and cardiovascular disease-related mortality, in an Asian cohort with type 2 diabetes mellitus. *Diabetes Metab.* **41**, 291–300 (2015).

122. Aune, D., Schlesinger, S., Norat, T., & Riboli, E. Body mass index, abdominal fatness, and the risk of sudden cardiac death: a systematic review and dose-response meta-analysis of prospective studies. *Eur. J. Epidemiol.* (2018). doi:10.1007/s10654-017-0353-9

123. InterAct Consortium *et al.* Long-term risk of incident type 2 diabetes and measures of overall and regional obesity: the EPIC-InterAct case-cohort study. *PLoS Med.* **9**, e1001230 (2012).

124. Seo, D.-C., Choe, S., & Torabi, M. R. Is waist circumference ≥102/88cm better than body mass index ≥30 to predict hypertension and diabetes development regardless of gender, age group, and race/ethnicity? Meta-analysis. *Prev. Med.* **97**, 100–8 (2017).

125. Hidayat, K., Du, X., Chen, G., Shi, M., & Shi, B. Abdominal obesity and lung cancer risk: systematic review and meta-analysis of prospective studies. *Nutrients* **8**, (2016).

126. Dong, Y. *et al.* Abdominal obesity and colorectal cancer risk: systematic review and meta-analysis of prospective studies. *Biosci. Rep.* **37**, (2017).

127. Emdin, C. A. *et al.* Genetic association of waist-to-hip ratio with cardiometabolic traits, type 2 diabetes, and coronary heart disease. *JAMA* **317**, 626–34 (2017).

128. Dale, C. E. *et al.* Causal associations of adiposity and body fat distribution with coronary heart disease, stroke subtypes, and type 2 diabetes mellitus: a Mendelian randomization analysis. *Circulation* **135**, 2373–88 (2017).

129. Luz, R. H., Barbosa, A. R., & D'Orsi, E. Waist circumference, body mass index and waist-height ratio: are two indices better than one for identifying hypertension risk in older adults? *Prev. Med.* **93**, 76–81 (2016).

130. Ntuk, U. E., Gill, J. M. R., Mackay, D. F., Sattar, N., & Pell, J. P. Ethnic-specific obesity cutoffs for diabetes risk: cross-sectional study of 490,288 UK biobank participants. *Diabetes Care* **37**, 2500–7 (2014).

131. Okada, R. *et al.* Upper-normal waist circumference is a risk marker for metabolic syndrome in normal-weight subjects. *Nutr. Metab. Cardiovasc. Dis.* **26**, 67–76 (2016).

132. Yusuf, S. *et al.* Obesity and the risk of myocardial infarction in 27,000 participants from 52 countries: a case-control study. *Lancet* **366**, 1640–9 (2005).

133. Canoy, D. *et al.* Body fat distribution and risk of coronary heart disease in men and women in the European Prospective Investigation Into Cancer and Nutrition in Norfolk cohort: a population-based prospective study. *Circulation* **116**, 2933–43 (2007).

134. Snijder, M. B. *et al.* Associations of hip and thigh circumferences independent of waist circumference with the incidence of type 2 diabetes: the Hoorn Study. *Am. J. Clin. Nutr.* **77**, 1192–7 (2003).

135. Yaghootkar, H. *et al.* Genetic evidence for a link between favorable adiposity and lower risk of type 2 diabetes, hypertension, and heart disease. *Diabetes* **65**, 2448–60 (2016).

136. Camhi, S. M. *et al.* The relationship of waist circumference and BMI to visceral, subcutaneous, and total body fat: sex and race differences. *Obesity (Silver Spring)* **19**, 402–8 (2011).

137. Lee, S. W. *et al.* Body fat distribution is more predictive of all-cause mortality than overall adiposity. *Diabetes. Obes. Metab.* **20**, 141–7 (2018).

138. Vasan, S. K. *et al.* Comparison of regional fat measurements by dual-energy X-ray absorptiometry and conventional anthropometry and their association with markers of diabetes and cardiovascular disease risk. *Int. J. Obes.* (2017). doi:10.1038/ijo.2017.289

139. Kim, D. *et al.* Body fat distribution and risk of incident and regressed nonalcoholic fatty liver disease. *Clin. Gastroenterol. Hepatol.* **14**, 132–8.e4 (2016).

140. Ebadi, M. *et al.* Subcutaneous adiposity is an independent predictor of mortality in cancer patients. *Br. J. Cancer* **117**, 148–55 (2017).

141. Xiao, J., Mazurak, V. C., Olobatuyi, T. A., Caan, B. J., & Prado, C. M. Visceral adiposity and cancer survival: a review of imaging studies. *Eur. J. Cancer Care (Engl).* (2016). doi:10.1111/ecc.12611

142. Li, C., Ford, E. S., Zhao, G., Balluz, L. S., & Giles, W. H. Estimates of body composition with dual-energy X-ray absorptiometry in adults. *Am. J. Clin. Nutr.* **90**, 1457–65 (2009).

143. Demerath, E. W. *et al.* Anatomical patterning of visceral adipose tissue: race, sex, and age variation. *Obesity (Silver Spring)* **15**, 2984–93 (2007).

144. Snijder, M. B. *et al.* Low subcutaneous thigh fat is a risk factor for unfavourable glucose and lipid levels, independently of high abdominal fat. The Health ABC Study. *Diabetologia* **48**, 301–8 (2005).

145. Staiano, A. E. & Katzmarzyk, P. T. Ethnic and sex differences in body fat and visceral and subcutaneous adiposity in children and adolescents. *Int. J. Obes.* **36**, 1261–9 (2012).

146. Pulit, S. L., Karaderi, T., & Lindgren, C. M. Sexual dimorphisms in genetic loci linked to body fat distribution. *Biosci. Rep.* **37**, (2017).

147. Ferguson, L. D. *et al.* Men across a range of ethnicities have a higher prevalence of diabetes: findings from a cross-sectional study of 500,000 UK Biobank participants. *Diabet. Med.* **35**, 270–6 (2018).

148. Regensteiner, J. G. *et al.* Sex differences in the cardiovascular consequences of diabetes mellitus: a scientific statement from the American Heart Association. *Circulation* **132**, 2424–47 (2015).

149. Go, A. S. *et al.* Heart disease and stroke statistics--2014 update: a report from the American Heart Association. *Circulation* **129**, e28–e292 (2014).

150. Benjamin, E. J. *et al.* Heart disease and stroke statistics–2017 update: a report from the American Heart Association. *Circulation* **135**, e146–e603 (2017).

151. Kelly, T. L., Wilson, K. E., & Heymsfield, S. B. Dual energy X-Ray absorptiometry body composition reference values from NHANES. *PLoS One* **4**, e7038 (2009).

152. Lee, M.-M., Jebb, S. A., Oke, J., & Piernas, C. Reference values for skeletal muscle mass and fat mass measured by bioelectrical impedance in 390,565 UK adults. *J. Cachexia. Sarcopenia Muscle* **11**, 487–96 (2020).

153. Fields, J. B., Merrigan, J. J., White, J. B., & Jones, M. T. Body composition variables by sport and sport-position in elite collegiate athletes. *J. strength Cond. Res.* (2018). doi:10.1519/JSC.0000000000002865

154. Rush, E. C., Freitas, I., & Plank, L. D. Body size, body composition and fat distribution: comparative analysis of European, Maori, Pacific Island and Asian Indian adults. *Br. J. Nutr.* **102**, 632–41 (2009).

155. Wells, J. C. K. Ecogeographical associations between climate and human body composition: analyses based on anthropometry and skinfolds. *Am. J. Phys. Anthropol.* **147**, 169–86 (2012).

156. Wells, J. C. K. Ethnic variability in adiposity and cardiovascular risk: the variable disease selection hypothesis. *Int. J. Epidemiol.* **38**, 63–71 (2009).

157. Kadowaki, S. *et al.* International comparison of abdominal fat distribution among four populations: the ERA-JUMP study. *Metab. Syndr. Relat. Disord.* **16**, 166–73 (2018).

158. Stults-Kolehmainen, M. A. *et al.* DXA estimates of fat in abdominal, trunk and hip regions varies by ethnicity in men. *Nutr. Diabetes* **3**, e64 (2013).

159. Stults-Kolehmainen, M. A., Stanforth, P. R., & Bartholomew, J. B. Fat in android, trunk, and peripheral regions varies by ethnicity and race in college aged women. *Obesity (Silver Spring)* **20**, 660–5 (2012).

160. Lovejoy, J. C., Smith, S. R., & Rood, J. C. Comparison of regional fat distribution and health risk factors in middle-aged white and African American women: the Healthy Transitions Study. *Obes. Res.* **9**, 10–16 (2001).

6

Same but Different

Fat Biology around the Body

Of Mice and Men

Despite significant advances in our understanding of fat biology, gaps remain—some considerably larger than others. In contrast to the imagery dominating contemporary Western media, relatively little attention has been paid to the biology of lower body adipose tissue, with the evidence base instead displaying a heavy bias towards abdominal fat (both subcutaneous and visceral depots). This historical preference likely developed for various reasons, some academic, others practical. Aside from central obesity being a strong predictor of metabolic and cardiovascular disease,[1] abdominal subcutaneous fat samples can be obtained fairly easily via biopsy under local anaesthetic while visceral fat can be acquired from individuals undergoing routine surgery. Subcutaneous abdominal and visceral fat have also received much academic attention because these depots can be studied in mice due to their broad biological similarities.

Mice have two main subcutaneous fat pads,[2] one located between the shoulder blades (i.e., cervical and axillary) and another located between the lumbar vertebrae that descends to the gluteal region (i.e., the inguinal pad); the latter supposedly represents the mouse equivalent of a bum or thighs (Figure 6.1). In addition to these subcutaneous depots, mice have visceral fat located in the peri-gonadal region (i.e., epididymal fat in males and peri-ovarian fat in females). Scientists have used mouse models to make innumerable important biomedical discoveries which translate to the human condition owing to similarities across species, and similarities in adipose biology are no exception. Indeed, human and mouse fat display similar gene expression profiles[3] (i.e., the pattern of active and inactive genes), undergo a similar pattern of aging-related redistribution,[4] and contain precursor

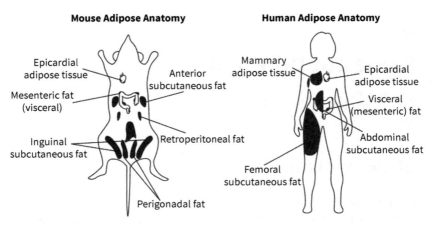

Figure 6.1 Comparison of mouse and human adipose anatomy.

cells (i.e., preadipocytes) that display many similar depot-specific functional properties.[2,5]

But as useful as these animal models are, mice *aren't* humans. For instance, peri-gonadal fat is amongst the most frequently studied depot in the literature and is often thought to be analogous to human visceral fat. However, this fat depot lacks portal vein drainage from the liver in mice, unlike omental and mesenteric fat in humans. This and other species-specific differences mean that not all findings translate easily, if at all, to the human condition.[2] This challenge is highlighted in the ongoing brown fat saga (see Chapter 4) with another case pertaining to the mechanism by which fat expands upon overfeeding. The 'AdipoChaser' transgenic mouse enables researchers to indelibly label adipocytes as they are generated throughout life.[6] Unquestionably an impressive piece of biological engineering, the AdipoChaser mouse's adipose tissue depots expand in a manner *opposite* to that observed in humans, thus undermining this tool's utility. Species-specific differences at the molecular, tissue, and anatomical levels mean it is unwise to extrapolate findings between species in the absence of direct comparison studies; the widespread use of mice coupled with the vanishingly rare number of direct comparative studies[2] means an overhaul in the way biomedical research is conducted is long overdue.

Where the River Flows

Representing the mechanism by which fat tissue connects to the rest of the body to receive and dispatch nutrients and hormones, blood flow and its regulation are crucial aspects of adipose biology which display regional variation. Blood flow through adipose tissue can change dynamically and dramatically under different physiological conditions, just as fatty acid handling can shift from storage to mobilization (see Chapter 3). Indeed, these two fundamental features of adipose biology, fatty acid flux and blood flow, are tightly co-ordinated in the healthy state. The regulation of adipose tissue blood flow is multi-faceted and complex,[7] which should be unsurprising given the convergence of numerous biological systems involved in co-ordinating the distinct biological responses to feeding, starvation, and exercise.

Blood flow to subcutaneous adipose tissue, which accounts for the vast majority (~85%) of human fat mass,[7] tends to be considerably higher in the abdomen compared to the lower body in the fasted state.[8] Adipose tissue blood flow often increases significantly when a meal is consumed,[9] although the magnitude of response varies considerably between individuals.[10] This co-ordinated response supports the efficient and timely storage of recently ingested nutrients (Figure 6.2), thus protecting non-adipose tissues (e.g., the liver, pancreas, and muscle) against prolonged exposure to excessively high levels of circulating fat (i.e., lipotoxicity), a situation which promotes ectopic fat accumulation that can result in tissue dysfunction and damage.[11] While blood flow increases to upper and lower body subcutaneous fat after the consumption of a meal, data suggest that there may be a greater increase to the latter depot in women.[12] This greater delivery of blood, and therefore nutrients, to bum and thigh fat might be one such mechanism that supports the generation and maintenance of the distinctive gynoid body shape in women.

Nutrient delivery and increased adipose tissue blood flow after a meal are tied together by insulin, the master nutrient storage signal.[13] Indeed, the post-meal increase in blood flow in subcutaneous (abdominal) fat is severely blunted in insulin-resistant individuals.[14,15] Insulin seems to regulate adipose tissue blood flow via indirect mechanisms,[16] with nitric oxide (a highly reactive, naturally occurring molecule which causes blood vessel dilation and is employed by Viagra to achieve its distinctive effect) and

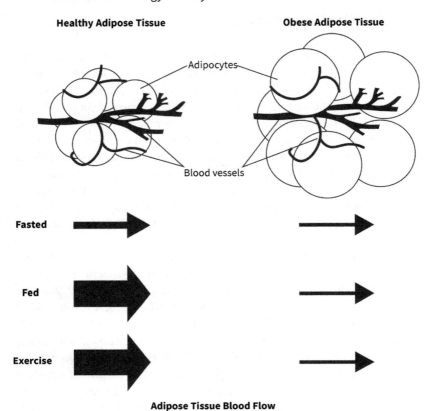

Figure 6.2 Blood flow in healthy and obese adipose tissue.

catecholamines (i.e., noradrenaline) released by the sympathetic nervous system representing key mediators.[17] But although increased blood flow enhances the delivery of nutrients, the actual uptake of fatty acids varies between adipose depots.

The post-meal increase in adipose blood flow is akin to widening the service road behind a row of shops; more trucks may be able to park, but the number of deliveries made is ultimately limited by each shop's staff and equipment. Similarly, dietary fatty acids carried in chylomicrons appear to be stored more efficiently in subcutaneous abdominal fat compared to that in the buttocks and thighs,[12,18] although there may be more uptake in the lower body in women.[12] The increased post-meal level of circulating insulin also suppresses fatty acid mobilization, although this effect varies between adipose depots. For instance, insulin completely suppresses lipolysis in lower body fat, but only partially in upper body fat, with visceral fat being particularly resistant to its anti-lipolytic effects[19] (imagine trying to fill different baths with water, one whose plug fits neatly whereas another is leaky).

The uptake of fatty acids by adipose tissue closely mirrors the blood flow it receives, but the delivery location for a dietary fatty acid may not necessarily be its final destination. Indeed, fatty acids undergo substantial re-distribution between subcutaneous fat in the abdomen, thighs, and buttocks over time.[20] Moreover, the short-term pattern of fatty acid uptake reportedly does not predict the regional pattern of fat expansion over the long-term.[21] This re-distribution may involve regional variation in the direct uptake of circulating free fatty acids liberated from adipose tissue via lipolysis in which those not used as metabolic fuel may return to their site of origin or be taken up by a different depot. Consistent with the typical body shapes, direct free fatty acid uptake is reportedly greater in abdominal fat in men,[22] whereas this process occurs to a greater extent in lower body fat in women.[23] Relatedly, adipose tissue displays regional preferences for fatty acids carried in specific types of lipoprotein. For instance, lower body subcutaneous fat efficiently collects fatty acids derived from the very low density lipoprotein particles released by the liver[24] (see Chapter 3). This observation has prompted the suggestion that the lower body fat depot acts as a metabolic 'sink' which accumulates fatty acids recycled by the liver, capturing them for long-term storage.

The regulation of adipose tissue blood flow is impaired in obesity and metabolic disease, with reduced insulin sensitivity playing a key role, regardless of the fat depot's size.[14] Adipose tissue in obese individuals receives a smaller, less dynamic blood supply compared to fat from healthy, lean individuals[25], with the post-meal blood flow increase being severely blunted in high-BMI individuals[10] (Figure 6.2). This reduced response might represent an early marker of increased insulin resistance,[26] so it follows that impairments to adipose blood flow are exacerbated in individuals with type 2 diabetes.[15,27] This phenomenon is not unique to adipose tissue though, as it also occurs in skeletal muscle.[28] In addition to decreased insulin action, reduced release and/or action of various signals such as the gut hormone glucose-dependent insulinotropic polypeptide[29] may also underpin impairments to post-meal adipose tissue blood flow in obesity and/or metabolic disease.[7]

Flowing Out

On the flip side, fatty acid mobilization and the associated blood flow display some notable depot-specific differences. Data derived from numerous experimental techniques indicate that subcutaneous abdominal fat is considerably more active than lower body fat and contributes the majority of free fatty acids in the circulation in men and women[30–32] at rest and during exercise.[33] This is consistent with the considerably lower blood flow[8] and slower turnover of fatty acids[34] reported in lower body fat compared to subcutaneous abdominal fat. The most striking regional differences in fatty acid mobilization, however, emerge when certain biochemical signals that stimulate this process are presented. For instance, adrenaline released by the adrenal gland upon exercise or stress exposure activates lipolysis specifically in subcutaneous abdominal fat, but has no effect in the lower body[35]; this effect is accompanied by a corresponding selective increase in blood flow to upper body fat.[36] This remarkable depot-specific effect to the same chemical signal is driven by greater expression of inhibitory adrenoceptors in gluteal adipocytes[37] which prevent adrenaline and other catecholamines from activating lipolysis in these cells and also limit blood flow increases.[38]

Lower body subcutaneous fat is not completely unresponsive or metabolically inert though. Blood flow to and lipolysis in subcutaneous adipose tissue in the leg can be increased in a localized manner by exercise.[39] However, lower body fat is usually reluctant to mobilize during extended periods of fasting/starvation, in which subcutaneous abdominal fat contributes the most during this period, followed by leg fat, with adipose tissue in the buttocks generally being spared.[40] However, this unwilling fat store can be compelled to give up the goods when exceptionally high calorie demands need to be met, with lactation being notable for its somewhat unique ability to induce lower body fat mobilization.[41,42] The reluctance of lower body fat to mobilize its energy stores in nearly every other situation suggests that supporting lactation is probably its main evolutionarily defined purpose (see Chapter 2), at least in women, which is understandable given the benefits that this process confers. The metabolic inertia displayed by lower body fat is also what makes it such an important player in determining overall metabolic health, as the locking away of fatty acids protects the rest of the body against the deleterious effects of lipotoxicity and ectopic fat accumulation. Whoever said that 'a moment on the lips, a lifetime on the hips' was a bad thing?

I Can't Believe It's Not Palmitoleate

Biochemical analyses have highlighted that the abundance of different fatty acid types varies between subcutaneous abdominal and gluteo-femoral fat,[43] as well as visceral fat[44]; think of how butter and margarine may look similar while having distinct molecular compositions. This situation raises the possibility that not only *how much* fat is mobilized may vary between depots, but also *what type* of fatty acids are mobilized. One notable example concerns palmitoleate, an unsaturated fatty acid released by adipose tissue that was originally identified in mice where it was found to enhance insulin sensitivity in skeletal muscle and the liver.[45] Looking to humans, circulating palmitoleate levels are reportedly higher in more insulin-sensitive individuals.[46] Moreover, palmitoleate is more abundant in lower body adipose tissue, the depot from which it is also released at a greater rate.[47] Before reaching for the nearest palmitoleate supplement, however, other reports suggest that circulating palmitoleate levels are elevated in individuals with fatty liver disease[48] who have a higher risk of developing cardiovascular and metabolic disease.[49] Evidently there is more to this complex story, but the notion that anatomically distinct adipose depots have different biochemical compositions in a way that may relate to health outcomes certainly warrants further exploration.

The Body Shop

These data paint a picture in which subcutaneous abdominal fat tissue is a highly active player, whereas lower body subcutaneous fat acts primarily as a largely quiescent long-term energy store that kicks into action in times of large energy demands. But how does this relate to health outcomes? When attempting to apply our knowledge of depot-specific adipose biology to the relationship between regional fat accumulation and metabolic/cardiovascular health (and disease), it can be useful to think of the body as a shop. A healthy, normal weight body would be like a well-run shop that perfectly balances inventory with sales, meaning the shelves and storeroom are always adequately stocked without being cluttered or overfilled. However, if the shop starts selling less, orders too much merchandise, or both, the finite storage space will be strained and threaten the shop's efficient operation. While some temporary overstocking may be manageable, prolonged accumulation will inevitably result in the shop becoming a cluttered, inefficient mess in which stocktaking becomes impossible and customers find it difficult, even dangerous, to conduct business. Eventually the dysfunctional set-up will reach a point where (potentially irreversible) damage is caused or an accident happens. The best way to bring order to this chaos involves reducing inventory (or increasing storage capacity).

This can be achieved if business picks up and more items are sold than delivered, at which point inappropriately stored items can be moved back to their rightful place and the strain on storage space is reduced. On the road to recovery, the shop obviously doesn't want to overshoot and deplete its inventory too much though. Amidst the complex workings of operating a business successfully, the shift from healthy to dysfunctional can result from a number of different factors acting independently or together, a situation akin to the multiple-hit theory in the development of cancer.[50] It is important to remember that at the heart of this situation, the surplus of goods relative to the shop's storage capacity represents the main factor putting the entire system under pressure. With that, it is worth noting that the set-up and storage capacity of an individual's 'biological shop' can vary considerably and might even change over time. Maintaining a well-run shop throughout its lifespan requires constant upkeep and vigilance.

Putting the Pieces Together

The striking relationship between (central) obesity and metabolic disease can be interpreted as a failure of subcutaneous fat to adequately store surplus calories and the resultant back-up and dysfunction of the metabolic energy storage system.[51] Continued excessive calorie consumption initially manifests as the expansion of subcutaneous (abdominal) adipose tissue whose function and insulin sensitivity decline in a self-reinforcing vicious cycle in which the ability to safely accommodate more calories is progressively impaired.[52] This metabolic dysfunction is exacerbated further by the knock-on effects of ectopic fat accumulation in the liver and muscle (i.e., lipotoxicity[11]). It follows that visceral fat is increasingly being viewed as a site of ectopic lipid accumulation, as expansion of this depot is often associated with deterioration of cardiovascular and metabolic health in a way that parallels the relationship observed for 'true' ectopic sites like the liver, pancreas, and skeletal muscle.[53]

Preferential fat deposition in subcutaneous fat goes hand in hand with greater insulin sensitivity,[54] a scenario associated with protection against visceral and ectopic fat expansion and a reduced risk of developing metabolic disease in men and women of all ages[55–57] (Figure 6.3). Moreover, the expansion of visceral fat mass reportedly reflects the degree of subcutaneous fat dysfunction[58] and can accurately predict the conversion of metabolically healthy obesity (see Chapter 5) to an unhealthy state.[59,60] The excessive accumulation of fat, particularly visceral and ectopic fat, can therefore be considered both a cause *and* effect of metabolic dysfunction. What represents

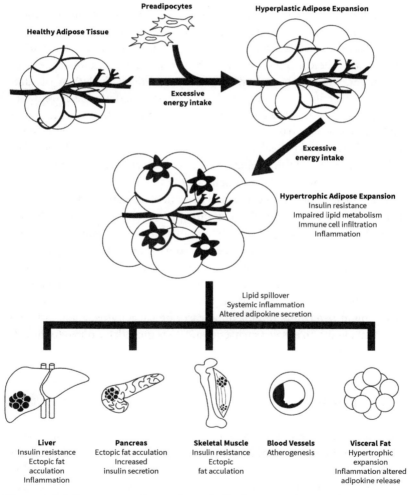

Figure 6.3 Adipose expansion and metabolic disease pathogenesis.

the trigger for (subcutaneous) adipose tissue to cease functioning properly remains ill-defined, however, and may not be embodied by a single event or molecule. What is clear though, is that an individual carrying an excessive quantity of calories relative to their body's safe maximal carrying capacity is key in perpetuating this destructive chain of events.

Personal Space

Just as the amount of storage and display space in a shop is limited, so too is the amount of fat that people can accumulate before they experience metabolic disease, which is neatly summarized in the notion of the *personal fat threshold*.[61] The concept of *embonpoint* ('in good condition') echoes this sentiment,[62] in which excessive fatness (*exces d'embonpoint*) or slenderness (*un embonpoint inutile*) have been viewed as undesirable extremes of an individual's possible weight spectrum. Historical notions that excessive embonpoint will corrupt beauty, sap the body's strength, weigh it down, and be detrimental to health, fertility, and intelligence[63] have played a key role in the modern framing and treatment of obesity as a disease with predominantly negative social connotations.[64]

A key determinant of the maximal amount of fat an individual can carry before they experience metabolic dysfunction requires introducing the notion of *expandability*[52] (i.e., the ability of fat to expand before it becomes dysfunctional), a property that emerges from the integrated biological processes within and between different depots to influence overall metabolic health. This set-up is complicated further by the fact that distinct fat depots behave differently plus the considerable differences between the sexes. So, what might determine the maximal carrying capacity/expandability of a given fat depot? To answer such a question, we must delve down to the cellular and molecular level.

Fit to Burst

One of the most important determinants of adipose tissue expandability pertains to the mechanism by which fat expands to accommodate excess calories. Either pre-existing mature adipocytes can swell (i.e., hypertrophy) or progenitor cells (i.e., preadipocytes) can be recruited to form new adipocytes (i.e., hyperplasia). Imagine the storage of fatty acids in adipocytes like the collection of rubbish; ideally bin bags would only get moderately full and there would be a number of spare bags to use for future rubbish collection (i.e., adipose hyperplasia). The worse-case scenario involves trying to collect too much rubbish, in which one runs out of bags and fills those available until they're overflowing (i.e., adipocyte hypertrophy associated with adipose dysfunction and ectopic fat accumulation). Adipose tissue expands using a combination of hypertrophy and hyperplasia, although different fat depots preferentially utilize one mechanism at the expense of the other. In humans, visceral fat seems to primarily expand via hypertrophy whereas subcutaneous adipose tissue does so via hyperplasia.[65,66] There is further variation, however, as subcutaneous abdominal adipocytes are predisposed to undergo hypertrophy whereas gluteo-femoral fat exhibits a preference for hyperplasia.[67] This pattern is consistent with the report that the formation rate of new preadipocytes and adipocytes is significantly higher in subcutaneous gluteal fat compared to that in the abdomen, at least in women.[68]

Using an inspired method to quantify cell turnover by measuring the incorporation of atmospheric radioactive carbon from above-ground nuclear bomb tests (1955–1963) into cellular DNA, it has been determined that approximately 10% of adipocytes in subcutaneous abdominal fat are renewed every year throughout adulthood in lean and obese individuals.[69] This means the entire cellular composition of an individual's adipose tissue is renewed every ten years. Moving beyond adipocyte quantity, a substantial body of evidence indicates that the related phenomenon of *adipocyte size* represents an important index of adipose tissue function and overall metabolic health.[70] Since the early studies performed in the 1970s,[71] it has become well-established that smaller adipocyte size is associated with favourable metabolic health status and vice versa.[70] Such data have led to the proposal that hyperplasia underpins metabolically favourable adipose expansion.[70,72] Conversely, adipose tissue with a reduced hyperplastic capacity will preferentially expand via adipocyte hypertrophy; the greater propensity of a depot to undergo hypertrophy might also be indicative of a smaller maximal carrying capacity.

Adipocyte size reflects how full and functional a fat depot is, with both of these features being closely related to metabolic and cardiovascular health more generally.[73] Indeed, subcutaneous (abdominal) adipocyte hypertrophy is a hallmark of adipose tissue from normal weight individuals who have type 2 diabetes[74] or have a hereditary predisposition to developing it.[75] The size of subcutaneous abdominal adipocytes is also inversely associated with overall insulin sensitivity and circulating adiponectin levels,[76] and can even predict the metabolic benefits of weight loss in overweight/obese individuals[77] (those carrying more smaller adipocytes experience better health outcomes). It should be noted that the absolute amount of fat an individual is carrying is not as important as how this relates to the maximal carrying capacity of their adipose tissue (as reflected by adipocyte number and size). It follows that being obese or not (according to BMI) is not so relevant to the development of metabolic/cardiovascular disease as whether an individual is carrying an excess amount of fat relative to their personal fat threshold.[61] Indeed, the relationship between adipocyte size and various aspects of metabolic health is independent of overall fat mass.[78]

Noting the aforementioned properties of the various fat depots, it is notable that adipose dysfunction primarily manifests as central fat accumulation,[58] regardless of BMI, sex, age, or ethnicity. Moreover, the degree to which healthy individuals lose insulin sensitivity when they gain fat upon overfeeding is closely related to the extent of subcutaneous adipocyte hypertrophy and expansion of visceral fat mass.[79] This already complex situation is further complicated, however, by the observation that the mechanism by which fat expands changes dynamically as it enlarges. Indeed, the initial phase of weight gain from a healthy baseline occurs via hyperplasia, but this shifts towards hypertrophy as further weight gain occurs and the individual transitions from normal weight to overweight, obese, and beyond.[80] So, how does adipocyte size relate to fat's carrying capacity and function?

Caught in a Mesh

The *extracellular matrix* is the biological scaffold which provides mechanical support to the cells embedded within, with its structure and composition also providing signals that direct the behaviour of the constituent cells. This structure's components are constantly being turned over and remodelled to co-ordinate the morphology (i.e., size and shape), number, and function of the resident cells with hormonal and nutritional signals it receives from the circulation and those emanating from within the fat depot itself. This dynamic remodelling involves highly regulated alterations to the expression and activity of structural components and degradative enzymes[81] as well as the immune system.[82] A mounting body of evidence also implicates this rather underappreciated structure in the development of obesity[83] and metabolic disease.[84] As one might expect, the composition and structure of the extracellular matrix displays regional variation,[85,86] although most data concern differences between upper body stores, particularly subcutaneous abdominal and visceral fat.[87]

Thinking of the adipose extracellular matrix as a house, remodelling is the biological equivalent of redecorating the rooms or re-arranging the furniture. Obviously, each house has a unique limit on the amount of available space, with these physical boundaries defining its maximal safe carrying capacity (i.e., personal fat threshold). If the number of residents exceeds the maximal capacity, living arrangements can go from comfortable, to cosy, to dangerously overcrowded. In this situation, *how* space is used is also crucial; neatly arranged, minimalistic furniture has a clear advantage over opulent, bulky furniture. It follows that the physical proportions of the residents will also influence how many can live comfortably in the same amount of space; just think of how living and working arrangements on a submarine are far from ideal for obese or very tall people.

But how does the extracellular matrix relate to adipose expansion? Extracellular matrix remodelling is essential for the process of adipogenesis[88,89] (i.e., the generation of new adipocytes), meaning this structure plays a key role in determining whether adipose expansion occurs via hyperplasia and/or hypertrophy. The importance of this structure was highlighted in an intriguing study in which visceral preadipocytes were carefully extracted from their resident extracellular matrix and transplanted into decellularized extracellular matrix from subcutaneous fat. The usually poor ability of visceral cells to differentiate into mature adipocytes was completely restored by the subcutaneous extracellular matrix,[90] indicating how important the immediate environment is to cellular function; if adipogenesis were akin to completing homework, the environment of visceral fat would be a torturously noisy and distracting household while subcutaneous fat would offer the quiet sanctuary of an empty library. The expression of many different genes encoding extracellular components changes in subcutaneous (abdominal) fat upon weight gain,[91] with these changes distinguishing adipose tissue from healthy/lean and obese individuals.[92] Mounting evidence also indicates that the quality and quantity of extracellular matrix that gets laid down during weight gain can change in such a way that manifests as *fibrosis*. Recalling the house analogy, fibrosis is like squeezing too much furniture into a confined space, turning the house into a dysfunctional clutter-fest.

Subcutaneous (abdominal) and visceral adipose tissue fibrosis is present in individuals who are obese and/or have metabolic disease.[93,94] Fibrosis makes adipose tissue stiffer, with the extent of stiffness being closely related to the degree of insulin resistance.[95] It has been proposed that fibrotic fat tissue has a reduced ability to expand, thereby increasing the likelihood of ectopic lipid deposition and metabolic dysfunction. For instance, subcutaneous (abdominal) fat of individuals genetically predisposed to developing metabolic disease (i.e., the currently normal weight, otherwise healthy children of obese and/or diabetic parents) reportedly exhibits increased fibrosis and adipocyte hypertrophy compared to lean, healthy controls.[75] Visceral fat fibrosis is also related to the risk of developing type 2 diabetes and cardiovascular disease.[96] Subcutaneous (abdominal) adipose tissue's greater capacity to expand than visceral fat is matched by a heightened ability to increase its capillary network than visceral fat, although this declines with obesity.[97] It is likely that altered extracellular matrix composition contributes to the inadequate and unresponsive adipose blood supply that supports the metabolic dysfunction associated with excessive fat accumulation.[7]

It appears that the extracellular matrix provides a mechanism linking adipose expandability to depot-specific fat biology, adipocyte size, and metabolic health.[52] This complex interplay is perhaps best illustrated in the remarkable case of a transgenic mouse deficient for collagen VI. Upon being fed a high-fat diet, this mouse's adipose tissue was capable of almost limitless expansion, a feature which protected these animals from the severe metabolic disturbances typically associated with such extreme levels of fatness[98]; this is like having a house with rubber walls. What was most notable about this case, however, was that expansion occurred mainly via adipocyte hypertrophy, which highlights the importance of context when considering adipocyte size (even though this specific gene's biology does not translate directly to humans[99–101]). Larger adipocyte size is usually associated with worse metabolic health outcomes, but this may depend on the degree by which the adipocyte is physically constrained, something which could take effect at different absolute sizes in different people. Exploring the biology of the extracellular matrix and its role in the relationship between expandability and metabolic health certainly requires further exploration. However, particular care is needed as adipose tissue biopsy technique, processing, and analysis (in addition to donor variation and experimental design) can influence a sample's properties and therefore the study outcome.[102]

As the extracellular matrix is turned over, some of the degradation products become something more than innocuous waste; some act as biological signals that act elsewhere in the body. One such example pertains to *endotrophin*, a breakdown product of collagen VI identified in mice that promotes adipose tissue fibrosis and exacerbates the metabolic derangements of high-fat feeding.[103] Moreover, endotrophin was found to enter the general circulation from adipose tissue and accumulate in breast tissue where it promoted the formation of mammary tumours.[104] Evidently such a discovery represents a potentially important mechanism in which signals emanating from (dysfunctional) adipose tissue raise the risk of developing certain cancers (and other diseases), thus providing a potential link between obesity and increased cancer risk that warrants exploring in humans, with endotrophin probably representing the tip of the iceberg.[105] Evidently the adipose extracellular matrix represents an understudied[106] yet fertile ground for study, rich with biological processes and potential therapeutic targets that await discovery.

Fat on Fire

Usually concerned with defending the body from external (i.e., microbes) and internal (e.g., cancerous cells) threats, the immune system also plays a key role in adipose remodelling. Repurposing its tools to degrade, dispose, and recycle the extracellular matrix as well as dead or dying cells, immune system activity can influence adipose function. A vast amount of data indicates that obesity and metabolic disease are associated with chronic inflammation[107] (i.e., persistent, inappropriate activation of the immune system). Many of the immune system's manoeuvres are co-ordinated by locally released signals, but these can leak into the general circulation to contribute to the persistent, low-level inflammatory state that negatively impacts overall metabolic health.[108,109] Whether this adipose inflammation is a cause or consequence remains unclear and highly contentious[110]; it could be both.

The term 'inflammation' has acquired predominantly negative connotations, but the impressive complexity involved means that this phenomenon should not be viewed as a binary either 'on' or 'off', but more like a light with a dimmer switch and several colour filters. Indeed, inflammation is absolutely required for the metabolically favourable remodelling and (hyperplastic) expansion of adipose tissue,[111] yet blockage of inflammatory signalling in humans can (partially) rescue insulin sensitivity.[112] However, evidence suggests that inflammatory signalling by adipocytes supports adipose function and metabolic health, whereas activation of adipose-based immune cells (e.g., macrophages), often by similar biological signals and pathways, has a deleterious effect on adipose function, insulin sensitivity, and metabolic health.[113] Attaining and maintaining good metabolic health requires carefully regulating the extent and type of inflammatory activity by various cell types within adipose tissue, just like students need a good teacher to direct their energy in a constructive direction.

A number of mechanisms link adipose tissue inflammation in obesity[114] and type 2 diabetes.[115] For example, inflammatory signals can act directly on adipocytes to cause insulin resistance,[109] prevent adipogenesis,[116,117] promote fibrosis,[113] and disrupt the generation of new blood vessels.[118] The expansion of fat mass is associated with increased overall levels of adipose inflammation, as highlighted by greater infiltration of activated white blood cells into adipose tissue,[119] as well as higher expression of immune response-related genes.[120,121] But this does not occur in a uniform manner throughout the body, with the extent and type of inflammatory signalling varying between different adipose depots in a way that closely relates to insulin sensitivity and metabolic health. Greater inflammation in subcutaneous (abdominal) and visceral fat is associated with more insulin resistance and worse health outcomes.[122] The relationship between visceral fat and inflammation runs deep though, as immune cell infiltration in subcutaneous abdominal and visceral fat is positively correlated with visceral fat accumulation.[123] The level of inflammation in subcutaneous[124] and visceral fat[125] also appears to be closely related to liver fat accumulation and liver fibrosis, with the latter also exhibiting a particularly strong association with the development of metabolic and cardiovascular disease.[126]

Based on the prevailing data and its protective effects against cardiovascular and metabolic disease development, it would be assumed that lower body subcutaneous fat would be less prone to inflammation. However, the expression and release of various pro-inflammatory signals by lower body fat have been reported to be higher,[127] lower,[128] and no different from subcutaneous abdominal fat, even after weight loss.[129,130] This has been confused further by reports that circulating levels of inflammatory signals can stay high even after substantial weight loss and the restoration of systemic insulin sensitivity,[131] with their expression in fat staying the same[132] or even increasing.[133] Evidently measuring only a handful of inflammatory signals can't provide the detailed, comprehensive picture required to understand the interplay between (depot-specific) adipose inflammation and metabolic health.[134] However, recent efforts with technology that can simultaneously measure numerous inflammatory signals are providing evidence that the secretory profile of inflammatory signals from adipose tissue differs between depots.[135] Moreover, these profiles can distinguish fat from healthy, lean individuals and those who are obese and/or have type 2 diabetes.[136] Although research is still in its early days, it is possible that further studies may lead to methods that could determine one's metabolic health status and future prospects, as well as develop novel treatments that harness the power of the immune system.

Life at the Extremes

The concepts of adipose expandability and personal fat threshold are useful in rationalizing seemingly paradoxical clinical cases. For instance, individuals with a reduced capacity for subcutaneous adipose tissue expansion (i.e., low personal fat threshold) may be predisposed to developing metabolic disease, even at a normal BMI. This predisposition may be due to ectopic lipid deposition which manifests as visceral fat expansion and lipid accumulation in the liver, pancreas, and muscle tissue. This is probably the case for lipodystrophy patients (see Chapter 7) and individuals who develop metabolic disease at a normal BMI (i.e., normal weight obesity; see Chapter 5). On the opposite end of the spectrum, individuals with a greater ability to expand their subcutaneous adipose tissue (i.e., high personal fat threshold) are able to accrue substantial amounts of fat without experiencing any metabolic disturbances.[137] This phenomenon likely applies to overweight or obese people who exhibit normal insulin sensitivity, even if this grace period of seemingly good health may cease at any time. Most importantly, however, is that it can be interpreted that the vast number of people developing metabolic and cardiovascular disease who are normal weight, overweight, obese, or heavier, are likely carrying an amount of fat that exceeds their *own* personal fat threshold. So, while these concepts are useful for understanding *how* different fat depots behave and interact in various clinical cases, we now need to examine the reasons pertaining to *why* fat behaves differently in anatomically distinct depots.

Many of the depot-specific properties observed at the tissue level are actually retained and exhibited at the cellular level *in vitro*.[138,139] This has led to the proposition that these cells retain an 'intrinsic memory' of their anatomical origin (think 'you can take the girl out of the city, but you can't take the city out of the girl'). Not all biological properties survive excision though, indicating that a cell's behaviour likely emerges from a complex interplay between its inherent properties and the local microenvironment[140] (comprising hormones, nutrients, neighbouring cells, the extracellular matrix, etc.). When considering adipose expansion at the cellular level, visceral fat may be predisposed to metabolically unfavourable hypertrophic expansion (in comparison to subcutaneous abdominal fat) due to a reduced progenitor cell pool. Indeed, visceral preadipocytes proliferate more slowly than subcutaneous abdominal cells[141] and are more susceptible to apoptosis[142] (i.e., programmed cell death). Despite some inconsistencies[140,143] (likely due to variation in the donor population, experimental design, and/or culture conditions[139]), visceral preadipocytes reportedly exhibit a much reduced ability to undergo *in vitro* adipogenesis compared to their subcutaneous counterparts.[144-146]

To Make a Fat Cell

Adipogenesis is the process in which preadipocytes undergo the radical transformation into a mature adipocyte. This tightly regulated, temporally co-ordinated multi-step process involves the sequential activation of numerous transcription factors (i.e., proteins which bind to DNA to turn genes on or off). Of these, peroxisome proliferator-activated receptor gamma (PPARG) is thought to be the 'master regulator' of adipogenesis[147] *in vivo* and *in vitro* in humans[148,149] and in mice.[150] The binding of specific molecular signals (i.e., fatty acids) to this transcription factor[151] sets a chain of events in motion that culminate in a preadipocyte differentiating into a mature adipocyte. If adipogenesis were a military operation, PPARG would be the General. PPARG attained the moniker of 'master regulator' following experiments in which artificially introducing this gene into mouse skin cells enabled them to turn into full-fledged adipocytes.[152] Conversely, transgenic mice deficient for PPARG are unable to generate adipose tissue and become lipodystrophic.[150]

Other transcription factors contribute to adipogenesis, with various members of the CCAAT/enhancer-binding protein (i.e., C/EBP) family being particularly prominent. These proteins act to regulate the levels of the other members of their family in addition to the various cellular components required to make a functional mature adipocyte. Adipogenesis involves a carefully co-ordinated rise and fall in the level of the various C/EBP proteins. The levels of C/EBP beta and delta rise[153] early in adipogenesis before falling after they stimulate the expression of C/EBP alpha[154] and PPARG.[155] After induction, C/EBP alpha promotes PPARG expression[156] while maintaining its own expression.[157] This interaction not only promotes the production of cellular machinery which defines the mature adipocyte, it also creates a self-perpetuating positive feedback loop that drives adipogenesis forward to terminal differentiation[158] and then locks the mature adipocyte state.[159] Adipogenesis is a bit like getting a satellite into space in which the satellite locks into a self-sustaining orbit after being released at the right altitude (Figure 6.4).

Much of the data pertaining to adipogenesis have been obtained from studies using a specific type of mouse-derived cell (i.e., 3T3-L1 preadipocytes). While the molecular minutiae of adipogenesis has not been as extensively characterized in human preadipocytes, data indicate that there are many similarities between the species.[160,161] However, significant differences have been reported for white[162,163] and brown[164] adipose tissue, meaning extrapolating between species in the absence of direct comparisons is risky. Further complexity is added when considering that adipogenesis might not be a single phenomenon, but actually several variations on a theme. While adipogenesis is fundamentally co-ordinated by transcription factors such as PPARG and the C/EBPs, preadipocytes and adipocytes from different adipose depots exhibit overlapping but distinct gene expression patterns, with such differences potentially underpinning the functional differences observed at the cellular and tissue level. Imagine adipocytes from different fat depots as distinct buildings in which the same

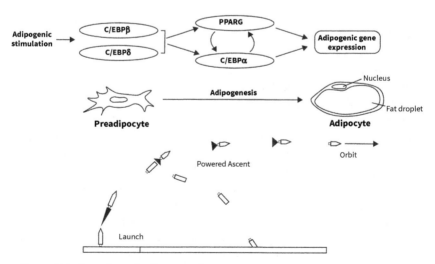

Figure 6.4 Overview of adipogenesis.

fundamental elements (e.g., rooms, doors, furniture, etc.) are arranged differently to fulfil different purposes. In other words, adipocytes from anatomically distinct adipose depots are the same but different.

The results of numerous studies comparing the pattern of gene expression between different adipose tissue depots provide compelling evidence that there are many similarities as well as striking differences. More specifically, the most differentially expressed genes between subcutaneous abdominal and gluteal/femoral depots[128,165–167] or visceral fat[3,168–171] regulate tissue development. The expression of certain differentially expressed genes also reportedly correlates with overall and regional fat mass.[3] Such differences in gene expression do not just passively reflect adipose tissue's anatomical location, like a set of genetic co-ordinates, but actually have functional consequences. For example, expression of the developmental regulator *TBX5* is limited to subcutaneous abdominal preadipocytes, and preventing its expression blocks adipogenesis.[128] Additionally, subcutaneous abdominal and gluteal preadipocytes have been found to exhibit opposite adipogenic responses upon presentation of the same growth factor.[172] Such results not only support the contention that adipogenesis refers to several anatomically distinct processes, but that differential gene expression—alone and in combination—plays a key role in determining fat's depot-specific functional properties. So, what underpins these differential gene expression patterns?

Leaving a Mark

Epigenetics refers to a number of molecular mechanisms that regulate gene expression, particularly DNA methylation, histone modification, and microRNAs (Figure 6.5). Each of these mechanisms has spawned their own sub-specialties within the burgeoning field of epigenetics. Epigenetics builds upon the foundational knowledge of fat development, accumulation, and regional distribution that conventional genetic analyses have provided, which are discussed in greater detail in Chapter 7. In this context, it is important to not get caught up in the molecular minutiae of epigenetic mechanisms and instead appreciate how the 'landscape' of epigenetic marks varies between different mature adipose depots as well as during transformative processes involving significant changes in gene expression (i.e., adipogenesis). Epigenetic regulation of gene expression via DNA methylation and histone modification is a complex and dynamic

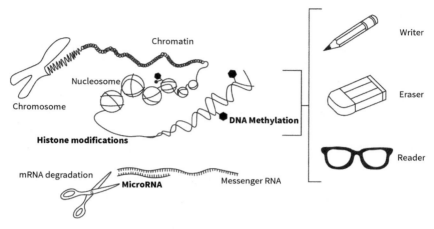

Figure 6.5 Epigenetic regulation of gene expression.

interplay between three broad categories of players; writers, erasers, and readers.[173]

DNA methylation refers to the 'tagging' of a nucleotide (i.e., the building block of DNA) with a 'methyl' chemical group that is typically associated with the switching *off* of the associated gene.[174] The genome-wide pattern of DNA methylation in human preadipocytes reportedly changes substantially during adipogenesis, with such changes being associated with the dramatic shift in the pattern of gene expression which occurs in differentiating cells.[175,176] This interplay is most clearly highlighted in reports that the DNA regions encoding key developmental regulators, such as PPARG,[177] tend to be heavily methylated in preadipocytes, but that a progressive 'de-methylation' and parallel increase in gene expression occurs during adipogenesis. As expected, the DNA methylation profile varies considerably between adipose depots, with specific differences reported between subcutaneous abdominal and visceral fat[178] as well as between upper and lower body subcutaneous fat.[128,179]

Adipose DNA methylation patterns also vary in accordance to metabolic health and obesity status. For instance, numerous studies have reported that DNA methylation patterns vary between visceral[180–182] and subcutaneous abdominal fat[183] taken from healthy individuals compared to those with metabolic disease. Other investigations have found that DNA methylation at specific genomic locations in subcutaneous abdominal and visceral fat are strongly associated with obesity[184,185] and metabolic disease[185,186], specifically in regions associated with adipogenesis, lipid metabolism, adipose tissue expansion, and inflammation.[184,187] The DNA methylation profile of adipose tissue also changes when fat mass and function improve, with significant epigenetic landscape shifts having been observed in subcutaneous abdominal[188] and visceral[189] fat after bariatric surgery-induced weight loss (see Chapter 7) and after a six-month exercise intervention.[190] DNA methylation appears to represent an important middle-man likely involved in co-ordinating adipose tissue's biological response to positive (i.e., exercise and weight loss) and deleterious (i.e., weight gain) stimuli.

Chromatin is another crucial aspect of the epigenetic landscape that undergoes considerable remodelling to support changes in gene expression of entire gene networks involved in adipogenesis and mature adipocyte function in health and disease. Chromatin is the highly sophisticated protein structure around which DNA is wrapped, with its arrangement determining whether a region of DNA is 'open' or 'closed' for business. Chemical modifications to the constituent histone proteins influence their structure to permit or deny access to the associated genomic region. At the molecular level, the outcome of this biological tug of war is determined by the balance of activity between enzymes that attach (writers) or remove (erasers) epigenetic marks that open or close chromatin structure and direct the action of 'readers' to determine whether a gene is expressed or not.[191]

The pattern of histone modifications undergoes significant remodelling during adipogenesis,[192] likely to support the associated widespread changes in gene expression. Several studies have highlighted that the expression levels of key co-ordinators of adipogenesis such as PPARG[193,194] and the members of the C/EBP family[194,195] are regulated by histone modifications. Associations between specific chromatin modifications in visceral fat have also been observed in relation to BMI and insulin sensitivity.[196] While much remains to be learned about histone modification's role in (regional) adipose function and dysfunction, there has been increasing interest in drugs that modify the action of specific histone-modifying enzymes (and therefore gene expression) as a novel approach to treat obesity and metabolic disease.[197]

Redirecting the Mail

The other main epigenetic regulatory mechanism likely involved in determining adipose tissue's depot-specific biology concerns the expression of *microRNAs*, which are small molecules that can modulate the expression of entire gene networks by targeting messenger RNA molecules for degradation.[198] DNA is essentially a database containing the blueprints for a cell and assembling a component involves making a copy of the original blueprint (i.e., messenger RNA), and then dispatching it to the manufacturing department via mail service. As the copied blueprints for a cellular component have an identifying tag (like a barcoded envelope), specific microRNAs can intercept and destroy the manufacturing order. As the instructions for distinct cellular components which act together (directly or indirectly) often share the same identifying tag, a single microRNA variant can regulate entire gene networks. Numerous microRNAs exist which influence multiple distinct but overlapping gene networks, meaning these molecules can exert far-reaching yet exquisitely precise control over the expression of many genes to enable a cell to rapidly shift its biological trajectory in response to any number of factors.

MicroRNAs appear to play a crucial role in supporting the substantial shift in gene expression that underpins adipogenesis,[199] with this cellular transformation not occurring if the expression of certain microRNAs is prevented.[200] Additionally, microRNAs have been implicated in the regulation of depot-specific gene expression (and therefore functional properties) as the expression profile of microRNAs varies considerably between subcutaneous fat from the abdomen and lower body[201] and visceral fat.[202] This contention is exemplified in the report that the exact same microRNA promoted adipogenesis in subcutaneous, but not visceral, preadipocytes.[203] Due to the highly specific yet broad-acting nature of these molecules, it is possible that they not only represent a novel treatment approach for obesity and metabolic disease, but can also act as biomarkers that can be used to identify disease risk and/or progression.[204,205]

It is important to note that while the different epigenetic mechanisms have important effects in isolation, extensive two-way interactions occur between the different 'dimensions' of gene expression regulation. Indeed, whether a gene is turned on or off at any given moment involves integrating (at least) DNA methylation, histone modification, and microRNA action, as well as transcription factor binding. And while each regulatory system makes a contribution, its relative importance may change depending on the scenario. For instance, recent data suggest that transcription factors play a primary role in co-ordinating gene expression early in adipogenesis, while the terminally differentiated state (i.e., mature adipocyte) is largely defined by histone modifications which stabilize the gene expression profile.[206] Epigenetic profiles may also influence how adipose tissue integrates external signals (e.g., hormones and nutrients) and what response it mounts.[207] Evidently a great deal remains to be learned about the role of epigenetics in adipose tissue function in health and disease, but it is clear that these mechanisms represent a great potential power waiting to be harnessed.

References

1. Cerhan, J. R. *et al.* A pooled analysis of waist circumference and mortality in 650,000 adults. *Mayo Clin. Proc.* **89**, 335–45 (2014).
2. Chusyd, D. E., Wang, D., Huffman, D. M., & Nagy, T. R. Relationships between rodent white adipose fat pads and human white adipose fat depots. *Front. Nutr.* **3**, 10 (2016).
3. Gesta, S. *et al.* Evidence for a role of developmental genes in the origin of obesity and body fat distribution. *Proc. Natl. Acad. Sci. U. S. A.* **103**, 6676–81 (2006).
4. Tchkonia, T. *et al.* Fat tissue, aging, and cellular senescence. *Aging Cell* **9**, 667–84 (2010).
5. Lee, M.-J., Wu, Y., & Fried, S. K. Adipose tissue heterogeneity: implication of depot differences in adipose tissue for obesity complications. *Mol. Aspects Med.* **34**, 1–11 (2013).
6. Wang, Q. A., Tao, C., Gupta, R. K., & Scherer, P. E. Tracking adipogenesis during white adipose tissue development, expansion and regeneration. *Nat. Med.* **19**, 1338–44 (2013).
7. Frayn, K. N. & Karpe, F. Regulation of human subcutaneous adipose tissue blood flow. *Int. J. Obes.* **38**, 1019–26 (2014).
8. Tan, G. D., Goossens, G. H., Humphreys, S. M., Vidal, H., & Karpe, F. Upper and lower body adipose tissue function: a direct comparison of fat mobilization in humans. *Obes. Res.* **12**, 114–18 (2004).
9. Karpe, F., Fielding, B. A., Ilic, V., Humphreys, S. M., & Frayn, K. N. Monitoring adipose tissue blood flow in man: a comparison between the 133xenon washout method and microdialysis. *Int. J. Obes.* **26**, 1 (2002).
10. Summers, L. K., Samra, J. S., Humphreys, S. M., Morris, R. J., & Frayn, K. N. Subcutaneous abdominal adipose tissue blood flow: variation within and between subjects and relationship to obesity. *Clin. Sci.* **91**, 679–83 (1996).
11. Engin, A. B. What is lipotoxicity? *Adv. Exp. Med. Biol.* **960**, 197–220 (2017).
12. Romanski, S. A., Nelson, R. M., & Jensen, M. D. Meal fatty acid uptake in adipose tissue: gender effects in nonobese humans. *Am. J. Physiol. Endocrinol. Metab.* **279**, E455–62 (2000).
13. Iozzo, P. *et al.* The interaction of blood flow, insulin, and bradykinin in regulating glucose uptake in lower-body adipose tissue in lean and obese subjects. *J. Clin. Endocrinol. Metab.* **97**, E1192–6 (2012).

14. Karpe, F. *et al.* Impaired postprandial adipose tissue blood flow response is related to aspects of insulin sensitivity. *Diabetes* 51, 2467–73 (2002).
15. Tobin, L., Simonsen, L., & Bülow, J. The dynamics of the microcirculation in the subcutaneous adipose tissue is impaired in the postprandial state in type 2 diabetes. *Clin. Physiol. Funct. Imaging* 31, 458–63 (2011).
16. Karpe, F. *et al.* Effects of insulin on adipose tissue blood flow in man. *J. Physiol.* 540, 1087–93 (2002).
17. Ardilouze, J.-L., Fielding, B. A., Currie, J. M., Frayn, K. N., & Karpe, F. Nitric oxide and beta-adrenergic stimulation are major regulators of preprandial and postprandial subcutaneous adipose tissue blood flow in humans. *Circulation* 109, 47–52 (2004).
18. Koutsari, C., Snozek, C. L. H., & Jensen, M. D. Plasma NEFA storage in adipose tissue in the postprandial state: sex-related and regional differences. *Diabetologia* 51, 2041–8 (2008).
19. Meek, S. E., Nair, K. S., & Jensen, M. D. Insulin regulation of regional free fatty acid metabolism. *Diabetes* 48, 10–14 (1999).
20. Mårin, P., Rebuffé-Scrive, M., & Björntorp, P. Uptake of triglyceride fatty acids in adipose tissue in vivo in man. *Eur. J. Clin. Invest.* 20, 158–65 (1990).
21. Votruba, S. B. & Jensen, M. D. Short-term regional meal fat storage in nonobese humans is not a predictor of long-term regional fat gain. *Am. J. Physiol. Endocrinol. Metab.* 302, E1078–83 (2012).
22. Shadid, S., Koutsari, C., & Jensen, M. D. Direct free fatty acid uptake into human adipocytes in vivo: relation to body fat distribution. *Diabetes* 56, 1369–75 (2007).
23. Koutsari, C., Ali, A. H., Mundi, M. S., & Jensen, M. D. Storage of circulating free fatty acid in adipose tissue of postabsorptive humans: quantitative measures and implications for body fat distribution. *Diabetes* 60, 2032–40 (2011).
24. McQuaid, S. E. *et al.* Femoral adipose tissue may accumulate the fat that has been recycled as VLDL and nonesterified fatty acids. *Diabetes* 59, 2465–73 (2010).
25. Spencer, M. *et al.* Adipose tissue extracellular matrix and vascular abnormalities in obesity and insulin resistance. *J. Clin. Endocrinol. Metab.* 96, E1990–8 (2011).
26. Dimitriadis, G. *et al.* Impaired postprandial blood flow in adipose tissue may be an early marker of insulin resistance in type 2 diabetes. *Diabetes Care* 30, 3128–30 (2007).
27. Jansson, P. A., Larsson, A., & Lönnroth, P. N. Relationship between blood pressure, metabolic variables and blood flow in obese subjects with or without non-insulin-dependent diabetes mellitus. *Eur. J. Clin. Invest.* 28, 813–18 (1998).
28. Lambadiari, V. *et al.* Increases in muscle blood flow after a mixed meal are impaired at all stages of type 2 diabetes. *Clin. Endocrinol.* 76, 825–30 (2012).
29. Asmar, M. *et al.* Glucose-dependent insulinotropic polypeptide has impaired effect on abdominal, subcutaneous adipose tissue metabolism in obese subjects. *Int. J. Obes.* 38, 259–65 (2014).

30. Jensen, M. D. & Johnson, C. M. Contribution of leg and splanchnic free fatty acid (FFA) kinetics to postabsorptive FFA flux in men and women. *Metabolism.* 45, 662–6 (1996).

31. Martin, M. L. & Jensen, M. D. Effects of body fat distribution on regional lipolysis in obesity. *J. Clin. Invest.* 88, 609–13 (1991).

32. Guo, Z., Hensrud, D. D., Johnson, C. M., & Jensen, M. D. Regional postprandial fatty acid metabolism in different obesity phenotypes. *Diabetes* 48, 1586–92 (1999).

33. Arner, P., Kriegholm, E., Engfeldt, P., & Bolinder, J. Adrenergic regulation of lipolysis in situ at rest and during exercise. *J. Clin. Invest.* 85, 893–8 (1990).

34. Mårin, P., Rebuffé-Scrive, M., Smith, U., & Björntorp, P. Glucose uptake in human adipose tissue. *Metabolism.* 36, 1154–60 (1987).

35. Jensen, M. D., Cryer, P. E., Johnson, C. M., & Murray, M. J. Effects of epinephrine on regional free fatty acid and energy metabolism in men and women. *Am. J. Physiol.* 270, E259–64 (1996).

36. Manolopoulos, K. N., Karpe, F., & Frayn, K. N. Marked resistance of femoral adipose tissue blood flow and lipolysis to adrenaline in vivo. *Diabetologia* 55, 3029–37 (2012).

37. Wahrenberg, H., Lönnqvist, F., & Arner, P. Mechanisms underlying regional differences in lipolysis in human adipose tissue. *J. Clin. Invest.* 84, 458–67 (1989).

38. Galitzky, J., Lafontan, M., Nordenström, J., & Arner, P. Role of vascular alpha-2 adrenoceptors in regulating lipid mobilization from human adipose tissue. *J. Clin. Invest.* 91, 1997–2003 (1993).

39. Heinonen, I. *et al.* Regulation of subcutaneous adipose tissue blood flow during exercise in humans. *J. Appl. Physiol.* 112, 1059–63 (2012).

40. Gjedsted, J. *et al.* Effects of a 3-day fast on regional lipid and glucose metabolism in human skeletal muscle and adipose tissue. *Acta Physiol.* 191, 205–16 (2007).

41. Lassek, W. D. & Gaulin, S. J. C. Changes in body fat distribution in relation to parity in American women: a covert form of maternal depletion. *Am. J. Phys. Anthropol.* 131, 295–302 (2006).

42. Kramer, F. M., Stunkard, A. J., Marshall, K. A., McKinney, S., & Liebschutz, J. Breast-feeding reduces maternal lower-body fat. *J. Am. Diet. Assoc.* 93, 429–33 (1993).

43. Jové, M. *et al.* Human omental and subcutaneous adipose tissue exhibit specific lipidomic signatures. *FASEB J.* 28, 1071–81 (2014).

44. Petrus, P. *et al.* Depot-specific differences in fatty acid composition and distinct associations with lipogenic gene expression in abdominal adipose tissue of obese women. *Int. J. Obes.* 41, 1295–8 (2017).

45. Cao, H. *et al.* Identification of a lipokine, a lipid hormone linking adipose tissue to systemic metabolism. *Cell* 134, 933–44 (2008).

46. Stefan, N. *et al.* Circulating palmitoleate strongly and independently predicts insulin sensitivity in humans. *Diabetes Care* 33, 405–7 (2010).

47. Pinnick, K. E. *et al.* Gluteofemoral adipose tissue plays a major role in production of the lipokine palmitoleate in humans. *Diabetes* 61, 1399–403 (2012).

48. Lee, J. J. *et al.* Palmitoleic acid is elevated in fatty liver disease and reflects hepatic lipogenesis. *Am. J. Clin. Nutr.* **101**, 34–43 (2015).

49. Merino, J. *et al.* Serum palmitoleate acts as a lipokine in subjects at high cardiometabolic risk. *Nutr. Metab. Cardiovasc. Dis.* **26**, 261–7 (2016).

50. Ashley, D. J. The two 'hit' and multiple 'hit' theories of carcinogenesis. *Br. J. Cancer* **23**, 313–28 (1969).

51. Smith, S. R. *et al.* Contributions of total body fat, abdominal subcutaneous adipose tissue compartments, and visceral adipose tissue to the metabolic complications of obesity. *Metabolism.* **50**, 425–35 (2001).

52. Carobbio, S., Pellegrinelli, V., & Vidal-Puig, A. Adipose tissue function and expandability as determinants of lipotoxicity and the metabolic syndrome. *Adv. Exp. Med. Biol.* **960**, 161–96 (2017).

53. Lim, S. & Meigs, J. B. Ectopic fat and cardiometabolic and vascular risk. *Int. J. Cardiol.* **169**, 166–76 (2013).

54. McLaughlin, T., Lamendola, C., Liu, A., & Abbasi, F. Preferential fat deposition in subcutaneous versus visceral depots is associated with insulin sensitivity. *J. Clin. Endocrinol. Metab.* **96**, E1756–60 (2011).

55. Alligier, M. *et al.* Visceral fat accumulation during lipid overfeeding is related to subcutaneous adipose tissue characteristics in healthy men. *J. Clin. Endocrinol. Metab.* **98**, 802–10 (2013).

56. Gyllenhammer, L. E., Alderete, T. L., Toledo-Corral, C. M., Weigensberg, M., & Goran, M. I. Saturation of subcutaneous adipose tissue expansion and accumulation of ectopic fat associated with metabolic dysfunction during late and post-pubertal growth. *Int. J. Obes.* **40**, 601–6 (2016).

57. Serra, M. C., Ryan, A. S., & Goldberg, A. P. Reduced LPL and subcutaneous lipid storage capacity are associated with metabolic syndrome in postmenopausal women with obesity. *Obes. Sci. Pract.* **3**, 106–14 (2017).

58. Bays, H. Central obesity as a clinical marker of adiposopathy; increased visceral adiposity as a surrogate marker for global fat dysfunction. *Curr. Opin. Endocrinol. Diabetes. Obes.* **21**, 345–51 (2014).

59. Hwang, Y.-C. *et al.* Visceral abdominal fat accumulation predicts the conversion of metabolically healthy obese subjects to an unhealthy phenotype. *Int. J. Obes.* **39**, 1365–70 (2015).

60. Kang, Y. M. *et al.* Visceral adiposity index predicts the conversion of metabolically healthy obesity to an unhealthy phenotype. *PLoS One* **12**, e0179635 (2017).

61. Taylor, R. & Holman, R. R. Normal weight individuals who develop type 2 diabetes: the personal fat threshold. *Clin. Sci.* **128**, 405–10 (2015).

62. In praise of embonpoint. *Lancet* **2**, 491–2 (1987).

63. Forth, C. E. *Fat: A Cultural History of the Stuff of Life.* Reaktion Books, 2019.

64. Eknoyan, G. A history of obesity, or how what was good became ugly and then bad. *Adv. Chronic Kidney Dis.* **13**, 421–7 (2006).

65. Rydén, M., Andersson, D. P., Bergström, I. B., & Arner, P. Adipose tissue and metabolic alterations: regional differences in fat cell size and number matter, but differently: a cross-sectional study. *J. Clin. Endocrinol. Metab.* **99**, E1870–6 (2014).

66. Drolet, R. *et al.* Hypertrophy and hyperplasia of abdominal adipose tissues in women. *Int. J. Obes.* **32**, 283–91 (2008).

67. Tchoukalova, Y. D. *et al.* Regional differences in cellular mechanisms of adipose tissue gain with overfeeding. *Proc. Natl. Acad. Sci. U. S. A.* **107**, 18226–31 (2010).

68. White, U. A., Fitch, M. D., Beyl, R. A., Hellerstein, M. K., & Ravussin, E. Differences in in vivo cellular kinetics in abdominal and femoral subcutaneous adipose tissue in women. *Diabetes* **65**, 1642–7 (2016).

69. Spalding, K. L. *et al.* Dynamics of fat cell turnover in humans. *Nature* **453**, 783–7 (2008).

70. Laforest, S., Labrecque, J., Michaud, A., Cianflone, K., & Tchernof, A. Adipocyte size as a determinant of metabolic disease and adipose tissue dysfunction. *Crit. Rev. Clin. Lab. Sci.* **52**, 301–13 (2015).

71. Björntorp, P. *et al.* Adipose tissue fat cell size in relation to metabolism in weight-stabile, physically active men. *Horm. Metab. Res.* **4**, 182–6 (1972).

72. Hoffstedt, J. *et al.* Regional impact of adipose tissue morphology on the metabolic profile in morbid obesity. *Diabetologia* **53**, 2496–503 (2010).

73. Ryden, M. & Arner, P. Cardiovascular risk score is linked to subcutaneous adipocyte size and lipid metabolism. *J. Intern. Med.* **282**, 220–8 (2017).

74. Acosta, J. R. *et al.* Increased fat cell size: a major phenotype of subcutaneous white adipose tissue in non-obese individuals with type 2 diabetes. *Diabetologia* **59**, 560–70 (2016).

75. Henninger, A. M. J., Eliasson, B., Jenndahl, L. E., & Hammarstedt, A. Adipocyte hypertrophy, inflammation and fibrosis characterize subcutaneous adipose tissue of healthy, non-obese subjects predisposed to type 2 diabetes. *PLoS One* **9**, e105262 (2014).

76. Hammarstedt, A., Graham, T. E., & Kahn, B. B. Adipose tissue dysregulation and reduced insulin sensitivity in non-obese individuals with enlarged abdominal adipose cells. *Diabetol. Metab. Syndr.* **4**, 42 (2012).

77. Eriksson-Hogling, D. *et al.* Adipose tissue morphology predicts improved insulin sensitivity following moderate or pronounced weight loss. *Int. J. Obes.* **39**, 893–8 (2015).

78. Weyer, C., Foley, J. E., Bogardus, C., Tataranni, P. A., & Pratley, R. E. Enlarged subcutaneous abdominal adipocyte size, but not obesity itself, predicts type II diabetes independent of insulin resistance. *Diabetologia* **43**, 1498–506 (2000).

79. McLaughlin, T. *et al.* Adipose cell size and regional fat deposition as predictors of metabolic response to overfeeding in insulin-resistant and insulin-sensitive humans. *Diabetes* **65**, 1245–54 (2016).

80. Arner, E. *et al.* Adipocyte turnover: relevance to human adipose tissue morphology. *Diabetes* **59**, 105–9 (2010).

81. Lin, D., Chun, T.-H., & Kang, L. Adipose extracellular matrix remodelling in obesity and insulin resistance. *Biochem. Pharmacol.* **119**, 8–16 (2016).

82. Choe, S. S., Huh, J. Y., Hwang, I. J., Kim, J. I., & Kim, J. B. Adipose tissue remodeling: its role in energy metabolism and metabolic disorders. *Front. Endocrinol.* **7**, 30 (2016).

83. Catalán, V., Gómez-Ambrosi, J., Rodríguez, A., & Frühbeck, G. Role of extracellular matrix remodelling in adipose tissue pathophysiology: relevance in the development of obesity. *Histol. Histopathol.* **27**, 1515–28 (2012).

84. Williams, A. S., Kang, L., & Wasserman, D. H. The extracellular matrix and insulin resistance. *Trends Endocrinol. Metab.* **26**, 357–66 (2015).

85. Mori, S., Kiuchi, S., Ouchi, A., Hase, T., & Murase, T. Characteristic expression of extracellular matrix in subcutaneous adipose tissue development and adipogenesis; comparison with visceral adipose tissue. *Int. J. Biol. Sci.* **10**, 825–33 (2014).

86. Roca-Rivada, A. *et al.* CILAIR-based secretome analysis of obese visceral and subcutaneous adipose tissues reveals distinctive ECM remodeling and inflammation mediators. *Sci. Rep.* **5**, 12214 (2015).

87. Pellegrinelli, V., Carobbio, S., & Vidal-Puig, A. Adipose tissue plasticity: how fat depots respond differently to pathophysiological cues. *Diabetologia* **59**, 1075–88 (2016).

88. Nakajima, I., Yamaguchi, T., Ozutsumi, K., & Aso, H. Adipose tissue extracellular matrix: newly organized by adipocytes during differentiation. *Differentiation* **63**, 193–200 (1998).

89. Nakajima, I., Muroya, S., Tanabe, R., & Chikuni, K. Extracellular matrix development during differentiation into adipocytes with a unique increase in type V and VI collagen. *Biol. cell* **94**, 197–203 (2002).

90. Grandl, G. *et al.* Depot specific differences in the adipogenic potential of precursors are mediated by collagenous extracellular matrix and Flotillin 2 dependent signaling. *Mol. Metab.* **5**, 937–47 (2016).

91. Alligier, M. *et al.* Subcutaneous adipose tissue remodeling during the initial phase of weight gain induced by overfeeding in humans. *J. Clin. Endocrinol. Metab.* **97**, E183–92 (2012).

92. Henegar, C. *et al.* Adipose tissue transcriptomic signature highlights the pathological relevance of extracellular matrix in human obesity. *Genome Biol.* **9**, R14 (2008).

93. Divoux, A. *et al.* Fibrosis in human adipose tissue: composition, distribution, and link with lipid metabolism and fat mass loss. *Diabetes* **59**, 2817–25 (2010).

94. Abdennour, M. *et al.* Association of adipose tissue and liver fibrosis with tissue stiffness in morbid obesity: links with diabetes and BMI loss after gastric bypass. *J. Clin. Endocrinol. Metab.* **99**, 898–907 (2014).

95. Lackey, D. E. *et al.* Contributions of adipose tissue architectural and tensile properties toward defining healthy and unhealthy obesity. *Am. J. Physiol. Endocrinol. Metab.* **306**, E233–46 (2014).

96. Michaud, A. *et al.* Relevance of omental pericellular adipose tissue collagen in the pathophysiology of human abdominal obesity and related cardiometabolic risk. *Int. J. Obes.* **40**, 1823–31 (2016).

97. Gealekman, O. *et al.* Depot-specific differences and insufficient subcutaneous adipose tissue angiogenesis in human obesity. *Circulation* **123**, 186–94 (2011).

98. Khan, T. *et al.* Metabolic dysregulation and adipose tissue fibrosis: role of collagen VI. *Mol. Cell. Biol.* **29**, 1575–91 (2009).

99. Dankel, S. N. *et al.* COL6A3 expression in adipocytes associates with insulin resistance and depends on PPARγ and adipocyte size. *Obesity (Silver Spring)* **22**, 1807–13 (2014).

100. McCulloch, L. J. *et al.* COL6A3 is regulated by leptin in human adipose tissue and reduced in obesity. *Endocrinology* **156**, 134–46 (2015).

101. Pasarica, M. *et al.* Adipose tissue collagen VI in obesity. *J. Clin. Endocrinol. Metab.* **94**, 5155–62 (2009).

102. Mutch, D. M. *et al.* Needle and surgical biopsy techniques differentially affect adipose tissue gene expression profiles. *Am. J. Clin. Nutr.* **89**, 51–7 (2009).

103. Sun, K. *et al.* Endotrophin triggers adipose tissue fibrosis and metabolic dysfunction. *Nat. Commun.* **5**, 3485 (2014).

104. Park, J. & Scherer, P. E. Adipocyte-derived endotrophin promotes malignant tumor progression. *J. Clin. Invest.* **122**, 4243–56 (2012).

105. Funcke, J.-B. & Scherer, P. E. Beyond adiponectin and leptin: adipose tissue-derived mediators of inter-organ communication. *J. Lipid Res.* **60**, 1648–84 (2019).

106. Divoux, A. & Clément, K. Architecture and the extracellular matrix: the still unappreciated components of the adipose tissue. *Obes. Rev.* **12**, e494–503 (2011).

107. Pirola, L. & Ferraz, J. C. Role of pro- and anti-inflammatory phenomena in the physiopathology of type 2 diabetes and obesity. *World J. Biol. Chem.* **8**, 120–8 (2017).

108. Gerner, R. R., Wieser, V., Moschen, A. R., & Tilg, H. Metabolic inflammation: role of cytokines in the crosstalk between adipose tissue and liver. *Can. J. Physiol. Pharmacol.* **91**, 867–72 (2013).

109. Lee, B.-C. & Lee, J. Cellular and molecular players in adipose tissue inflammation in the development of obesity-induced insulin resistance. *Biochim. Biophys. Acta* **1842**, 446–62 (2014).

110. Blüher, M. Adipose tissue inflammation: a cause or consequence of obesity-related insulin resistance? *Clin. Sci.* **130**, 1603–14 (2016).

111. Wernstedt Asterholm, I. *et al.* Adipocyte inflammation is essential for healthy adipose tissue expansion and remodeling. *Cell Metab.* **20**, 103–18 (2014).

112. Esser, N., Paquot, N., & Scheen, A. J. Anti-inflammatory agents to treat or prevent type 2 diabetes, metabolic syndrome and cardiovascular disease. *Expert Opin. Investig. Drugs* **24**, 283–307 (2015).

113. Zhu, Q. *et al.* Suppressing adipocyte inflammation promotes insulin resistance in mice. *Mol. Metab.* **39**, 101010 (2020).

114. Sun, S., Ji, Y., Kersten, S., & Qi, L. Mechanisms of inflammatory responses in obese adipose tissue. *Annu. Rev. Nutr.* **32**, 261–86 (2012).

115. Kohlgruber, A. & Lynch, L. Adipose tissue inflammation in the pathogenesis of type 2 diabetes. *Curr. Diab. Rep.* **15**, 92 (2015).

116. Liu, L. F. *et al.* Adipose tissue macrophages impair preadipocyte differentiation in humans. *PLoS One* **12**, e0170728 (2017).

117. Isakson, P., Hammarstedt, A., Gustafson, B., & Smith, U. Impaired preadipocyte differentiation in human abdominal obesity: role of Wnt, tumor necrosis factor-alpha, and inflammation. *Diabetes* **58**, 1550–7 (2009).

118. Saltiel, A. R. & Olefsky, J. M. Inflammatory mechanisms linking obesity and metabolic disease. *J. Clin. Invest.* **127**, 1–4 (2017).

119. Travers, R. L., Motta, A. C., Betts, J. A., Bouloumié, A., & Thompson, D. The impact of adiposity on adipose tissue-resident lymphocyte activation in humans. *Int. J. Obes.* **39**, 762–9 (2015).

120. Klimcáková, E. *et al.* Worsening of obesity and metabolic status yields similar molecular adaptations in human subcutaneous and visceral adipose tissue: decreased metabolism and increased immune response. *J. Clin. Endocrinol. Metab.* **96**, E73–82 (2011).

121. Klimcakova, E. *et al.* Macrophage gene expression is related to obesity and the metabolic syndrome in human subcutaneous fat as well as in visceral fat. *Diabetologia* **54**, 876–87 (2011).

122. Bigornia, S. J. *et al.* Relation of depot-specific adipose inflammation to insulin resistance in human obesity. *Nutr. Diabetes* **2**, e30 (2012).

123. Michaud, A., Drolet, R., Noël, S., Paris, G., & Tchernof, A. Visceral fat accumulation is an indicator of adipose tissue macrophage infiltration in women. *Metabolism* **61**, 689–98 (2012).

124. du Plessis, J. *et al.* Association of adipose tissue inflammation with histologic severity of nonalcoholic fatty liver disease. *Gastroenterology* **149**, 635–48.e14 (2015).

125. Cancello, R. *et al.* Increased infiltration of macrophages in omental adipose tissue is associated with marked hepatic lesions in morbid human obesity. *Diabetes* **55**, 1554–61 (2006).

126. Kranendonk, M. E. G. *et al.* Inflammatory characteristics of distinct abdominal adipose tissue depots relate differently to metabolic risk factors for cardiovascular disease: distinct fat depots and vascular risk factors. *Atherosclerosis* **239**, 419–27 (2015).

127. Evans, J. *et al.* Depot- and ethnic-specific differences in the relationship between adipose tissue inflammation and insulin sensitivity. *Clin. Endocrinol.* **74**, 51–9 (2011).

128. Pinnick, K. E. *et al.* Distinct developmental profile of lower-body adipose tissue defines resistance against obesity-associated metabolic complications. *Diabetes* **63**, 3785–97 (2014).

129. You, T. *et al.* Regional adipose tissue hormone/cytokine production before and after weight loss in abdominally obese women. *Obesity (Silver Spring)* **22**, 1679–84 (2014).

130. Mališová, L. *et al.* Expression of inflammation-related genes in gluteal and abdominal subcutaneous adipose tissue during weight-reducing dietary intervention in obese women. *Physiol. Res.* **63**, 73–82 (2014).

131. Solá, E. *et al.* Parameters of inflammation in morbid obesity: lack of effect of moderate weight loss. *Obes. Surg.* **19**, 571–6 (2009).

132. Hagman, D. K. *et al.* The short-term and long-term effects of bariatric/metabolic surgery on subcutaneous adipose tissue inflammation in humans. *Metabolism.* **70**, 12–22 (2017).

133. Salas-Salvadó, J. *et al.* Subcutaneous adipose tissue cytokine production is not responsible for the restoration of systemic inflammation markers during weight loss. *Int. J. Obes.* **30**, 1714–20 (2006).
134. Dam, V., Sikder, T., & Santosa, S. From neutrophils to macrophages: differences in regional adipose tissue depots. *Obes. Rev.* **17**, 1–17 (2016).
135. Spoto, B. *et al.* Pro- and anti-inflammatory cytokine gene expression in subcutaneous and visceral fat in severe obesity. *Nutr. Metab. Cardiovasc. Dis.* **24**, 1137–43 (2014).
136. Unamuno, X. *et al.* Adipokine dysregulation and adipose tissue inflammation in human obesity. *Eur. J. Clin. Invest.* e12997 (2018). doi:10.1111/eci.12997
137. Cuthbertson, D. J. *et al.* What have human experimental overfeeding studies taught us about adipose tissue expansion and susceptibility to obesity and metabolic complications? *Int. J. Obes.* **41**, 853–65 (2017).
138. Karpe, F. & Pinnick, K. E. Biology of upper-body and lower-body adipose tissue--link to whole-body phenotypes. *Nat. Rev. Endocrinol.* **11**, 90–100 (2015).
139. Tchkonia, T. *et al.* Mechanisms and metabolic implications of regional differences among fat depots. *Cell Metab.* **17**, 644–56 (2013).
140. Tchoukalova, Y. D. *et al.* Sex- and depot-dependent differences in adipogenesis in normal-weight humans. *Obesity (Silver Spring)* **18**, 1875–80 (2010).
141. Tchkonia, T. *et al.* Abundance of two human preadipocyte subtypes with distinct capacities for replication, adipogenesis, and apoptosis varies among fat depots. *Am. J. Physiol. Endocrinol. Metab.* **288**, E267–77 (2005).
142. Niesler, C. U., Siddle, K., & Prins, J. B. Human preadipocytes display a depot-specific susceptibility to apoptosis. *Diabetes* **47**, 1365–8 (1998).
143. Van Harmelen, V., Röhrig, K., & Hauner, H. Comparison of proliferation and differentiation capacity of human adipocyte precursor cells from the omental and subcutaneous adipose tissue depot of obese subjects. *Metabolism.* **53**, 632–7 (2004).
144. Adams, M. *et al.* Activators of peroxisome proliferator-activated receptor gamma have depot-specific effects on human preadipocyte differentiation. *J. Clin. Invest.* **100**, 3149–53 (1997).
145. Hauner, H., Wabitsch, M., & Pfeiffer, E. F. Differentiation of adipocyte precursor cells from obese and nonobese adult women and from different adipose tissue sites. *Horm. Metab. Res. Suppl.* **19**, 35–9 (1988).
146. Tchkonia, T. *et al.* Fat depot origin affects adipogenesis in primary cultured and cloned human preadipocytes. *Am. J. Physiol. Regul. Integr. Comp. Physiol.* **282**, R1286–96 (2002).
147. Shao, X. *et al.* Peroxisome proliferator-activated receptor-γ: master regulator of adipogenesis and obesity. *Curr. Stem Cell Res. Ther.* **11**, 282–9 (2016).
148. Rosen, E. D., Walkey, C. J., Puigserver, P., & Spiegelman, B. M. Transcriptional regulation of adipogenesis. *Genes Dev.* **14**, 1293–307 (2000).
149. Fajas, L. *et al.* E2Fs regulate adipocyte differentiation. *Dev. Cell* **3**, 39–49 (2002).
150. Rosen, E. D. *et al.* PPAR gamma is required for the differentiation of adipose tissue in vivo and in vitro. *Mol. Cell* **4**, 611–17 (1999).

151. Hallenborg, P. *et al.* The elusive endogenous adipogenic PPARγ agonists: lining up the suspects. *Prog. Lipid Res.* **61**, 149–62 (2016).
152. Tontonoz, P., Hu, E., & Spiegelman, B. M. Stimulation of adipogenesis in fibroblasts by PPAR gamma 2, a lipid-activated transcription factor. *Cell* **79**, 1147–56 (1994).
153. Tang, Q. Q. & Lane, M. D. Activation and centromeric localization of CCAAT/enhancer-binding proteins during the mitotic clonal expansion of adipocyte differentiation. *Genes Dev.* **13**, 2231–41 (1999).
154. Tang, Q.-Q., Zhang, J.-W., & Daniel Lane, M. Sequential gene promoter interactions of C/EBPbeta, C/EBPalpha, and PPARgamma during adipogenesis. *Biochem. Biophys. Res. Commun.* **319**, 235–9 (2004).
155. Zuo, Y., Qiang, L., & Farmer, S. R. Activation of CCAAT/enhancer-binding protein (C/EBP) alpha expression by C/EBP beta during adipogenesis requires a peroxisome proliferator-activated receptor-gamma-associated repression of HDAC1 at the C/ebp alpha gene promoter. *J. Biol. Chem.* **281**, 7960–7 (2006).
156. Wu, Z. *et al.* Cross-regulation of C/EBP alpha and PPAR gamma controls the transcriptional pathway of adipogenesis and insulin sensitivity. *Mol. Cell* **3**, 151–8 (1999).
157. Timchenko, N. *et al.* Autoregulation of the human C/EBP alpha gene by stimulation of upstream stimulatory factor binding. *Mol. Cell. Biol.* **15**, 1192–202 (1995).
158. Rosen, E. D. Molecular mechanisms of adipocyte differentiation. *Ann. Endocrinol.* **63**, 79–82 (2002).
159. Park, B. O., Ahrends, R., & Teruel, M. N. Consecutive positive feedback loops create a bistable switch that controls preadipocyte-to-adipocyte conversion. *Cell Rep.* **2**, 976–90 (2012).
160. Todoric, J. *et al.* Cross-talk between interferon-γ and hedgehog signaling regulates adipogenesis. *Diabetes* **60**, 1668–76 (2011).
161. Moreno-Navarrete, J. M. *et al.* Study of lactoferrin gene expression in human and mouse adipose tissue, human preadipocytes and mouse 3T3-L1 fibroblasts. Association with adipogenic and inflammatory markers. *J. Nutr. Biochem.* **24**, 1266–75 (2013).
162. Gagnon, A., Foster, C., Landry, A., & Sorisky, A. The role of interleukin 1 in the anti-adipogenic action of macrophages on human preadipocytes. *J. Endocrinol.* **217**, 197–206 (2013).
163. Ruiz-Ojeda, F. J., Rupérez, A. I., Gomez-Llorente, C., Gil, A., & Aguilera, C. M. Cell models and their application for studying adipogenic differentiation in relation to obesity: a review. *Int. J. Mol. Sci.* **17**, (2016).
164. Zuriaga, M. A., Fuster, J. J., Gokce, N., & Walsh, K. Humans and mice display opposing patterns of 'browning' gene expression in visceral and subcutaneous white adipose tissue depots. *Front. Cardiovasc. Med.* **4**, 27 (2017).
165. Passaro, A. *et al.* Gene expression regional differences in human subcutaneous adipose tissue. *BMC Genomics* **18**, 202 (2017).
166. Rehrer, C. W. *et al.* Regional differences in subcutaneous adipose tissue gene expression. *Obesity (Silver Spring)* **20**, 2168–73 (2012).

167. Karastergiou, K. *et al.* Distinct developmental signatures of human abdominal and gluteal subcutaneous adipose tissue depots. *J. Clin. Endocrinol. Metab.* **98**, 362–71 (2013).

168. Gerhard, G. S. *et al.* Gene expression profiling in subcutaneous, visceral and epigastric adipose tissues of patients with extreme obesity. *Int. J. Obes.* **38**, 371–8 (2014).

169. Kim, B. *et al.* Gene expression profiles of human subcutaneous and visceral adipose-derived stem cells. *Cell Biochem. Funct.* **34**, 563–71 (2016).

170. Vohl, M.-C. *et al.* A survey of genes differentially expressed in subcutaneous and visceral adipose tissue in men. *Obes. Res.* **12**, 1217–22 (2004).

171. Tchkonia, T. *et al.* Identification of depot-specific human fat cell progenitors through distinct expression profiles and developmental gene patterns. *Am. J. Physiol. Endocrinol. Metab.* **292**, E298–307 (2007).

172. Denton, N. F. *et al.* Bone morphogenetic protein 2 is a depot-specific regulator of human adipogenesis. *Int. J. Obes.* **43**, 2458–2468 (2019).

173. Syding, L. A., Nickl, P., Kasparek, P., & Sedlacek, R. CRISPR/Cas9 epigenome editing potential for rare imprinting diseases: a review. *Cells* **9**, 993 (2020).

174. Jones, P. A. Functions of DNA methylation: islands, start sites, gene bodies and beyond. *Nat. Rev. Genet.* **13**, 484–92 (2012).

175. van den Dungen, M. W., Murk, A. J., Kok, D. E., & Steegenga, W. T. Comprehensive DNA methylation and gene expression profiling in differentiating human adipocytes. *J. Cell. Biochem.* **117**, 2707–18 (2016).

176. Broholm, C. *et al.* Human adipogenesis is associated with genome-wide DNA methylation and gene-expression changes. *Epigenomics* **8**, 1601–17 (2016).

177. Fujiki, K., Kano, F., Shiota, K., & Murata, M. Expression of the peroxisome proliferator activated receptor gamma gene is repressed by DNA methylation in visceral adipose tissue of mouse models of diabetes. *BMC Biol.* **7**, 38 (2009).

178. Macartney-Coxson, D. *et al.* Genome-wide DNA methylation analysis reveals loci that distinguish different types of adipose tissue in obese individuals. *Clin. Epigenetics* **9**, 48 (2017).

179. Gehrke, S. *et al.* Epigenetic regulation of depot-specific gene expression in adipose tissue. *PLoS One* **8**, e82516 (2013).

180. Crujeiras, A. B. *et al.* Genome-wide DNA methylation pattern in visceral adipose tissue differentiates insulin-resistant from insulin-sensitive obese subjects. *Transl. Res.* **178**, 13–24.e5 (2016).

181. Guénard, F. *et al.* Differential methylation in visceral adipose tissue of obese men discordant for metabolic disturbances. *Physiol. Genomics* **46**, 216–22 (2014).

182. Guénard, F. *et al.* Genetic regulation of differentially methylated genes in visceral adipose tissue of severely obese men discordant for the metabolic syndrome. *Transl. Res.* **184**, 1–11.e2 (2017).

183. Arner, P. *et al.* The epigenetic signature of systemic insulin resistance in obese women. *Diabetologia* **59**, 2393–405 (2016).

184. Keller, M. *et al.* Genome-wide DNA promoter methylation and transcriptome analysis in human adipose tissue unravels novel candidate genes for obesity. *Mol. Metab.* **6**, 86–100 (2017).

185. Wahl, S. *et al.* Epigenome-wide association study of body mass index, and the adverse outcomes of adiposity. *Nature* **541**, 81–6 (2017).

186. Volkov, P. *et al.* A genome-wide mQTL analysis in human adipose tissue identifies genetic variants associated with DNA methylation, gene expression and metabolic traits. *PLoS One* **11**, e0157776 (2016).

187. Barajas-Olmos, F. *et al.* Altered DNA methylation in liver and adipose tissues derived from individuals with obesity and type 2 diabetes. *BMC Med. Genet.* **19**, 28 (2018).

188. Dahlman, I. *et al.* The fat cell epigenetic signature in post-obese women is characterized by global hypomethylation and differential DNA methylation of adipogenesis genes. *Int. J. Obes.* **39**, 910–19 (2015).

189. Benton, M. C. *et al.* An analysis of DNA methylation in human adipose tissue reveals differential modification of obesity genes before and after gastric bypass and weight loss. *Genome Biol.* **16**, 8 (2015).

190. Rönn, T. *et al.* A six months exercise intervention influences the genome-wide DNA methylation pattern in human adipose tissue. *PLoS Genet.* **9**, e1003572 (2013).

191. Zhou, Y., Peng, J., & Jiang, S. Role of histone acetyltransferases and histone deacetylases in adipocyte differentiation and adipogenesis. *Eur. J. Cell Biol.* **93**, 170–7 (2014).

192. Saidi, N. *et al.* Dynamic changes of epigenetic signatures during chondrogenic and adipogenic differentiation of mesenchymal stem cells. *Biomed. Pharmacother.* **89**, 719–31 (2017).

193. Wang, L. *et al.* Histone H3K9 methyltransferase G9a represses PPARγ expression and adipogenesis. *EMBO J.* **32**, 45–59 (2013).

194. Jang, M.-K., Kim, J.-H., & Jung, M. H. Histone H3K9 demethylase JMJD2B activates adipogenesis by regulating H3K9 methylation on PPARγ and C/EBPα during adipogenesis. *PLoS One* **12**, e0168185 (2017).

195. Lee, K.-H., Ju, U.-I., Song, J.-Y., & Chun, Y.-S. The histone demethylase PHF2 promotes fat cell differentiation as an epigenetic activator of both C/EBPα and C/EBPδ. *Mol. Cells* **37**, 734–41 (2014).

196. Castellano-Castillo, D. *et al.* Human adipose tissue H3K4me3 histone mark in adipogenic, lipid metabolism and inflammatory genes is positively associated with BMI and HOMA-IR. *PLoS One* **14**, e0215083 (2019).

197. Sharma, S. & Taliyan, R. Histone deacetylase inhibitors: future therapeutics for insulin resistance and type 2 diabetes. *Pharmacol. Res.* **113**, 320–6 (2016).

198. Mohr, A. M. & Mott, J. L. Overview of microRNA biology. *Semin. Liver Dis.* **35**, 3–11 (2015).

199. McGregor, R. A. & Choi, M. S. MicroRNAs in the regulation of adipogenesis and obesity. *Curr. Mol. Med.* **11**, 304–16 (2011).

200. Esau, C. *et al.* MicroRNA-143 regulates adipocyte differentiation. *J. Biol. Chem.* **279**, 52361–5 (2004).

201. Rantalainen, M. *et al.* MicroRNA expression in abdominal and gluteal adipose tissue is associated with mRNA expression levels and partly genetically driven. *PLoS One* **6**, e27338 (2011).

202. Klöting, N. *et al.* MicroRNA expression in human omental and subcutaneous adipose tissue. *PLoS One* 4, e4699 (2009).

203. Yu, J. *et al.* Expression profiling of PPARγ-regulated microRNAs in human subcutaneous and visceral adipogenesis in both genders. *Endocrinology* 155, 2155–65 (2014).

204. Ji, C. & Guo, X. The clinical potential of circulating microRNAs in obesity. *Nat. Rev. Endocrinol.* 15, 731–43 (2019).

205. Ortega, F. J. *et al.* MiRNA expression profile of human subcutaneous adipose and during adipocyte differentiation. *PLoS One* 5, e9022 (2010).

206. Sarusi Portuguez, A. *et al.* Hierarchical role for transcription factors and chromatin structure in genome organization along adipogenesis. *FEBS J.* 284, 3230–44 (2017).

207. Siersbæk, R. *et al.* Molecular architecture of transcription factor hotspots in early adipogenesis. *Cell Rep.* 7, 1434–42 (2014).

7
Defining Your Shape
The Determinants of Body Fat Distribution

Genetics

Genetics has played an instrumental role in the natural world since time immemorial. Representing one of the primary mechanisms employed by natural selection, all members of the animal and plant kingdoms have been influenced to some extent by the inclusion/exclusion of specific characteristics encoded by genes passed (or not) down the generations. Building upon the groundwork laid by the Augustinian friar Gregor Mendel during the nineteenth century as he studied 'trait inheritance' in plants,[1] the field of genetics has flourished into a scientific marvel that sits at the interface between biology, biochemistry, and information technology. Technological advancements mean scientists and clinicians are now able to collect and analyze samples on a previously unthinkable and unattainable scale, but what does the 'genetics of obesity and body fat distribution' actually mean?

Do These Genes Make Me Look Fat?

Evidence accumulated over decades indicates that there is more than a sliver of truth to the retort 'it's my genes' that is often proffered in response to a taunt about someone's weight. Various studies indicate body mass, body mass index (BMI), and fat mass are all highly heritable traits,[2,3] meaning genetic factors (i.e., genotype) make a strong contribution to these physical features (i.e., phenotypes). Heritability is a key concept in genetics that refers to the proportion of variation in a physical attribute that can be attributed to genetic factors. This can be quantified by comparing the similarity of a physical attribute between mono- or dizygotic twins (who have all or half of their genetic background in common, respectively) to the similarity between unrelated individuals (who are genetically dissimilar).

The data are compelling,[4] with heritability estimates for body size (according to BMI) ranging from ~45%[5] to ~80%.[6] This variable, but overall high degree of heritability is most clearly demonstrated by the finding that the BMI of adopted children correlates more with their biological rather than adopted parents' BMI.[7] The heterogeneity in heritability estimates has been found to vary according to age,[4,8] sex,[9] and ethnicity,[10] as well as factors like rapid economic growth,[11] meaning our genes interact with our dynamic (internal and external) environment throughout life. Not all things heritable are molecular in nature though; we also inherit (to some extent) our parent's eating habits, diets, physical activity levels, and even appetites.[12] Both nature and nurture matter.

The story is very similar for body fat distribution (according to waist/hip circumference, waist-hip ratio (WHR), and dual-energy X-ray absorptiometry (DXA) data). Waist circumference heritability is estimated at ~30%[13] to ~80%[3,14] whereas WHR heritability is reportedly ~30%[15] to ~70%,[2] with the contribution of these genetic factors varying according to age,[3] sex,[16] and ethnicity.[17] The high heritability of body fat distribution is exemplified by the finding that the pattern of regional fat expansion upon overfeeding is strikingly similar in identical twins.[18] Further complexity is added by the observation that regional fat mass heritability may not be homogenous; the Quebec family study reported that the heritability estimate for visceral fat mass was 56%, but 42% for subcutaneous fat mass.[19] It appears that we have our parents to thank (or not) for their substantial contribution to our past, current, and future physical form.

Building on the high heritability of body size and shape, there has been a large push to identify the underlying genes, with this pursuit primarily taking the form of genome-wide association studies (GWAS). Approximately 100 genomic loci are significantly associated with increased BMI[20] and ~50 with WHR[21] (independent of overall fatness). On the opposite end of the scale, genomic loci associated with low BMI have also been identified,[22] meaning thinness also has a genetic element. Alpha-ketoglutarate-dependent dioxygenase (more commonly known as *fat mass and obesity associated/FTO)* is one of the most famous genomic loci as it was the first to be associated with an increased risk of obesity, an effect it achieves by altering food intake and preference in a complex, yet subtle manner.[23] In terms of fat distribution, a number of genomic loci have also been significantly associated with subcutaneous abdominal and visceral fat mass.[16] Some of these GWAS hits only affect men or women,[16] while others are ethnicity-specific.[24] The important contribution of adipose distribution and function to metabolic health was further emphasized in a recent meta-analysis in which a number of genomic loci were associated with both greater fat mass and reduced cardiometabolic disease risk. More specifically, these genomic hits were associated with enhanced *peripheral* fat storage (i.e., in lower-body subcutaneous stores) as well as processes relating to adipocyte differentiation and function, insulin-glucose signalling, and inflammation.[25] GWAS hits have also been identified for lean mass[26] (as measured via DXA). Despite this success in dissecting the genetics underpinning obesity and diabetes,[27] it has proven difficult to translate these 'hits' into tangible molecular mechanisms[28]; there is also a striking inability to square the GWAS data with heritability estimates.

The Invisible Hand

Heritability studies indicate that genetic factors apparently explain up to 80% of the variation in overall and regional adiposity between individuals. However, the combined contribution of the currently identified genomic loci explains only 2.7% of the variance for BMI[20] and 1.4% of WHR.[21] This incongruence has led to the term 'the missing heritability' being coined,[29] and also prompted the proposal that the high heritability of body size and shape are explained by factors that may not be picked up by GWAS. For instance, 'genetic susceptibility' proffers that a number of coincident genetic variants interact to predispose (or prevent) the development of a certain biological outcome[30] upon exposure to specific environmental conditions; in other words, 'genetics loads the gun, but the environment pulls the trigger.'[31] Alternatively, copy number variants (i.e., replications or deletions of entire chromosomal segments which can affect the 'dose' of genes an individual may receive[32]) are not usually picked up in GWAS, but may contribute to the missing heritability. Epigenetic mechanisms like DNA methylation (see Chapter 6) have also been implicated.[33] Regardless of one's genetic risk of becoming obese or developing metabolic disease, however, anyone can benefit from consuming a healthier diet[34] and/or exercise.[35]

Analysis of the biological pathways in which GWAS hits operate suggests that the central nervous system plays a crucial role in determining an individual's susceptibility to obesity.[20] Indeed, one's genetic predisposition for obesity may reside in their head, more specifically in appetite and satiety regulation. Without necessarily being deterministic, it may be the case that some people have a genetic background that makes them more susceptible to overeating, with this genetic potential likely to be fulfilled when living in an environment laden with calorie-rich food.[36,37] But before everyone absolves their individual or society's responsibility and blames their genes for their weight, much remains to be learned about the nature and size of the genetic contribution to appetite and satiety, two complex phenomena that can be overridden by behavioural responses (e.g., willpower to ignore hunger) and environmental factors (e.g., food type and availability). These genetic factors may also contribute to perturbed neuronal control of energy expenditure which predisposes carriers to obesity.[38]

Conversely, the ~50 genomic loci significantly associated with body fat distribution predominantly relate to fat metabolism and development.[21] Although much work remains to delineate the biology associated with these genomic loci,[39] it appears that the genetics underpinning *where* we put on fat are distinct from those which influence *how much* fat we accumulate, even if their overall effect size is rather small and complex in the general population. The true power of genetics to affect overall and regional fat mass is truly exemplified, however, in rare disorders such as monogenic (i.e., caused by a mutation in a single gene) obesity and congenital lipodystrophy, respectively.

Hungry Hungry Mice

No-one could have possibly predicted that studying the colour of a mouse's fur coat would have provided some of the most important insights into (mammalian) appetite regulation. A mouse's coat colour is regulated by agouti, a small protein produced by hair follicles which acts in pigment-producing melanocytes (i.e., a skin cell type) to promote the production of yellow-red phaeomelanin at the expense of brown-black eumelanin.[40] It achieves this by preventing alpha-melanocyte-stimulating hormone (α-MSH) from binding to its surface receptor on melanocytes, thereby blocking brown-black eumelanin production.[41] Agouti usually produces a specific pattern of coat colouration in which black hairs are surrounded by a yellow band. However, scientists noticed that transgenic mice carrying specific mutations in the *agouti* gene had a wholly yellow coat and also developed severe obesity and type 2 diabetes.[42] Further analyses have since identified that these genetic mutations cause agouti protein levels to dramatically increase,[43] thereby completely blocking the α-MSH-directed production of brown-black eumelanin. So, how do pigmentation and obesity intersect?

The original observation of the obese yellow mouse was made during the early 1900s, but a published description of this particular mouse strain didn't emerge for several decades.[44] Interest was renewed during the 1970s and 1980s, at which point genetic technology advancements enabled the discovery of mutations in the *agouti* gene that were responsible for a ravenous appetite which invariably resulted in mice becoming severely obese.[45] Further work highlighted that the α-MSH receptor family (i.e., melanocortin receptors; MCRs) upon which agouti protein acts is present in skin cells and the appetite-regulating area of the hypothalamus in the brain.[46,47] As expected, injecting α-MSH analogues into the brains of mice to activate MCRs potently suppresses appetite, whereas co-administration of an agouti protein analogue blocks this effect and increases appetite.[48] Genetic inactivation of MC4R (which conveys an appetite-suppressing effect when activated by α-MSH) has the same effect as increasing agouti protein levels; mice develop a ravenous appetite and become obese.[49] But how do mice and men compare?

In this case, they're quite similar; human versions of the agouti protein[50] (i.e., agouti-related protein, AgRP), as well as the MCRs on which it acts,[51] have been identified. Spurred on by these findings, genetic analysis of patients affected by early-onset, hyperphagic (large appetite) severe obesity during the late 1990s and early 2000s resulted in the identification of several genetic mutations within the *MC4R* gene.[52–54] It is now known that *MC4R* mutations are present in 1–2.5% of obese people, making them the most common genetic factor associated with obesity described to date,[55] with several loci located near to the *MC4R* gene being significantly associated with increased waist circumference.[55] Men and women with *MC4R* mutations typically experience sexual dysfunction[56] in addition to obesity, further emphasizing the link between reproductive health and energy metabolism. Given this background, various anti-obesity drugs which target MC4R (and/or mimic AgRP action) are being developed.[57]

Dangerously Low Fat

Congenital lipodystrophy disorders involve the partial or complete loss of adipose tissue and provide a powerful, often tragic demonstration of the relationship between overall and regional fat mass with metabolic health. However, the inspiring Tom Staniford has not let his diagnosis with mandibular dysplasia with deafness and progeroid features (MDP syndrome)—an exceptionally rare disorder comprising generalized lipodystrophy, deafness, and an under-developed jawbone—hold him back from becoming a successful para-cyclist.[58] Generalized lipodystrophies involve total loss of adipose tissue, with patients typically experiencing severe metabolic complications such as type 2 diabetes, raised circulating blood lipids, and non-alcoholic fatty liver disease,[59] all of which arise because fatty acids have nowhere to be stored safely. Partial fat loss tends to have a smaller impact on one's health, with the severity often reflecting both the anatomical location affected and extent of loss. For instance, familial partial lipodystrophy of the Dunnigan variety (FPLD) is defined by loss of fat in the lower body coupled with expansion of upper body adipose tissue[60] and is associated with severe metabolic consequences.[61] As expected, however, when upper body fat is lost but lower body fat remains unaffected, as in the rare Barraquer-Simons syndrome, metabolic complications are usually mild and can even be absent.[62]

Detailed investigation has highlighted that the lipodystrophies typically arise from mutations in genes involved in various aspects of adipose biology.[63] For example, congenital generalized lipodystrophy type 1 (CGL1) is associated with mutations in the 1-acylglycerol-3-phosphate O-acyltransferase 2 (AGPAT2) gene.[64] AGPAT2 is an enzyme which facilitates the formation of a signalling molecule required for normal adipocyte function and triacylglycerol synthesis. AGPAT2 mutations primarily affect subcutaneous and visceral adipose tissue involved in metabolic homeostasis, while mechanically important fat tissue in the palms, soles, eye sockets, and scalp remains unaffected.[65] Patients with CGL2 have a similar generalized deficiency of metabolically important fat to that observed in individuals with CGL1, but they also lose mechanically important fat.[65] So, while CGL1 and CGL2 appear to be similar, they are distinct. CGL2 results from mutations in *Seipin*, the gene which encodes a protein crucially involved in lipid droplet synthesis and adipogenesis.[63] Evidently disrupting a seemingly fundamental piece of cellular machinery to adipose function can still manifest in a depot-specific manner, a phenomenon which is perhaps best displayed by the various types of congenital partial lipodystrophy.

The aforementioned FPLD is caused by mutations in LMNA,[66] the gene which encodes the ubiquitous lamin A/C protein that contributes to the nuclear envelope (i.e., the structure which surrounds a cell's nucleus).

Given that the vast majority of cells in the body have a nucleus (barring red blood cells), why disruption to this seemingly fundamental protein's function should manifest in such an unusual manner that specifically affects fat tissue is a great unsolved mystery in medicine. Equally mystifying is the discovery that numerous mutations within the *PPARG* gene have been associated with partial, not generalized, lipodystrophy disorders given that *PPARG* supposedly acts as the 'master regulator of adipogenesis.'

Rear View

The congenital lipodystrophies are not the only indicators that genetics play an important role in determining body fat distribution. Another piece of compelling evidence comes in the distinctive shape of the members of the Khoisan tribe of South Africa (called the Hottentot by early White settlers) and, to a lesser extent, the Pygmies of Central Africa. *Steatopygia* is defined by the substantial and selective accumulation of fat on the buttocks and thighs that makes them protrude outwards in a conspicuous, and potentially impractical, manner.[67] Likely underpinned by a complex genetic architecture, the reportedly high prevalence of steatopygia among the Khoisan people and their descendants represents a clear example of how social attitudes toward body shape, sexual selection, and fat biology can intersect.

The remarkable steatopygic shape of the Khoisan women has not gone unnoticed through history, with fascination in this feature morphing into a tragic tale of colonial exploitation that started in the late 1700s and only concluded in the early 2000s. Sarah Baartman was born in South Africa's Eastern Cape in 1789 to a difficult early life in which she endured domestic servitude and various personal tragedies. She thought her luck had changed upon meeting English ship surgeon William Dunlop and entrepreneur Hendrik Cesars, who convinced her to travel to England in order to take part in shows. Despite being illiterate, she was coerced into signing a contract and soon found herself being exploited in freak shows, parading around on stage for the gawking masses as the 'Hottentot Venus.'[68] Her popularity would later dwindle in London at which point she moved to France and managed to rekindle some kind of celebrity while mingling with eminent artists and scientists before dying at the young age of 26.

As if her tragically short, hard life wasn't troubling enough, the naturalist Georges Cuvier (with whom she had danced at a party) made a plaster cast of her distinctive body before dissecting it. Preserving her skeleton and pickling her brain and genitals in jars, her remains and the sculpture of her body went on public display in Paris's Museum of Man until 1974. Sarah Baartman's protracted degradation only concluded upon Nelson Mandela's election as President of South Africa and his request to have her remains and plaster cast repatriated. After years of discussion, the French government finally agreed and returned Sarah Baartman home in March 2002. This sorry episode of exploitation and humiliation finally concluded when Sarah's remains were buried in Hankey, Eastern Cape province, in August 2002, 192 years after she had left for Europe.[1]

Drugs

Drugs can affect overall and regional fat mass in both beneficial and harmful ways, with the latter often manifesting as an unintended side-effect. The major drug class known to promote metabolically favourable changes to body fat distribution are the *thiazolidinediones* (TZDs). TZDs are used as insulin-sensitizing agents in the treatment of type 2 diabetes.[69] These drugs activate PPARG to directly promote adipogenesis in addition to widespread effects on lipid metabolism. The TZD-induced increase in insulin sensitivity often occurs in conjunction with weight gain, but how can this be? Far from being a paradox, TZD use is associated with subcutaneous fat expansion,[70] a phenomenon which is sometimes accompanied by the simultaneous retraction of visceral[71] and/or intra-muscle fat.[72] TZDs appear to improve patients' metabolic health by artificially enhancing their subcutaneous fat's expandability (by promoting hyperplastic expansion) and therefore function, an effect which allows their 'backed-up' energy storage system to clear and ectopic fat to redistribute, enabling the rescue of insulin sensitivity. TZDs have also proven useful in the treatment of certain forms of lipodystrophy,[73] with disease tractability reflecting the underlying molecular pathology.[74]

For all of their beneficial effects on metabolic health, however, these drugs have unfortunately been mired in controversy over their side-effects which can include fluid retention, heart failure, bone fractures, and an increased risk of bladder cancer; these effects likely reflect the activation of

---

[1] A detailed account of Sarah Baartman's life is documented in 'The Hottentot Venus: The Life and Death of Saartjie Baartman' by Rachel Holmes.

PPARG in non-adipose tissues.[69] While the TZDs have not been the runaway success that clinicians and scientists would have liked, they currently represent the single class of drug that induces the beneficial re-distribution of body fat to alleviate metabolic disease. Even though the current generation of PPARG activators are far from ideal (although new, improved versions are being developed[75]), they are living proof that body fat distribution modification represents a viable therapeutic strategy that can confer substantial metabolic and cardiovascular health benefits and warrants further exploration.

Many other drugs modify overall and/or regional fat mass in a way that precipitates negative health consequences. For instance, some of the older anti-retroviral drugs used to treat HIV/AIDS proved to be a double-edged sword, as although they have drastically reduced HIV-associated mortality, their use is associated with cardiovascular and metabolic disturbances.[76] HIV patients treated with these anti-retroviral drugs often experience some form of fat atrophy (i.e., loss of adipose tissue) which typically affected the face and extremities, as well as caused fat re-distribution in which abdominal, predominantly visceral, depots expanded in conjunction with ectopic fat accumulation in the liver and skeletal muscle.[77] The nucleoside reverse transcription inhibitors (which negatively affect adipogenesis[78]) appear to be the main culprits responsible for this fat atrophy.[79] Other anti-retroviral drugs, specifically protease inhibitors, can precipitate (partial) lipodystrophies in which lower body subcutaneous fat wastes away while subcutaneous abdominal and visceral fat expands[80]; such changes are associated with an increased risk of developing metabolic and cardiovascular disease. Why these drugs exert such distinctly localized effects remains a matter of intrigue.

The Price of Freedom?

Antipsychotic medication used to treat psychiatric conditions like schizophrenia often causes serious metabolic side effects. While these powerful drugs can stabilize otherwise debilitating symptoms and enable patients to lead relatively independent lives, use of antipsychotic drugs is strongly associated with accelerated weight gain, insulin resistance, type 2 diabetes, abnormal blood lipids, and an increased risk of developing cardiovascular disease, with these symptoms usually manifesting within six months of initiating therapy.[81] It is not entirely clear how antipsychotic medication precipitates such severe metabolic side-effects, but evidence suggests that the broad neuronal effects of these potent drugs perturb appetite and satiety regulation, as well as that of resting metabolic rate, to promote the development of obesity.[82] These drugs also disrupt adipogenesis, lipogenesis, adipokine secretion, lipolysis, and insulin sensitivity.[83] These metabolic symptoms are often managed with conventional treatments (e.g., metformin and statins), although efforts have been made to identify predisposing genetic factors that enable the tailoring of drug regimens to minimize side effects.[84] The powerful, broad-acting nature of antipsychotic medication nonetheless carries a high risk of causing side-effects though, metabolic or otherwise.

Managing the Munchies

Several recreational drugs have a reputation for their effects on fat mass, with such effects potentially being amongst the various reasons people consume them. *Nicotine* from tobacco smoking or vaping is typically associated with some degree of weight loss, primarily due to its appetite-suppressing effects.[85] Representing a highly unlikely, otherwise unhealthy, and probably ineffectual proposition, it has been suggested that nicotine vaping could represent a novel approach to promote weight loss amid the global obesity crisis.[86] *Cocaine* is another stimulant that some individuals use to induce and maintain weight loss,[87] with some evidence suggesting that cocaine directly alters adipose biology.[88]

The *amphetamines* represent another class of drug that, similar to nicotine, act as a stimulant and exert a powerful appetite-suppressing effect.[89] Amphetamine-derived appetite suppressants, such as phentermine, are used clinically to treat obesity, although not all have been deemed safe or successful due to their cardiovascular side effects, as highlighted by the Servier benfluorex (sold as Mediator) scandal in France. An unhealthy relationship between industry and regulators, complex bureaucracy, and dubious scientific practices combined with high-stakes business decisions resulted in Mediator causing between 500 and 2000 avoidable deaths over the 33 years it was on the market, despite numerous warning signs that it should have been pulled many years earlier.[90]

On the opposite end of the spectrum, *marijuana* is well-known for its appetite-*promoting* effects.[91] Using this underlying biology, an anti-obesity drug known as rimonabant was developed to block the naturally occurring endocannabinoids positive contribution to appetite regulation. As rimonabant disrupts endocannabinoid signalling throughout the brain, however, it not only reduced people's appetite, but also precipitated dramatic adverse effects on mood and emotion regulation (including suicidal thoughts).[92] Such side-effects meant it was soon pulled from the market and shelved. Despite failing to safely manipulate endocannabinoid signalling to suppress appetite, there is the potential that the appetite-promoting effects of marijuana could be harnessed to alleviate clinical conditions such as wasting syndromes that can affect cancer and HIV/AIDS patients.[93]

Suppressing appetite does represent a viable approach to weight loss, although *how* such an effect is achieved is crucial to its success. *Lorcaserin* acts on a specific serotonin receptor in the brain to selectively reduce an individual's appetite and therefore food intake.[94] Is lorcaserin the magic bullet that the medical profession has been searching for? Not quite.[95] While reportedly promoting weight loss without negatively impacting cardiovascular health[96] (i.e., stroke or heart attack), the FDA requested that lorcaserin be withdrawn from the market in February 2020 due to data suggesting it may increase the risk of developing cancer.[97] Given its beleaguered situation, it seems unlikely that lorcaserin represents a viable and cost-effective option in the global battle against obesity.

Glucocorticoids

The glucocorticoids are steroid hormones released by the adrenal gland that are vital for life and influence the biology of nearly every type of cell in our bodies. Glucocorticoid action is complex and wide-ranging, with these hormones being most famous for their role in co-ordinating the evolutionarily honed, multi-faceted 'fight or flight' response to stress. Responsible for the rapid mobilization of energy (e.g., acute cortisol infusion promotes fat mobilization from upper and lower body subcutaneous fat in humans[98–100]) to support the extrication of oneself from a threatening situation, these effects are undoubtedly beneficial on a short-term basis. However, a substantial amount of evidence indicates that prolonged exposure to stress, and therefore elevated glucocorticoid levels, is harmful to our health. This situation is associated with a distinctive shift in body fat distribution towards central obesity that is accompanied by an increased risk of developing metabolic and cardiovascular disease. Indeed, there is a growing consensus that the glucocorticoids play an important role in the global (central) obesity crisis, as they represent a mechanism that links metabolic health and body fat distribution to lifestyle[101] and even our emotional state.[102]

A Crucial Discovery

Cushing's disease is a distinctive clinical condition that exemplifies glucocorticoid biology. It was originally described in 1912 by the pioneering American neurosurgeon Harvey Cushing (1869–1939) after he encountered the patient Minnie G. in 1910. This young woman presented with a novel and unique combination of symptoms that included 'painful obesity, hypertrichosis (i.e., excessive hair growth), and amenorrhea (i.e., cessation of periods) with overdevelopment of secondary sexual characteristics accompanying a low grade of hydrocephalus and increased cerebral tension.'[103] Harvey Cushing made the link between these symptoms and her elevated levels of cortisol, the primary glucocorticoid in humans. While the exact cause of Minnie's case was never conclusively resolved, Cushing published an account in 1932 stating his firm belief that, although her symptoms and those of similar cases closely resembled those of patients with adrenal tumours, her disease was probably caused by a tumour affecting the function of the pituitary gland (i.e., a small hormone-secreting gland that protrudes from the hypothalamus in the brain) that resulted in elevated circulating cortisol levels.[103,104] The Soviet neurologist Nikolai Itsenko (1889–1954) independently confirmed this proposition in 1924,[105] with his contribution being recognized in some Eastern European and Asian countries by the addition of his name to the condition's title (i.e., Itsenko-Cushing disease).

While Cushing's disease is quite rare, the symptoms that patients experience are not. In fact, the same array of symptoms driven by a pituitary tumour in Cushing's disease can be recapitulated by the use of exogenous glucocorticoids. A key component of the modern medical toolbox, glucocorticoids are routinely used to treat inflammatory conditions (e.g., asthma, rheumatoid arthritis, and eczema), as well as to suppress the immune system to prevent post-transplantation rejection.[106] The plethora of symptoms experienced by patients with Cushing's syndrome reflect the wide range of organs and tissues that glucocorticoids influence (Figure 7.1), with the most distinctive features reflecting their effects on adipose tissue; weight gain as central obesity, fat accumulation behind the neck

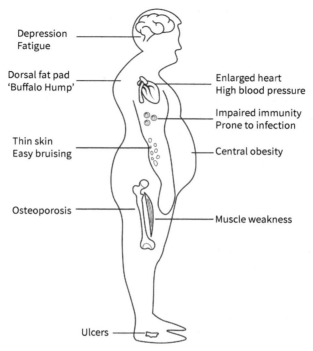

Figure 7.1 Cushing's syndrome symptoms.

which forms a 'buffalo hump', and a 'moon face' resulting from fat accretion around the side of the face.[107]

The distinctive pattern of fat re-distribution which accompanies Cushing's syndrome typically involves expansion of upper body fat stores, particularly visceral fat, in conjunction with the wasting of lower body subcutaneous fat.[108,109] This selective expansion of upper body fat stores is often accompanied by adipose inflammation and adipocyte hyper-trophy[110] (associated with adipose dysfunction[111]) which increases one's risk of developing metabolic and cardiovascular diseases (i.e., type 2 diabetes, non-alcoholic fatty liver disease, and atherosclerosis[112]). There has been a sustained push to understand the biology underpinning Cushing's syndrome, but pinning down the exact mechanisms responsible has proven to be challenging due to the delicate and dynamic nature of glucocorticoid action.

An Essential but Mysterious Ingredient

Consistent with the weight gain that typically accompanies prolonged exposure to elevated glucocorticoid levels, abundant evidence indicates these chemicals are required for (*in vitro*) adipogenesis.[113] Identifying glucocorticoids as one of the crucial ingredients for turning cultured precursor cells into mature adipocytes represents an important scientific milestone that has since enabled many researchers to study adipose cell biology, particularly the process of adipogenesis. Despite the striking fat re-distribution phenotype exhibited by Cushing's disease patients, however, there is a relative paucity of data examining the depot-specific actions of glucocorticoids, particularly why lower body subcutaneous fat wastes away.[101] Of the limited information available though, these hormones reportedly exert striking depot-specific effects on entire gene networks involved in vital processes such as adipogenesis in abdominal subcutaneous and visceral fat.[114,115]

While glucocorticoids apparently play an important role in adipogenesis, the preferential expansion of upper body fat stores in Cushing's syndrome appears to manifest from glucocorticoid-dependent changes in regional fatty acid handling. In fact, the current data paint a somewhat paradoxical picture in which glucocorticoids promote adipogenesis *in vitro* (so one would expect fat cell number to increase), yet subcutaneous abdominal and visceral fat in Cushing's syndrome patients expands via hypertrophy[110] (suggesting adipogenesis is inhibited).

With respect to fatty acid storage, glucocorticoids interact with insulin to increase the levels and activity of lipoprotein lipase[116–118] (see Chapter 3). This synergistic interaction between hormones occurs in subcutaneous and visceral abdominal adipose tissue and could promote the preferential expansion of upper body fat.[116,118,119] Glucocorticoids also synergize with insulin to increase the expression and activity of genes involved in *de novo* lipogenesis (DNL; i.e. the synthesis of fatty acids—see Chapter 3) in human adipose tissue.[114,120,121] As glucocorticoids seem to activate this biological pathway to a significantly greater extent in visceral fat compared to abdominal subcutaneous fat,[114,121] this phenomenon could link central fat accumulation with adipocyte hypertrophy[101] (even if DNL only makes a minor contribution in adipose tissue under most circumstances[122,123]).

But how can cortisol cause fat mobilization *and* accumulation? This is not entirely clear, but as with many things in life, it seems that time and place are key. However, even with the best resources, experimental designs, and boundless enthusiasm of researchers and study participants, the slippery nature of glucocorticoids makes them difficult to study. Their highly context-specific actions make it challenging not only to replicate findings, but also to translate results between *in vitro* and *in vivo* contexts.[124] These difficulties are exacerbated by the observation that glucocorticoids can modify the action of other lipolytic hormones such as adrenaline.[125] Moreover, *time* makes an important contribution to the complex tapestry of glucocorticoid biology as these hormones often invoke complex compensatory mechanisms which typically diminish future responses to hormone exposure.[126] With so many moving parts, it is easy to see why studying the effects of glucocorticoids can be difficult to perform and interpret.

Top of the Morning

Circulating cortisol levels follow a 24-hour cyclical pattern in which they typically rise and peak early in the morning before slowly declining through the day,[127] with stressful events stimulating extra pulses that are overlaid on this background pattern. The early cortisol peak is associated with increased lipolysis,[128] suggesting cortisol prepares the body for the 'stress' of waking by mobilizing its fuel stores. This recurrent dynamic pattern of circulating glucocorticoid levels has played an instrumental role in the evolution of modern humans as a predominantly diurnal species (i.e., active during the day). These regularly fluctuating glucocorticoid levels play a crucial role in many aspects of our biology by acting as a calibrating signal that synchronizes our peripheral tissues and organs to the central biological clock in our brain (i.e., the suprachiasmatic nucleus in the hypothalamus) which is entrained to the time of the chronological day by light.[129]

Many different types of illness are accompanied by disturbances to the normal 24-hour pattern of circulating cortisol. The seemingly disparate array of complex clinical conditions unified by disrupted glucocorticoid secretion patterns include psychiatric disorders[130] (e.g., anxiety, depression, and insomnia), and metabolic and cardiovascular disease.[131] It has been known since at least the 1970s[132] that Cushing's syndrome patients often display highly abnormal patterns of cortisol secretion.[133] Moreover, data suggests these hormones may link the psychological stress, sleep disturbances, and altered appetite that define Cushing's syndrome patients and centrally obese individuals.[134]

While disturbed patterns of circulating glucocorticoid levels could be merely coincidental, a body of evidence indicates that the duration and timing of glucocorticoid treatment often has a profound impact on an individual's health.[135] Although difficult to achieve, replicating the endogenous secretion pattern is associated with the best clinical outcomes; treatment regimens that cause persistently high levels of exogenous glucocorticoid are often associated with metabolic derangements, impaired bone health, and even cardiovascular death.[135] Relatedly, the circadian pattern of glucocorticoid levels may contribute to the significantly higher mortality rates among trauma patients admitted during the night (when cortisol levels are low and the body is less able to handle stress) compared to the daytime.[136]

Entry Denied

Amidst this maelstrom of moving parts, *pre-receptor metabolism* is another factor that influences glucocorticoid action via local activation and inactivation[101,124] (Figure 7.2). It can be helpful to envision the cell's nucleus as an exclusive nightclub; the bioactive glucocorticoid cortisol (i.e., an appropriately dressed partygoer) can only have a biological effect (i.e., modify gene expression) if it gets into the nucleus. Inactive glucocorticoid metabolites (i.e., inappropriately dressed would-be partygoers) initially refused entry can undergo a structural modification (i.e., outfit change) to become active; this conversion is catalyzed by the enzyme 11β-hydroxysteroid dehydrogenase (HSD) type 1. This glucocorticoid re-activation is countered by 11β-HSD type 2, the enzyme which converts active cortisol into inactive cortisone in humans, much like a subversive agitator placed in the crowd rendering would-be revellers ineligible for entry. Finally, there are synthetic glucocorticoids not recognized by any enzymes that act as independent rogues, coming and going as they please.

Pre-receptor metabolism influences how much active hormone is present within a cell at any given time and contributes to the highly context-specific nature of glucocorticoid action, particularly between adipose tissue depots. For instance, 11β-HSD type 1 (which increases active cortisol levels) expression and activity are reportedly higher in visceral compared to subcutaneous abdominal fat.[137] Higher expression of this enzyme in visceral fat has also been found to be correlated with larger adipocyte size, independent of overall fat mass,[138] meaning this enzyme may link adipose expandability, regional fat mass, and metabolic health. Additionally, transgenic mice engineered to have elevated levels of 11β-HSD type 1 in

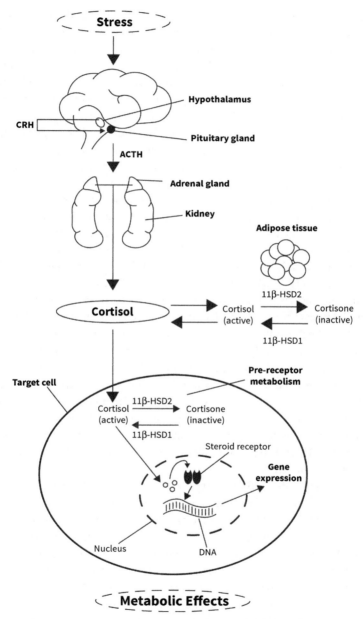

Figure 7.2 The stress response and pre-receptor glucocorticoid metabolism.

adipose tissue become obese and develop serious metabolic and cardiovascular complications that are heavily reminiscent of Cushing's syndrome.[139] On the contrary, selectively deleting 11β-HSD type 1 from adipose tissue produces mice which are lean, highly insulin-sensitive, and protected from diet-induced obesity.[140] Moreover, adipose tissue plays a crucial role in this interplay as deleting the 11β-HSD type 1 gene from the liver does not protect mice from developing these Cushing-like symptoms.[141]

The similarities in metabolic and anthropometric phenotype between Cushing's syndrome patients and individuals who develop central obesity in the general population has prompted the suggestion that pathologically elevated local glucocorticoid action due to increased 11β-HSD type 1 activity in adipose tissue represents a major process common to these groups.[142,143] While a novel indicator of long-term glucocorticoid metabolism—cortisol levels in hair follicles—suggests that circulating cortisol levels are indeed elevated in obesity,[144] altered local glucocorticoid metabolism in adipose tissue may actually represent the missing link to regional fat accumulation. Indeed, 11β-HSD type 1 expression is higher in obese subcutaneous abdominal and visceral fat, with enzyme levels correlating positively with overall fatness, waist circumference, insulin resistance, and adipocyte size.[145-147] Such results have spurred the development of 11β-HSD type 1 inhibitors to treat Cushing's syndrome and central obesity-related metabolic disease. Several molecules have been developed that show some efficacy in improving metabolic dysfunction in type 2 diabetic patients, but their small glucose-lowering effect precluded further commercial development.[148] It remains unclear whether these drugs would be more effective in combination with lifestyle interventions and/or other pharmacological agents, but 11β-HSD type 1 inhibition represents an interesting therapeutic approach to pursue.[149]

On the flip side, 11β-HSD type 2 (which inactivates cortisol) is inhibited by glycyrrhetic acid, a naturally occurring compound present in liquorice. Inhibiting this enzyme tilts the balance in favour of activating glucocorticoid signalling, something which is not associated with beneficial or desirable effects. Indeed, individuals have been admitted to hospital due to kidney problems after consuming excessive quantities of liquorice, and therefore glycyrrhetic acid. This is because 11β-HSD type 2 protects the kidney (and other tissues) against cortisol activating the mineralocorticoid receptor, a related but distinct receptor involved in co-ordinating salt and water balance; this receptor is activated by the steroid hormone aldosterone. Inhibition of 11β-HSD type 2 by glycyrrhetic acid results in inappropriate activation of this receptor by excess levels of cortisol, thereby leading to water retention and increased potassium excretion by the kidney, a situation which can damage the heart and even cause temporary weakness of all four limbs.[150] Despite such negative effects, glycyrrhetic acid is readily consumed around the world as the main sweet-tasting component of liquorice—having evolved from the ancient Egyptian drink 'erk soos' to the family of liquorice products spanning liquorice sticks, Pontefract cakes, Belgian beers, and even flavoured tobacco twists.

Comfort in Calories

The glucocorticoid-driven 'fight or flight' stress response plays a crucial part in maximizing our chances of our survival in the face of extreme adversity. While useful in acute life-threatening circumstances, the stress response is ill-suited to handle many of modern humanity's existential threats which often involve chronic psychological stress[151] and typically manifest as anxiety and/or depression; between stressors stemming from family, relationships, work, finances, one's place in society, crime, the COVID-19 pandemic, and local and global politics, it's no wonder anxiety and depression are so common.[152] It is unsurprising that chronic stress, anxiety, and depression are all strongly associated with the development of central obesity, metabolic dysfunction, and an increased risk of premature death.[153] Aside from their biochemical effects to prime our bodies to handle stress, glucocorticoids exert a potent influence over our appetite.

Consistent with many people's personal experiences and/or observations, extensive evidence indicates that psychological stress is associated with altered food intake and dietary choices, with stressed individuals often eating more than required and opting for highly palatable foods rich in fat and sugar.[154] As the consumption of highly palatable foods can stimulate the release of endogenous opioids/endorphins[155] (i.e., naturally occurring 'feel-good' hormones) which can dampen stress response activity,[156] this dietary adaptation may temporarily alleviate one's psychological stress,[157] albeit at the cost of promoting the compulsive overeating of highly calorific food.[158] Why many of us turn to ice cream or chocolate for comfort is not certain, but it may represent an evolutionary vestige that promotes short-term gratification as a brief reprieve from our stress and/or a primitive drive to stock up, or even expand, our energy reserves in case our already stressful circumstances take a turn for the worse.

Evidently this stress response is deleterious in the long-term, however enjoyable that decadent treat may be in the short-term. The metabolic consequences of overeating and obesity are clear, but persistently elevated glucocorticoid levels resulting from chronic psychological stress can exacerbate this already-hazardous situation by directing upper body fat expansion. The calorie-rich environment of the industrialized world means it is very easy to fall into a vicious cycle of overeating and worrying, in which body weight and health concerns can easily be added to the original psychological stressor.[159] The vicious cycle of stress-driven overeating can be difficult to break, although exercise[160] and relaxation/meditation[161] can be effective methods for managing stress, breaking the habit of comfort eating, and mitigating the effects of weight gain. More structural changes at the societal level are also critical to increase the feasibility of such individual lifestyle/behavioural strategies, especially given that most people's decisions will also be shaped in part by various social determinants of health (e.g., occupation, education, race, gender, ethnicity, etc.). Whatever the underlying source and focus of intervention, modern medicine may have harnessed the unique power of the glucocorticoids to tame crippling inflammatory diseases and make organ transplantation a reality, but the world's bulging waistline and worsening health should be a stark reminder of the dark side of these enigmatic hormones.

Sex Steroids

The sex steroids, specifically the *androgens* and *oestrogens*, make a key contribution to the distinctive patterns of regional fat distribution displayed by men and women. Both classes of sex steroid are present in men and women, albeit in different proportions; androgens (e.g., testosterone released by the testes) predominate in men whereas oestrogens (from the ovaries) are the primary sex steroid in women. While these hormones are most famous for co-ordinating sexual development and reproductive function, they also exert wide-ranging effects on our immune[162] and cardiovascular[163] systems, skeletal muscle,[164] bones,[165] and brain.[166] More pertinently, the sex steroids act on adipose tissue to instigate and maintain the body composition and shape which define the archetypal male and female bodies.

Adult men and women display striking differences in body composition and regional fat accumulation that result from divergent developmental trajectories that arise during puberty (see Chapter 5). While several genetic variants are significantly associated with sex-specific patterns of fat accumulation,[167] sex steroid action is primarily responsible for generating and maintaining the android and gynoid patterns of regional fat distribution. Before delving into the science, it is worth noting that this knowledge base is not as well developed as it could be due to the under-representation, even exclusion, of women in biomedical research. Men and women are not the same as biological sex influences many aspects of health and disease[168]; sex-specific differences exist in the risk, timing, pathogenesis (e.g., cancer and obesity[169]), symptoms, and outcomes of many diseases (e.g., cardiovascular events, cancer, and mortality related to metabolic disease[170]).

Several areas of biomedical research underplay or overlook the potential effects of biological sex by using cell lines, animal models, and/ or human participants representing only one sex. This means that a great deal of data cannot be used to determine whether or not numerous phenomena are applicable to both sexes.[171] There have been numerous efforts to raise awareness of this representation gap which emphasize the scientific merit and public health benefits of closing it.[172,173] Attention to gender-based social roles and expectations, which in turn can be shaped by numerous social factors (e.g., class, ethnicity, religion), that can influence health has also been lacking in most biomedical research.[174,175] Obtaining a truly comprehensive understanding of human biology in men and women will take time, changing research practices, and broader analytical frameworks.

The Basis of Female Sex Differences

Adipose tissue is a key site of sex steroid metabolism which can exert local and systemic effects.[176] Sex steroids affect adipose biology by binding to oestrogen[177] and androgen[178] receptors on the surface of adipocytes. Investigations using *in vitro* systems have identified several potential mechanisms which may underpin these hormones' distinctive influence over regional fat accumulation and metabolic health. For instance, oestradiol promotes the proliferation of male and female preadipocytes, but (abdominal) subcutaneous cells are more sensitive to the proliferation-promoting effects of oestradiol than their omental (i.e., visceral) counterparts, while female cells are more sensitive than male cells.[179] This effect is consistent with the well-established trend that women have more subcutaneous fat (and less visceral fat) than men.[180]

The effects of oestrogens on adipogenesis are less clear-cut, with the current body of data on this important topic being surprisingly small and somewhat contradictory (e.g., oestrogens promote adipogenesis in mouse cells[181] yet inhibit it in human cells[182]), a situation which has raised concern in the research community.[183] Oestrogens can also affect the production and release of certain adipokines like leptin. For instance, oestrogen treatment increased circulating levels of leptin in women[184]; this finding adds meaning to the positive association between circulating leptin and oestrogen levels[185] and may help explain why leptin levels are considerably higher in women,[186] a difference which cannot be entirely explained by women carrying proportionately more fat than men.

Oestrogens contribute to the development and maintenance of the gynoid fat distribution pattern by modifying fatty acid handling in adipose tissue. Oestrogen administered during exercise promoted the mobilization of fatty acids from abdominal subcutaneous fat, but had a negligible effect on their release from subcutaneous fat in the thighs and buttocks.[187] The reluctance of lower body fat depots to mobilize their fatty acid stores, particularly in women, is supported by the higher levels of a specific type of adrenergic receptor; this receptor inhibits activation of the lipolysis machinery[188] and its expression levels are enhanced by oestrogen.[189]

Oestrogen biology is complicated by the two classes of 'classical' oestrogen receptor (ER), namely the alpha (α) and beta (β) forms. Both of these receptor types are present in adipocytes, but their relative proportions vary between different fat depots in a sex-specific manner.[190-192] As oestrogen binding to these receptors leads to activation of distinct biological pathways within the target cell, the same hormone at the same concentration can have different effects in different parts of the body (e.g., how much leptin a particular adipose depot produces[193]). What's more, the relative proportion of these receptors in adipose tissue can change, even as a result of oestrogen action itself.[191] This phenomenon may explain the inconsistent effects of oestrogen in the laboratory (e.g., during adipogenesis[194]) and also contribute to various complex mechanisms relating regional oestrogen action and adipose biology to metabolic health.[195]

Changing of the Seasons

The potent effect of oestrogen on adipose biology is most clearly demonstrated in menopause, the phenomenon in which endogenous oestrogen production by the ovaries ceases. Given the broad-acting nature of oestrogen, many different biological systems are affected by this natural hormonal decline. Among the various changes, however, the most distinctive involves a shift from the gynoid towards an increasingly android pattern of body fat distribution[196] and the parallel adoption of an increasingly masculine metabolic and cardiovascular disease risk profile. Before considering the changing pattern of body fat distribution, it is important to note that post-menopausal women tend to have a greater overall fat mass compared to their pre-menopausal counterparts,[197] a finding which probably aligns with many people's personal experiences, observations, and/or fears. This fat mass expansion may be the result of many things including reduced energy expenditure at rest[198] and during exercise,[199] and possibly even increased expression of enzymes which catalyze DNL.[200] Such observations add weight to the widely held belief that it is more difficult to keep the pounds off after menopause while reinforcing the potent influence of oestrogen on fat metabolism.

As post-menopausal women gain weight, their upper body fat depots tend to expand at the expense of lower body fat stores,[201] which is the opposite of how their pre-menopausal bodies would have handled the same weight gain. In terms of fatty acid uptake, oestrogen reportedly suppresses lipoprotein lipase activity[202]; while circulating oestrogen levels decline in menopause, it has been proposed that greater local production of oestrogen in thigh fat of post-menopausal women results in reduced lower body fat accumulation. What is most concerning about the gynoid-to-android fat distribution pattern, however, is the expansion of visceral fat.[198] This complex process likely involves various depot-specific mechanisms, such as higher lipoprotein lipase activity in visceral compared to subcutaneous fat.[203]

Visceral fat expansion predicts worse metabolic health outcomes (see Chapter 6), and this is no different in post-menopausal women.[204] Contrarily, greater amounts of lower body subcutaneous fat is associated with better metabolic health in post-menopausal women.[205] Such findings reinforce that a gynoid body shape appears to be beneficial regardless of age. So, surely maintaining this fat distribution pattern should have favourable health consequences? With oestrogen playing an instrumental role in maintaining this body shape, it makes implicit sense to simply replace it as naturally occurring levels decline during menopause; this rationale underpinned the development of hormone replacement therapy (HRT).

The Elixir of Youth?

Before considering the biological effects of administering oestrogen to post-menopausal women, it is important to consider that the medicalization of menopause and related treatments has proven controversial. Menopause is fundamentally a natural phenomenon that has increasingly been framed as a 'disease state' (particularly in the West) in which women become 'oestrogen deficient' and need to be treated accordingly.[206] It is interesting to note that such meanings are not ubiquitous, as cultural anthropologist Margaret Lock's seminal work on menopause in Japan suggests. Lock reported very different experiences of, and social meanings pertaining to menopause in North American versus Japanese women, such that this transition was viewed more as a natural part of aging in Japan, rather than a disease-like state.[207] Whatever your stance, the gynoid-to-android redistribution of fat starts with the oestrogen decline in menopause, and this process can be halted, or even reversed by HRT.

Hormone replacement therapy-treated post-menopausal women exhibit a body fat distribution pattern similar to their pre-menopausal counterparts, in which they store a greater proportion of total fat in their lower body as subcutaneous leg fat[208] and have reduced central (according to waist circumference and WHR[209]) and visceral[210] fat accumulation. Upon its advent, such striking effects stoked enthusiasm that HRT represented an intervention which could prevent a woman's youthful feminine shape being lost by the onward march of time and preserve the associated beneficial effects on metabolic and cardiovascular disease. Ageist notions of femininity aside, things have not transpired to be as straightforward or positive as many originally hoped.

After the widespread adoption of HRT during the early 1990s, data that emerged later in the decade prompted a cause for concern.[211] Despite the beneficial effects that HRT reportedly exerted on body fat distribution and blood lipid profile, the results of the Heart and Estrogen/Progestin Replacement Study (HERS) highlighted that HRT did not reduce coronary heart disease and was actually associated with an increased number of thromboembolic (blood clotting) and gallstone-related events.[212] This result was the tip of the iceberg though, with the current body of accumulated data clearly indicating that HRT is associated with an increased risk of having a heart attack, stroke, and venous thromboembolism, as well as gallbladder disease, although it does have beneficial effects on osteoporosis.[213]

Such results prompted a profession-wide re-evaluation of the widespread use of HRT in women going through the menopausal transition.

The HRT 'craze' has now passed and, although such treatment is still available, the medical profession now seems to advocate for a far more discriminating and measured approach to its use.[214] Given its side-effects, the clinical guidelines unsurprisingly state that HRT should not be used to prevent cardiovascular disease in post-menopausal women.[215] Given that HRT promotes the metabolically favourable gynoid fat distribution pattern, its negative cardiovascular effects are somewhat counter-intuitive. While much remains to be learned about the interplay between menopause, body fat distribution, and metabolic/cardiovascular disease risk, it seems that the same hormone can have distinct effects at different stages of life.[216] HRT may not be the panacea everyone wished it were, but it can effectively alleviate menopausal symptoms in a subgroup of women who have a particularly difficult time and decide (with their doctor) that the benefits outweigh the risks.

The relationship between menopause and cardiovascular disease outcomes in women remains unclear,[215] although menopause before age 45 is consistently associated with an increased risk.[217] With respect to metabolic disease, the rate of type 2 diabetes is lower in women at all ages, although the gap between men and women closes with increasing age.[218] Overall, the data suggest that menopause is not inherently bad for metabolic health, but that it represents the time when hormonal support for the metabolically favourable gynoid fat distribution pattern ceases. The ensuing gynoid-to-android fat re-distribution is accompanied by the acquisition of an increasingly masculine risk profile with respect to cardiovascular and metabolic disease. However, as central obesity, not menopausal status, appears to be the key factor that predicts metabolic disease risk,[219] encouraging physical activity and appropriate weight loss in (post-menopausal) women should remain the primary focus to improve health outcomes.[215,220]

Bellies and Babies

Polycystic ovary syndrome (PCOS) is a fairly common, highly complex, yet poorly understood endocrine disorder which mainly affects overweight/obese women. It has been proposed that dysfunctional fat supports a vicious cycle of disturbed steroid hormone metabolism which manifests as infertility, central obesity, and metabolic disease,[221] in addition to distressing symptoms such as acne, facial hair growth, and alopecia (spot baldness).[222,223] Adipose tissue's site at the interface between metabolic and reproductive biology is further reinforced by the report that many genetic loci significantly associated with obesity are also associated with indices of infertility and reproductive health.[224]

Looking beyond PCOS primarily affecting overweight and obese women, the extent of upper body fat accumulation is strongly associated with PCOS incidence and severity,[225,226] metabolic health disturbance,[227] and circulating androgen levels.[228] The profile of adipokines released by subcutaneous abdominal and visceral fat in women with PCOS also becomes more 'masculine.'[229] This altered pattern of adipokines from dysfunctional, obese adipose tissue can act in concert with the pathologically elevated levels of androgens to deleteriously affect fertility.[230] Weight loss currently represents the most effective and sustainable approach to addressing the various aspects of PCOS.[231]

Distilling Male Sex Differences

The androgen sex steroids (such as testosterone and its derivatives) are responsible for driving male sexual development and promoting upper body fat accumulation. Androgens influence adipose biology at a number of different levels to precipitate changes in body fat distribution, although these phenomena can be difficult to study owing to the numerous moving parts (recall that adipose tissue can interconvert steroids; testosterone metabolism reportedly varies between fat depots[232]) and challenges involved in replicating the *in vivo* environment *in vitro*.[233] Androgens exert complex effects on adipogenesis,[234] with studies suggesting testosterone may promote adipocyte hypertrophy by inhibiting adipogenesis in subcutaneous abdominal and visceral fat.[235,236] Androgens also influence the release of adipokines, with testosterone notably acting on adipocytes to reduce the expression and release of insulin-sensitizing adiponectin.[237] This fits with the observation that elevated testosterone levels are associated with reduced circulating adiponectin levels[238] and may help explain why women tend to have higher adiponectin levels and are generally more insulin-sensitive than men despite carrying a proportionately greater fat mass.

Another Elixir of Youth?

Just as women experience menopause, men have to contend with the consequences of declining testosterone levels that occur with aging, even if the associated effects/symptoms don't manifest as conspicuously or receive the same level of public attention. Declining testosterone levels are associated with a loss of skeletal muscle mass and weight gain in subcutaneous and visceral depots,[239] effects which have a negative impact on mobility, physical strength, and metabolic health.[240] Just as HRT emerged for the management of menopausal symptoms, testosterone treatment has been put forward as an approach to slow or reverse the age-related negative changes to body composition which affect older men. Testosterone treatment seems to turn the clock back as it prevents skeletal muscle mass loss in older men[241,242] and has generally favourable effects on body fat distribution in which visceral fat expansion is slowed,[241] overall fat mass is reduced,[243,244] and insulin sensitivity increases.[244]

But before declaring that testosterone/androgens are the elixir of youth—just as oestrogen was deemed previously—much remains to be learned. While beneficial effects on body composition and fat distribution might be observed, it is unclear whether they translate to better long-term health outcomes.[245,246] It is also unclear whether testosterone therapy raises the risk of developing other health problems that would not have otherwise occurred (e.g., prostate or testicular cancer). And even if testosterone therapy 'works', who should benefit? What constitutes being 'testosterone-deficient'? Interesting times lie ahead as the medical profession increasingly operates as though the natural process of aging falls within their jurisdiction as a quasi-disease state[247] (similar to male pattern baldness and erectile dysfunction). As we continue to bolster our understanding of sex steroid action, there is another group that can provide some powerful, unique insights; individuals undergoing transsexual procedures.

Body Modification

Long-term sex steroid administration is associated with significant changes in body composition and fat distribution that align with their effects and usually manifest during puberty (Figure 7.3). Testosterone given to female-to-male transsexuals is accompanied by a shift from the gynoid-to-android

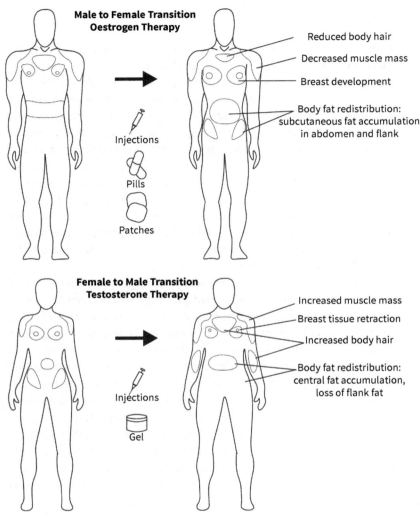

Figure 7.3 Body fat distribution changes in sex reassignment hormone therapy.

fat distribution pattern, a process in which overall fat mass, particularly subcutaneous fat,[248] tends to decrease while visceral fat expands.[249] This fat re-distribution tends to result in an expansion of the waist and is often accompanied by increased lean mass (mainly skeletal muscle) and

a masculinization of bone geometry.[250] Conversely, oestrogen administered to facilitate male-to-female transitions promotes fat re-distribution
that is associated with a general increase in overall fat mass, fat accumulation in the buttocks and thighs, and a reduction in lean mass.[251] Significant
body shape changes towards the affirmed sex can be achieved at any life
stage, but changes occur to a far greater extent the younger the transition
process is started.[252] Amid the wide-ranging and complex implications of
transsexual procedures, clinicians also have to contend with the additional
burden of minimizing the long-term effects on their patient's metabolic and
cardiovascular health. Current data suggest that steroid-induced body fat
distribution changes are associated with the expected metabolic health outcomes,[253] although more information is required to accurately determine
the long-term health prospects (e.g., cardiovascular outcomes[254]).

Androgens consumed for bodybuilding purposes are primarily used
for their ability to greatly enhance one's capacity to build lean mass as well
as for their effects on fat loss. However, their use in this context is associated with a complex series of insidious changes to the cardiovascular
system[255] and lipoprotein metabolism[256] that can put an individual's life
in jeopardy, ironically at a time when their physical appearance would
suggest they represent the epitome of health. And even if one manages
to avoid developing cardiovascular disease or worse, there's a high likelihood that these drugs will exert profound and irreversible adverse effects
on one's fertility.[257] Perhaps more feared than heart disease or infertility
among bodybuilders (as well as adolescents and overweight/obese men)
is *gynaecomastia*. In this situation, there is increased enzymatic conversion of androgens into oestrogens, often in fat tissue. This altered hormonal ratio promotes ductal tissue growth and local fat accumulation that
ultimately culminates in what are sometimes referred to as 'man boobs.'
In sum, the effects of these hormones can be profound, yet our understanding is rather rudimentary; there is a whole world to explore given
that sex steroids influence aspects of human biology as diverse as appetite regulation[258] to the number of white blood cells in adipose tissue,[259]
to their interplay with other hormones (e.g., glucocorticoids[260,261]).
Who knows, maybe careful manipulation of androgen[262] or oestrogen[263]
biology represents the novel approach that will turn the tide in the global
fight against obesity (and potentially infertility). But before any such fu-
turistic therapy possibly exists, many of us will have to make do with lifestyle (and/or societal) interventions.

Exercise and Diet

Beer Gut

The cultural phenomenon of the 'beer belly' reflects the common belief that drinking alcohol in the form of beer specifically promotes abdominal fat accumulation and waist circumference expansion. While many powerful images have permeated the media to reinforce the association between beer drinking and large bellies, the scientific basis for this connection is less compelling. On the one hand, robust evidence suggests that increased beer drinking is associated with a larger waist circumference,[264] although this relationship seems to be almost entirely driven by a general increase in body weight.[265] This is consistent with reports that increased alcohol consumption is associated with tangible, often deleterious, changes to body composition and fat distribution in various populations. For instance, greater alcohol intake has been associated with reduced subcutaneous abdominal but increased visceral fat mass in a Korean population.[266] Higher alcohol intake has also been associated with greater overall and central fat mass in a large European population,[267] particularly amongst men, and a cohort of elderly Australians,[268] while frequent binge drinking was associated with increased fat mass and poorer physical fitness in young military recruits.[269]

On the other hand, researchers who performed a meta-analysis of nearly 50 studies were unable to confidently draw conclusions about the relationship between alcohol consumption and overall and regional fat mass.[270] Such a result is perhaps unsurprising given the difficulty of obtaining robust data on dietary patterns in the real-world as many people don't report accurately, wittingly or otherwise; actual effects may also be masked by confounding factors such as exercise and dietary changes that go undocumented. Overall, the current evidence base does not suggest that alcohol has special properties which enable it to selectively promote abdominal fat accumulation. Instead, consuming excess calories in the form of calorie-dense alcoholic drinks, particularly beer, seems to drive overall weight gain which manifests as abdominal fat expansion, particularly in men; it is likely—but remains to be confirmed—whether individuals would develop the same protruding gut after over-indulging on sugary sweets or pasta as beer.

Sickly Sweet

Sugar is another prime nutritional villain, with *fructose* currently representing a focus of fascination and ire in the academic and public realms. Fructose is a specific sugar that has captured the public's attention since the advent of high-fructose corn syrup—a foodstuff which has infiltrated the recipes of many products in American supermarkets and increasingly other parts of the world. Fructose's omnipresence is certainly controversial, but this has been exacerbated by the scientific proposition that its unique biochemical properties directly cause liver fat accumulation. Fructose is unlike other carbohydrates as it provokes much less insulin secretion from the pancreas.[271] Moreover, when fructose is absorbed by liver cells, it passes unimpeded into the *de novo* lipogenesis pathway; a body of experimental data (often involving mice) suggests that this particular biochemical property predisposes those who consume it to developing fatty liver disease and metabolic disturbances.[272] Moreover, fructose reportedly has the potential to cause cellular stress, inflammation, and dysfunction in hepatocytes at high doses.[273] Coupling these properties with its infiltration of the global food chain, it has been easy to point the finger at fructose as a key perpetrator in the central obesity and diabetes pandemic. However, data from numerous epidemiological studies and dietary interventions indicate that fructose causes no more liver fat accumulation in humans than any other energy-dense nutrient when consumed in equivalent quantities.[274]

Excessive sugar consumption, regardless of what type, looms large as one of the main threats to public health around the world. The word 'excessive' should be particularly emphasized; sugar is not inherently toxic, but does cause deleterious health consequences if consumed in excess quantities[275] (in which a complex interplay between many factors will define an individual's threshold for safe sugar consumption). Reducing overall sugar consumption—particularly by removing the vast quantities stealthily added by the world's highly industrialized food production methods—represents one of the most effective strategies that would trim the world's waistline and drastically improve our collective health.[276]

One of the main ways in which substantial amounts of sugar enter our body, often far more than we realize, is through the consumption of sugar-sweetened beverages. Increased consumption of sugar-sweetened drinks is strongly associated with the development of central obesity as well as metabolic and cardiovascular disease in people of all ages.[277] While genetic background might modify overall[278] and regional fat accumulation[279] driven by sugar-sweetened beverage consumption, the associated effect size of such gene-diet interactions is almost negligible.[280] With the consumption of sugar-sweetened beverages also being a good indicator of poor dietary quality,[281] the massive global consumption of sugar and sugar-sweetened beverages paints a bleak picture of the world's health prospects. Seeking to address some of these challenges at a population and societal level, public health practitioners, policy makers, and various social scientists (e.g., medical sociologists) have increasingly called for interventions such as taxes or bans on certain sugary foods (e.g., soda taxes), as well as greater regulation of advertisements.

Fatally Fatty?

Fat is another nutrient whose relationship with the public, just like sugar, has been tumultuous. In terms of the relationship between fat consumption and (regional) fat accumulation, the relationship between dietary fat intake and body composition is ambiguous in children[282] and adults, particularly women.[283] Reducing one's fat intake often results in a small but detectable amount of weight loss though.[284] Relatedly, current evidence does not support the common assertion that fat consumption specifically/directly causes adipose expansion; total calorie consumption, rather than dietary fat (or sugar), is the crucial factor in the development of obesity[285] and pathological liver fat accumulation in humans.[286]

Understanding the relationship between fat biochemistry and health outcomes is complicated by the different types of fatty acid to contend with (Chapter 3). For example, increased consumption of saturated fat (in butter, processed meats, and baked goods) is associated with worse cardiovascular health, whereas replacing these calories with mono- or polyunsaturated fat (but not carbohydrate) has a beneficial effect, however small.[287] Note that having a high socioeconomic status helps considerably in reaping the health benefits of the polyunsaturated fatty acid-rich Mediterranean diet,[288] likely by facilitating one's ability to maintain such a diet compared to someone of lower socioeconomic status living in a 'food desert' who has far fewer dietary options. Perhaps unsurprisingly, the majority of people who develop non-alcoholic fatty liver disease apparently over-consume total and saturated fat as well as simple carbohydrates, and have a reduced intake of dietary fibre and polyunsaturated omega-3 fatty acids.[289] It has also been reported that both high and low carbohydrate diets are reportedly associated with increased mortality, with minimal risk observed with 50–55% carbohydrate intake; the source of nutrients plays an important modifying role though, as low-carbohydrate diets favouring plant-based protein and fat (e.g., vegetables, nuts) have lower mortality rates than their animal protein and fat-favouring (e.g., chicken, beef) counterpart.[290]

Dieting is a common and effective way of losing weight; maintaining the weight loss is difficult, although it can be achieved through intensive behavioural modification programmes involving emotional and nutritional counselling that can also reduce the need for bariatric surgery.[291] It is not clear whether continuous or intermittent calorie restriction is more effective,[292,293] but both are able to induce significant weight loss that confers wide-ranging health benefits, so whichever method the individual prefers and adheres to will be the best.[294] There are also promising data which indicate that very-low calorie diets (i.e., fewer than 800 kcal per day) can induce massive weight loss that alleviates, or even reverses, metabolic and cardiovascular disease, with such transformational results persisting with the appropriate training and support.[295] Once again, one's ability to take such steps such as changing one's diet or receiving support from health care professionals will depend on various social factors (e.g., social class, proximity and access to healthcare services, etc.).

The Wonder Drug

Representing the other half of 'lifestyle', physical activity and exercise are strongly encouraged by the medical profession and various governments around the world due to their many health benefits. Exercise truly deserves the 'wonder drug' moniker having proven to be effective in disease prevention and management. Exercise slows the progression and alleviates the symptoms of various chronic diseases[296,297] including type 2 diabetes,[298] coronary heart disease,[299] and depression.[300] Additionally, its positive health effects can be attained by any group at any age in any state of health, meaning children and adolescents,[35] adults,[301] postmenopausal women,[220] and elderly people[302] all stand to benefit. As with lifestyle changes around diet, one's ability to engage in physical activity are shaped and constrained by social factors such as where one lives, time available for exercise, access to gyms or other safe places to exercise, etc.

Sticking to an exercise regimen is associated with favourable changes to body composition (i.e., reduced fat mass and increased lean mass and bone density) and improved physical fitness[303] and metabolic health,[304] with these positive changes being most striking and profound in overweight and obese individuals. In terms of exercise type, meta-analyses indicate that aerobic exercise, especially in conjunction with resistance training, is an effective way of sustainably reducing overall (and central) obesity as well as liver fat mass in obese adolescents[305] and type 2 diabetes patients.[306] In other words, exercise is one thing everyone should be doing. But does exercise affect body fat distribution?

Cutting Waist

Ectopic fat mass seems to be the crucial factor linking fat mass, distribution, and function with overall metabolic and cardiovascular health. Indeed, loss of visceral fat mass has been identified as the key parameter that is independently associated with improvements in various risk factors for cardiovascular and metabolic disease.[307] Similar associations have also been detected for liver fat mass,[308] which is closely correlated to visceral fat mass.[309] However, visceral and liver fat accumulation are consequences of subcutaneous fat dysfunction and increased insulin resistance that underpins metabolic and cardiovascular disease.[310] Consequently, reductions in ectopic fat mass are closely associated with beneficial changes in metabolic health, although this probably reflects improvements to subcutaneous fat function and insulin sensitivity in metabolically important organs like the liver and skeletal muscle. This is illustrated by the report that exercise can reduce liver and visceral fat accumulation in the absence of weight loss, with such changes being associated with improved insulin sensitivity in obese adolescents.[311]

So, in answer to the question posed originally, yes, exercise can change body fat distribution. However, these changes are apparently guided by the underlying depot-specific properties of adipose tissue. Experimental data from a weight-loss study involving obese individuals highlighted that the abdomen was the region where the greatest fat loss occurred, followed by the legs and then the arms.[312] A study of regional weight loss (in post-menopausal women) also suggested that upper body fat mass was preferentially lost upon participation in an exercise programme.[313] When people lose weight, visceral fat preferentially retracts upon modest weight loss,[314] but subcutaneous fat mass reduction is far greater in absolute terms. However, the extent of visceral fat loss is linked strongly to subcutaneous fat loss.[315] As fat mass is lost, depot-specific cellular properties also come into play. Indeed, changes in abdominal fat mass predominantly occur via expansion and retraction of a relatively stable number of cells, whereas gluteo-femoral fat expands via hyperplasia and then retracts via reduced cell size. This scenario means repeated weight gain–loss cycles could lead to increased cell number,[316] a situation which could promote future weight (re)gain and make weight maintenance more difficult. However, no exercise intervention can induce the specific reduction of visceral fat, or any other depot for that matter (so-called 'spot reduction'). Indeed, training a muscle group will strengthen it and increase its endurance, but abdominal crunches don't preferentially mobilize abdominal fat[317] in the same way that squats won't selectively shift gluteo-femoral fat.[318]

A wealth of evidence indicates that a combination of aerobic and resistance exercise is most effective in reducing liver fat mass in children[319] and adults.[320] With respect to the latest trend in fitness, a recent meta-analysis reported that high-intensity interval training (HIIT) confers the same benefits as moderate-intensity continuous training on body mass and composition, total cholesterol, and other metabolic parameters, albeit achieved through shorter bouts of intense exercise.[321] HIIT has been found to better increase an individual's VO_2 max (i.e., maximal oxygen intake) than moderate intensity continuous exercise.[322] Bottom-line, doing exercise in whatever form suits the individual confers broad health benefits.

Our understanding of how the benefits of exercise manifest remains relatively modest though. Exercise-induced weight loss is associated with reduced subcutaneous (abdominal) adipocyte size,[323] with such improvements to fat function likely involving various epigenetic mechanisms[324] (e.g., DNA methylation[325]), the modulation of adipose tissue inflammation,[326] and the release of hormones that beneficially integrate multiple organs.[327] Although it is unlikely that we will ever be able to derive all of the benefits of exercise without actually performing it, understanding the mechanisms involved might provide some new leads in the development of therapeutic agents which can enhance physical fitness, metabolic health, and body composition.

What factors affect an individual's response to exercise interventions are currently unclear. For instance, women (but not men) with a genetic background associated with central obesity were found to respond less well to weight loss interventions.[328] Although statistically significant, it is unlikely that the size of this effect (i.e., 15g of fat per genetic risk variant) is of any clinical relevance, nor does it provide a compelling case to suggest the benefits of exercise can be negated by one's genes; they might mean the difference between a gold and silver medal though. On the contrary, individuals carrying the BMI-increasing *FTO* genetic variant respond as well to weight loss interventions as non-carriers.[329] Exercise is hard work though, and numerous societies have a predilection for specific body shapes and quick-fixes; it is perhaps unsurprising that cosmetic procedures to attain the seemingly unattainable have grown in popularity over the past few decades. But does surgically modifying one's body shape by changing regional fat mass confer the associated health benefits?

Surgery

Once deemed a vainglorious, self-indulgent practice reserved for the rich and famous, such a view of cosmetic surgery has been challenged by the vast and growing number of people who have gone under the knife. The decision to partake is complex and multi-faceted, involving factors such as media consumption, self-esteem, life satisfaction, sex life, and religiosity.[330] Other contributing factors include social interactions and peer pressure built around the internalization of the 'thin ideal'[331] (as perpetuated by the media and social attitudes), as well as an individual's materialistic tendencies, self-objectification, and willingness to capitalize on their deemed sexual attractiveness.[332] Whatever the justification, it will probably emanate from a desire to escape society's negative perspective of fat and the parallel belief that attaining what better resembles society's conception of the ideal female or male form, however problematic, will translate to an increase in social and/or economic standing. Unsurprisingly, adipose tissue represents the main target of many cosmetic procedures which cut away their (excess) fat and sculpt whatever remains into a supposedly more desirable shape.

An Ugly Start

The surgical removal of fat (i.e., lipectomy) was the earliest surgical option for treating obesity that was employed for a combination of health, mobility, and aesthetic reasons. Some of the earliest reports outlining abdominal lipectomies date back to the early 1900s, with one prominent report by

Dr H. E. Castle from 1911 describing how he excised a considerable amount of pendulous abdominal subcutaneous fat from a severely obese women.[333] However, the first attempt to remodel body fat for aesthetic reasons dates back to the 1920s when the French surgeon Dr Charles Dujarier attempted to enhance the apparently unsightly ankles and knees of Mademoiselle Geoffre, an aspiring young model.[334]

Representing a watershed moment in the history of medicine and cosmetic surgery, the operation itself was a complete disaster. Dr Dujarier removed an excessively large piece of skin and soft tissue (i.e., fat) before stitching the wound up too tightly, causing the wound to turn gangrenous and require amputation. Such a catastrophic outcome prompted Mademoiselle Geoffre to take Dr Dujarier to court. The effect of this lawsuit extended far beyond a 200,000-franc penalty to Dr Dujarier as plastic surgery was effectively outlawed thereafter. While this might have sounded the death knell for the fledgling field of cosmetic surgery, the case was revisited two years later. The court upheld Dr Dujarier's sentence, but relieved the ban on plastic surgery, thus declaring it legitimate on the condition that the patient's informed consent was obtained. Dr Dujarier died shortly after this second ruling and was unable to witness the flourishing of the surgical field he'd singlehandedly founded and nearly destroyed.

Many other attempts to sculpt the body's shape followed after the field received this green light, with the thighs representing the primary focus of the pioneering surgeons and their willing patients. This explorative period was defined by many flawed and botched surgical procedures that produced all-manner of post-operative deformities and potentially life-threatening complications[335] including tissue necrosis, infections, and haematomas (i.e., solid swellings of clotted blood). This protracted season of flawed experimental butchery was brought to a close in 1975 when the father-and-son cosmetic surgeons Arpad and Giorgio Fischer developed the modern technique of liposuction, which has since become the world's most popular method for the localized removal of subcutaneous fat[336] (Figure 7.4). Also focusing on the outer thigh, these surgeons pioneered the use of a blunt-tipped hollow cannula attached to a suction source which is inserted at multiple incision sites to get 'criss-cross' coverage of the target site, an approach which provides much better and more predictable aesthetic results with fewer complications.

After the inception of modern liposuction, two Parisian surgeons named Illouz and Fournier modified the equipment required for the Fischers' technique and extended the procedure to the whole body during the late 1970s

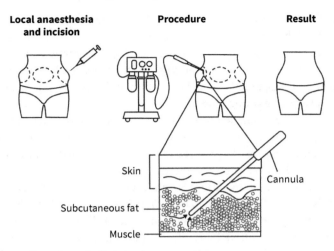

Figure 7.4 Overview of a liposuction procedure.

and 1980s.[337] Blunt cannulas of different sizes were developed for use on different parts of the body: the largest for use on the flanks, hips, and buttocks; a middle one for knees, ankles, and the abdomen; and a small one for the face. All of these cannulas also had a reduced diameter compared to their older counterparts to reduce the damage to nerves as well as blood and lymphatic vessels during the often quite vigorous and physically involved procedure.

As the modern incarnation of the liposuction technique became established around the world, particularly in the US and France, the American Society of Liposuction was formed in 1982 to unify the surgical training.[338] However, concerns that the technique was mostly performed under general anaesthetic weighed on the minds of its practitioners for a combination of safety and entrepreneurial reasons. In 1987, Jeffrey Klein, a Californian dermatologist, offered a solution in his method of performing liposuction under large volumes of dilute local anaesthesia that obviated the need for sedation or general anaesthesia and their associated risks and costs.[339] Now it was possible to (deliriously) watch your belly vanish before your very eyes!

Not all technological developments have been successful though. One variant involved using ultrasound emitted from the cannula tip to mechanically and thermally disrupt the target fat tissue and make it easier to remove while preserving the delicate nervous and vascular structures.

While sounding good in theory, the widespread adoption of ultrasonic liposuction in South America and Europe was quickly reversed after mounting reports that the procedure caused burns, skin sloughing/shedding, and seromas (i.e., the accumulation of clear fluid in post-operative wounds).[340] The latest development in liposuction technology utilizes observations from the early 1990s that adipocytes burst upon exposure to a laser beam, leaking their oily contents into the surrounding tissue fluid that can be easily removed via suction.[341] Owing to its precision and ability to stimulate cartilage remodelling within adipose tissue, laser-assisted liposuction is often used to sculpt areas in the body or face of lipodystrophy patients.[342]

Form, Not Function

The simplicity, versatility, and precision of the liposuction technique make it a highly effective and popular cosmetic procedure used for body sculpting and contouring around the world. The safety record for the actual procedure is largely good with a low risk of major complications when the procedure is performed in isolation.[343] Remarkably, however, little data exists on the effects of such procedures on long-term metabolic and cardiovascular health. We are thus left placing our bets and taking a guess as to whether removing subcutaneous fat from the abdomen and/or thighs would have a beneficial, neutral, or negative effect on one's metabolic health.

Based on the limited amount of evidence available, liposuction might have any of these effects. One prominent study of women (some with type 2 diabetes) who underwent liposuction to reduce their abdominal obesity found that the ~20% reduction in total fat mass induced by the procedure had absolutely *no effect* on various metabolic and cardiovascular disease risk factors measured three months after the operation.[344] Indeed, their fasting blood glucose, lipid, and insulin levels as well as blood pressure did not change, nor did the insulin sensitivity of their fat, liver, or muscle. Consistent with such findings, another study reported that the removal of considerable amounts of abdominal subcutaneous fat from obese women via liposuction had no tangible effect on insulin sensitivity, despite inducing a considerable reduction in circulating leptin levels.[345]

Other studies have reported small but statistically significant improvements to various metabolic parameters following liposuction (e.g., fasting glucose levels).[346-349] However, these and other studies were performed quite soon after the procedure (between one and six months), meaning the post-operative inflammatory response and healing process could have influenced the results. In contrast to these reports of beneficial, if marginal, effects observed shortly after the procedure, it has been reported that a liposuction-induced reduction of abdominal fat mass had no effect on a plethora of cardiovascular and metabolic disease risk factors up to four years after the operation, at which point the significant weight loss had been retained.[350] Achieving the same magnitude of weight loss from a liposuction procedure via any other method (particularly diet or exercise, but also bariatric surgery) would have exerted truly transformational effects on one's health.

So, what are the metabolic effects of cutting out substantial chunks of subcutaneous abdominal fat? A recent meta-analysis (which noted the conflicting literature) reported that abdominal lipectomy appears to have no significant effect on an individual's long-term metabolic health.[351] That means that if someone is already on their way to developing metabolic disease, having an abdominal lipectomy will not change their trajectory.[352] Instead, this technique appears to be most suited for addressing the aesthetic and physically incapacitating symptoms of (morbid) obesity. That doesn't mean that these fat removal procedures have no effect though. On the contrary, mounting data suggest that removing abdominal subcutaneous fat via liposuction[353] or lipectomy[354] is followed by fat re-growth[355] and/or re-distribution, often in a less metabolically favourable manner (i.e., adipocyte hypertrophy) that often involves the expansion of visceral stores.[356]

Cut It Out

While excising subcutaneous abdominal fat has neutral or negative effects on metabolic health, what about other parts of the body? As highlighted by Mademoiselle Geoffre's case, many individuals wish to have their legs contoured and sculpted. Compared to subcutaneous abdominal liposuction and lipectomy (which are essentially the same thing, albeit via different means), there is even less data on the effects of removing subcutaneous fat from the thighs and buttocks; what is available suggests that this might be a dangerous game to play. One notable study highlighted that femoral lipectomy (i.e., fat removal from the thigh) in women had a direct negative impact on fatty acid handling after a meal, meaning it took considerably longer to clear dietary fat from the bloodstream[357] - this could contribute to the development of atherosclerosis.[358] What's more, the removal of thigh fat was followed by expansion of abdominal fat stores.[359] As noted by the authors, the body vigorously defends its fat stores—as expected given its evolutionary heritage—such that the surgical removal of fat is reminiscent of the mythical Hydra whose heads grow back upon being cut off.

Other lipectomy procedures have provided additional insights into the depot-specific biology of human adipose tissue. For instance, a study of obese type 2 diabetes patients found that an omentectomy (in which the sheet of visceral fat which occupies the space around the liver, intestines, and stomach is removed) had no effect on insulin sensitivity,[360] consistent with visceral fat accumulation being consequential/correlative rather than causative in metabolic disease. Numerous reports have noted how supplementing gastric bypass surgery with an omentectomy does not enhance the well-established beneficial metabolic and cardiovascular effects of the former.[361–363]

The opportunity to better understand the short- and long-term health consequences and biology of procedures that alter body fat distribution should absolutely be taken. The numerous and growing group of people who have undertaken liposuction and similar procedures represent a unique and relatively untapped resource that could help answer various burning scientific and clinical questions that would otherwise be too expensive, impractical, or even unethical to address.[364] Moreover, a recent meta-analysis brought together the entire scientific literature on fat reduction interventions in the context of metabolic health in 2015 and pooled data from a total of 271 patients.[351] In that same year, a whopping 222,051 liposuction procedures were performed in the US alone according to the American Society of Plastic Surgeons.[365] Given the vast number of people undertaking such cosmetic procedures, potentially more than once in their lifetime, it is crucial that those electing to undertake non-essential surgery are aware of all of the risks—including, but certainly not limited to, what might happen on the operating table. Cosmetic surgery may have become relatively normalized in some modern societies, but the decision to go under the knife is not to be taken lightly.

The need to understand the long-term health consequences also applies to other (non-invasive) fat reduction technologies such as cryolipolysis, radiofrequency, low-level laser therapy, and high-intensity focused ultrasound. These techniques induce subcutaneous adipocyte death to reduce fat mass, facilitate body contouring, and alleviate cellulite[366] with a low complication rate.[367] In contrast to fat removal procedures (e.g., liposuction and lipectomy), the fat contained within the undesirable adipocytes remains within the body during these non-invasive procedures. But where does it go? This is not entirely clear, but the liver likely plays a role in processing the liberated fatty acids. Whether violently releasing the contents of adipocytes is a metabolically benign process is not clear, but a handful of (very) small-scale studies suggest that the vast majority of these procedures are probably safe,[368] an effect which probably derives from the typically small volumes of fat targeted. In sum, fat removal procedures don't appear to confer many, if any, health benefits as they apparently address a symptom, not a cause, of metabolic disease—even if they can make someone look like a picture of health.

Not all interventions centre around fat removal. The shape of the lower body can also be modified through an increasingly popular cosmetic procedure known colloquially as the 'Brazilian butt lift.' This technique involves taking subcutaneous fat removed via liposuction (usually from the abdomen) from an individual and transplanting it to the subcutaneous fat and intramuscular layers of their buttocks.[369] Compared to other cosmetic procedures, this transformation has been notable for its significantly higher mortality rate, which is due to a number of complications including pulmonary fat embolisms[370] (in which the grafted fat dislodges from the buttock and blocks blood flow to the lungs), although this may be reduced by injecting transplanted fat into the deep muscle.[371] In terms of examining long-term consequences, the focus has fallen primarily on whether the augmentation persists, with one notable study reporting that the graft volume typically shrinks by ~20% twelve months post-procedure.[372] Much like other cosmetic procedures, the long-term health consequences of procedures that modify metabolically important adipose tissue are unclear and await deeper investigation. This patient population provides a unique opportunity to delve into depot-specific fat biology; would augmenting lower body fat reduce cardiovascular and metabolic disease risk, or would the abdominal origin of the transplanted fat negate any potential benefit? Such augmentation (as well as reduction) raises equally interesting questions about differential socio-cultural meanings around body shape that may influence demand for such interventions in some contexts or groups but not others.

A Medical Miracle

Hoovering, cutting, or zapping fat in a cosmetic clinic aren't the only ways that surgery can modify body fat distribution. *Bariatric surgery* is another intervention that is often accompanied by profound beneficial effects on metabolic and cardiovascular health. Remarkably, however, this approach doesn't involve directly modifying fat tissue. Bariatric surgery refers to a handful of different surgical techniques which involve modifying the anatomy of the gastrointestinal tract in a way that reduces the size of one's stomach and/or surface area in the small intestine available for food absorption[373] (Figure 7.5). These anatomical modifications were originally devised to simply limit the amount of food that could be consumed as well

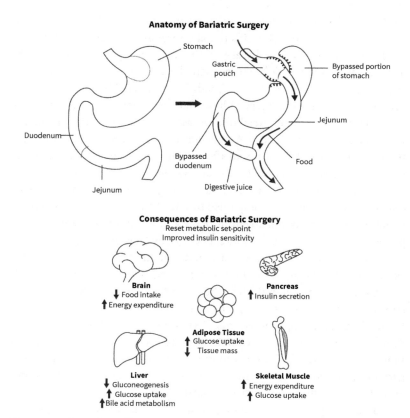

Figure 7.5 Overview of bariatric surgery anatomy and its consequences.

as the number of calories that could be absorbed, thereby inducing a negative energy balance; an individual expending more calories than they consume would therefore lose weight. A mounting body of evidence indicates, however, that bariatric procedures induce a far greater degree of weight loss than can be explained by the altered mechanics involved in food digestion and absorption.

Bariatric surgery has exploded in the media due to a number of high-profile individuals publicly undertaking gastric bypass surgery to assist in their weight loss (including the actress Roseanne Barr, singer Etta James, and the footballer Diego Maradona who has undertaken two procedures). Gastric bypass procedures are typically reserved for morbidly obese individuals (i.e., BMI >40kg/m^2) when all other attempts to manage or reverse their weight gain and metabolic disease (e.g., type 2 diabetes) have failed. Bariatric surgery induces far greater improvements in weight loss in adults[374] and children/adolescents[375] compared to any other non-surgical intervention; it is also highly effective at improving, or even resolving, type 2 diabetes[376] and fatty liver disease.[377] The effect of surgery-induced weight loss on male[378] and female[379] reproductive health remains less clear though, as irreversible damage may have already been inflicted by the time of surgery. In sum, bariatric surgery induces massive weight loss and the alleviation, if not remission, of metabolic disease in the vast majority of patients who undertake the procedure. As with any health procedure, such implications are limited to those who can afford such a procedure, or for whom the procedure is covered by their healthcare system/insurance plan.

Currently available data on bariatric surgery suggest that the post-operation weight loss is accompanied by a re-distribution of fat away from metabolically unfavourable central obesity to an increasingly gynoid fat pattern of fat distribution (in which upper body fat preferentially recedes), with improvements in various metabolic parameters (e.g., insulin sensitivity) being strongly associated with the degree of fat redistribution.[380] Visceral and ectopic fat in the liver, heart, and pancreas also tend to retract considerably following surgery,[381] albeit to different proportions (e.g., there is usually greater proportional loss of visceral compared to epicardial fat mass[382]). This reduction in ectopic fat mass—particularly from fat and muscle—and fat redistribution, reportedly persists for a long time after surgery (at least two years), even in the absence of further changes in overall weight[383]; such effects are really life-transforming.

Bariatric surgery seems to prompt a systemic change in a patient's body that essentially 'resets' their metabolic status and insulin sensitivity (i.e., their 'set point'[384]), dissociating it from their current less healthy body composition and fat distribution pattern. The ensuing chain of events leads to the body's physical form aligning with that of its 'perceived' metabolic status (i.e., toward a more healthy normal weight). Improvements in insulin sensitivity are largely restored in fat and skeletal muscle[385] as well as in the liver[386] fairly shortly after surgery (in a matter of weeks), well before any significant weight loss has occurred. Adipokine levels also change, albeit in unpredictable ways between individuals,[387] with leptin levels typically decreasing with weight loss while insulin-sensitizing adiponectin levels rise.[388]

Vascular function and health also improve, often manifesting as a clinically significant reduction in cardiovascular disease risk.[389] Circulating levels of inflammatory factors that promote insulin resistance and increased blood pressure also decline,[390] although local inflammation of adipose tissue does not change considerably post-operatively[391,392]; the quality, but not quantity, of immune system activity in adipose tissue may change to support beneficial fat remodelling and the restoration of fat function though. Overall, the loss and redistribution of fat, as well as the restoration of its function, are thought to contribute significantly toward the improvements in metabolic and cardiovascular health that most patients experience.[393] What acts as the initiating signal(s) in this complex chain of events currently remains a mystery, although its identification offers the tantalizing prospect of providing patients with the benefits of bariatric surgery in the form of a mass-producible drug.

Bowels, Brains, and Bacteria

The anatomical modification that bariatric surgery imposes on the gastrointestinal tract not only changes the mechanics of food digestion and absorption, but also the release of gut hormones which modulate digestion, enhance insulin-directed nutrient storage, and influence appetite. Bariatric surgery has been associated with favourable changes in the levels of various gut hormones (which read like an alphabet soup of acronyms such as PYY, GLP-1, and GIP). which co-ordinate post-operative improvements in systemic insulin sensitivity[394,395] and appetite control.[396,397] The resetting of one's appetite also plays a key role in inducing and maintaining weight loss in obese patients whose brains have become 'numb' to satiety signals (e.g., leptin) and lost the ability to feel full, or at least full enough to stop eating.[398]

Synergizing with hormonal changes, the presence of just a few mouthfuls of food in the small stomach pouch of a post-bariatric surgery patient stimulates an overwhelming battery of neuronal signals which indicate fullness,[399] thus making drastic reductions in food intake achievable to facilitate the weight loss process. Bariatric surgery also prompts the reconfiguration of food-associated thought processes; post-operative patients tend to experience a greatly reduced frequency of food cravings and an appetite that is less influenced by emotions,[400] with some patients even perceiving sweet flavours as less palatable.[401] It has also been reported that bariatric surgery increases resting and post-meal energy expenditure,[402] thus exerting an additional slow calorie-burning effect that facilitates weight loss and the restoration of metabolic health.[403]

Bariatric surgery is also associated with changes to the gut microbiota[404] (i.e., the innumerable bacteria which inhabit our intestinal tract). Data from the burgeoning field that explores such bacteria indicate that changes to gut microbiota and the metabolites they produce are associated with diseases ranging from obesity, type 2 diabetes, and fatty liver disease[405,406] to anxiety and depression,[407] inflammatory conditions such as irritable bowel syndrome,[408] and type 1 diabetes.[409] The public's fascination with this topic has grown in recent years, with the notion of faecal transplantation representing a possible treatment for *Clostridium difficile* infections proving to be particularly captivating.[410] Spurred on by this prospect, there are substantial ongoing efforts to harness this unique biology to treat all manner of diseases. Current data indicate that bariatric surgery can induce a significant re-configuring of the types of bacteria that inhabit the gut,[411,412] and that certain reconfigurations of the bacterial population correlate with metabolic health improvements.[413] While impressive and fascinating, it is not currently clear what contribution this phenomenon makes to the post-operative recovery.[414]

Bile acid metabolism also changes significantly following bariatric surgery. These cholesterol-based molecules aid in fat digestion by dispersing large fat droplets into numerous smaller droplets (see Chapter 3). They are, however, somewhat unique in that they are re-absorbed from the gut and transported back to the liver to be reclaimed and recycled.[415] Bile acid metabolism is disturbed in obesity[416] and metabolic disease (e.g., non-alcoholic fatty liver disease[417]), with this effect likely being co-ordinated by the action of bile acids on their receptors present on metabolically important tissues such as the liver[418] and potentially the brain.[419] Restoration of bile acid biology appears to contribute to the health improvements that follow bariatric surgery,[420] meaning synthetic versions may represent a useful treatment for the metabolic complications of obesity.[421] Indeed, GLP-1 receptor activators—which mimic the naturally occurring gut hormone whose low levels rise considerably following bariatric surgery—now represent a major class of drugs used to effectively manage type 2 diabetes and obesity.[422]

Making the Best of a Bad Situation

Understanding the mechanisms underpinning the improvements to metabolic health following bariatric surgery is certainly important. However, identifying which factors predict the best responses to this intervention (i.e., disease remission compared to weight regain and ongoing treatment[423]) has a greater immediate practical benefit, particularly when medical resources are being stretched beyond breaking point. The chances of post-operative success are bolstered by routine pre-operative interventions involving diet, exercise, and/or drugs.[424] Increasing evidence suggests that analyses of pre-operative body composition[425] and body fat distribution[426] (via WHR or DXA) may be more useful than BMI when used in conjunction with measures of metabolic health to identify the best prospects within the pool of candidates eligible for bariatric surgery. The pre-operative structure of fat is also a good predictor of an individual's response to bariatric surgery. For instance, individuals whose subcutaneous abdominal fat tissue is more fibrotic tend to lose significantly less weight and have a reduced improvement to their metabolic health after bariatric surgery.[427,428] There is also an increasing appreciation that certain psychological characteristics and social conditions are important in predicting whether the transformational effects of surgery will manifest and/or endure.[429]

Follow-up studies of post-operative patients provide further compelling evidence that emphasizes the robust relationship between body fat distribution and metabolic health. Indeed, bariatric surgery patients who experience the greatest fat redistribution to metabolically favourable subcutaneous stores, particularly to the lower body, tend to show the largest improvements in insulin sensitivity.[393] Moreover, individuals who retain visceral and ectopic fat tend to experience the lowest rates of improvements to metabolic and cardiovascular health.[430] In addition to drastic improvements to metabolic and cardiovascular health, bariatric surgery reportedly exerts positive effects on fatty liver disease,[431,432] as well as a number of types of cancer,[433] including those affecting the breast,[434] endometrium,[435] and colon[436] (i.e., diseases whose risk are increased by obesity).

A great deal of work remains to be done to conclusively identify the effects of bariatric surgery on patients' long-term health, but current data indicate strongly that this procedure improves and saves lives.[437] Bariatric surgery may constitute a modern medical miracle, and although it is not cheap and demand outstrips supply, there is a strong economic case for expanding access due to the significant health benefits it confers at an acceptable cost.[438] As a downstream intervention it does nothing to curtail the growing obese population though, and care should be taken to not undermine preventative policies which may have broader benefits beyond obesity as well (e.g., environmental benefits from changing food manufacturing practices).

References

1. Weiling, F. Historical study: Johann Gregor Mendel 1822–1884. *Am. J. Med. Genet.* **40**, 1–25; discussion 26 (1991).
2. Souren, N. Y. *et al.* Anthropometry, carbohydrate and lipid metabolism in the East Flanders Prospective Twin Survey: heritabilities. *Diabetologia* **50**, 2107–16 (2007).
3. Malis, C. *et al.* Total and regional fat distribution is strongly influenced by genetic factors in young and elderly twins. *Obes. Res.* **13**, 2139–45 (2005).
4. Elks, C. E. *et al.* Variability in the heritability of body mass index: a systematic review and meta-regression. *Front. Endocrinol.* **3**, 29 (2012).
5. Herskind, A. M., McGue, M., Sørensen, T. I., & Harvald, B. Sex and age specific assessment of genetic and environmental influences on body mass index in twins. *Int. J. Obes. Relat. Metab. Disord.* **20**, 106–13 (1996).
6. Hur, Y.-M. *et al.* Genetic influences on the difference in variability of height, weight and body mass index between Caucasian and East Asian adolescent twins. *Int. J. Obes.* **32**, 1455–67 (2008).
7. Stunkard, A. J., Foch, T. T., & Hrubec, Z. A twin study of human obesity. *JAMA* **256**, 51–4 (1986).
8. Poulsen, P., Vaag, A., Kyvik, K., & Beck-Nielsen, H. Genetic versus environmental aetiology of the metabolic syndrome among male and female twins. *Diabetologia* **44**, 537–43 (2001).
9. Song, M. *et al.* Longitudinal analysis of genetic susceptibility and BMI throughout adult life. *Diabetes* **67**, 248–55 (2018).
10. Graff, M. *et al.* BMI loci and longitudinal BMI from adolescence to young adulthood in an ethnically diverse cohort. *Int. J. Obes.* **41**, 759–68 (2017).

11. Min, J., Chiu, D. T., & Wang, Y. Variation in the heritability of body mass index based on diverse twin studies: a systematic review. *Obes. Rev.* 14, 871–82 (2013).

12. Wardle, J. & Carnell, S. Appetite is a heritable phenotype associated with adiposity. *Ann. Behav. Med.* 38 Suppl. 1, S25–30 (2009).

13. Nelson, T. L., Vogler, G. P., Pedersen, N. L., & Miles, T. P. Genetic and environmental influences on waist-to-hip ratio and waist circumference in an older Swedish twin population. *Int. J. Obes. Relat. Metab. Disord.* 23, 449–55 (1999).

14. Rose, K. M., Newman, B., Mayer-Davis, E. J., & Selby, J. V. Genetic and behavioral determinants of waist-hip ratio and waist circumference in women twins. *Obes. Res.* 6, 383–92 (1998).

15. Selby, J. V *et al.* Genetic and behavioral influences on body fat distribution. *Int. J. Obes.* 14, 593–602 (1990).

16. Sung, Y. J. *et al.* Genome-wide association studies suggest sex-specific loci associated with abdominal and visceral fat. *Int. J. Obes.* 40, 662–74 (2016).

17. Liu, C.-T. *et al.* Genome-wide association of body fat distribution in African ancestry populations suggests new loci. *PLoS Genet.* 9, e1003681 (2013).

18. Bouchard, C. *et al.* The response to long-term overfeeding in identical twins. *N. Engl. J. Med.* 322, 1477–82 (1990).

19. Pérusse, L. *et al.* Familial aggregation of abdominal visceral fat level: results from the Quebec family study. *Metabolism* (1996). doi:10.1016/S0026-0495(96)90294-2

20. Locke, A. E. *et al.* Genetic studies of body mass index yield new insights for obesity biology. *Nature* 518, 197–206 (2015).

21. Shungin, D. *et al.* New genetic loci link adipose and insulin biology to body fat distribution. *Nature* 518, 187–96 (2015).

22. Riveros-McKay, F. *et al.* Genetic architecture of human thinness compared to severe obesity. *PLOS Genet.* 15, e1007603 (2019).

23. Loos, R. J. F. & Yeo, G. S. H. The bigger picture of FTO: the first GWAS-identified obesity gene. *Nat. Rev. Endocrinol.* 10, 51–61 (2014).

24. Yoneyama, S. *et al.* Generalization and fine mapping of European ancestry-based central adiposity variants in African ancestry populations. *Int. J. Obes.* 41, 324–31 (2017).

25. Huang, L. O. *et al.* Genome-wide discovery of genetic loci that uncouple excess adiposity from its comorbidities. *Nat. Metab.* 3, 228–43 (2021).

26. Zillikens, M. C. *et al.* Large meta-analysis of genome-wide association studies identifies five loci for lean body mass. *Nat. Commun.* 8, 80 (2017).

27. Visscher, P. M. *et al.* 10 years of GWAS discovery: biology, function, and translation. *Am. J. Hum. Genet.* 101, 5–22 (2017).

28. Müller, M. J. *et al.* The case of GWAS of obesity: does body weight control play by the rules? *Int. J. Obes.* (2018). doi:10.1038/s41366-018-0081-6

29. Maher, B. Personal genomes: the case of the missing heritability. *Nature* 456, 18–21 (2008).

30. Pigeyre, M., Yazdi, F. T., Kaur, Y., & Meyre, D. Recent progress in genetics, epigenetics and metagenomics unveils the pathophysiology of human obesity. *Clin. Sci.* **130**, 943–86 (2016).

31. Olden, K. & White, S. L. Health-related disparities: influence of environmental factors. *Med. Clin. North Am.* **89**, 721–38 (2005).

32. Manolio, T. A. *et al.* Finding the missing heritability of complex diseases. *Nature* **461**, 747–53 (2009).

33. Trerotola, M., Relli, V., Simeone, P., & Alberti, S. Epigenetic inheritance and the missing heritability. *Hum. Genomics* **9**, 17 (2015).

34. Ericson, U. *et al.* Dietary and genetic risk scores and incidence of type 2 diabetes. *Genes Nutr.* **13**, 13 (2018).

35. Marson, E. C., Delevatti, R. S., Prado, A. K. G., Netto, N., & Kruel, L. F. M. Effects of aerobic, resistance, and combined exercise training on insulin resistance markers in overweight or obese children and adolescents: a systematic review and meta-analysis. *Prev. Med.* **93**, 211–18 (2016).

36. Llewellyn, C. H. & Fildes, A. Behavioural susceptibility theory: Professor Jane Wardle and the role of appetite in genetic risk of obesity. *Curr. Obes. Rep.* **6**, 38–45 (2017).

37. Konttinen, H. *et al.* Appetitive traits as behavioural pathways in genetic susceptibility to obesity: a population-based cross-sectional study. *Sci. Rep.* **5**, 14726 (2015).

38. Turcot, V. *et al.* Protein-altering variants associated with body mass index implicate pathways that control energy intake and expenditure in obesity. *Nat. Genet.* **50**, 26–41 (2018).

39. Schleinitz, D., Böttcher, Y., Blüher, M., & Kovacs, P. The genetics of fat distribution. *Diabetologia* **57**, 1276–86 (2014).

40. Bultman, S. J., Michaud, E. J., & Woychik, R. P. Molecular characterization of the mouse agouti locus. *Cell* **71**, 1195–204 (1992).

41. Lu, D. *et al.* Agouti protein is an antagonist of the melanocyte-stimulating-hormone receptor. *Nature* **371**, 799–802 (1994).

42. Klebig, M. L., Wilkinson, J. E., Geisler, J. G., & Woychik, R. P. Ectopic expression of the agouti gene in transgenic mice causes obesity, features of type II diabetes, and yellow fur. *Proc. Natl. Acad. Sci. U. S. A.* **92**, 4728–32 (1995).

43. Miller, M. W. *et al.* Cloning of the mouse agouti gene predicts a secreted protein ubiquitously expressed in mice carrying the lethal yellow mutation. *Genes Dev.* **7**, 454–67 (1993).

44. Bray, G. A. Hereditary adiposity in mice: human lessons from the yellow and obese (OB/OB) mice. *Obes. Res.* **4**, 91–5 (1996).

45. Shimizu, H., Shargill, N. S., Bray, G. A., Yen, T. T., & Gesellchen, P. D. Effects of MSH on food intake, body weight and coat color of the yellow obese mouse. *Life Sci.* **45**, 543–52 (1989).

46. Jacobowitz, D. M. & O'Donohue, T. L. alpha-Melanocyte stimulating hormone: immunohistochemical identification and mapping in neurons of rat brain. *Proc. Natl. Acad. Sci. U. S. A.* **75**, 6300–4 (1978).

47. Ollmann, M. M. *et al.* Antagonism of central melanocortin receptors in vitro and in vivo by agouti-related protein. *Science* **278**, 135–8 (1997).

48. Fan, W., Boston, B. A., Kesterson, R. A., Hruby, V. J., & Cone, R. D. Role of melanocortinergic neurons in feeding and the agouti obesity syndrome. *Nature* **385**, 165–8 (1997).

49. Huszar, D. *et al.* Targeted disruption of the melanocortin-4 receptor results in obesity in mice. *Cell* (1997). doi:10.1016/S0092-8674(00)81865-6

50. Wilson, B. D. *et al.* Structure and function of ASP, the human homolog of the mouse agouti gene. *Hum. Mol. Genet.* **4**, 223–30 (1995).

51. Fong, T. M. *et al.* ART (protein product of agouti-related transcript) as an antagonist of MC-3 and MC-4 receptors. *Biochem. Biophys. Res. Commun.* **237**, 629–31 (1997).

52. Farooqi, I. S. *et al.* Dominant and recessive inheritance of morbid obesity associated with melanocortin 4 receptor deficiency. *J. Clin. Invest.* **106**, 271–9 (2000).

53. Vaisse, C. *et al.* Melanocortin-4 receptor mutations are a frequent and heterogeneous cause of morbid obesity. *J. Clin. Invest.* **106**, 253–62 (2000).

54. Hinney, A. *et al.* Several mutations in the melanocortin-4 receptor gene including a nonsense and a frameshift mutation associated with dominantly inherited obesity in humans. *J. Clin. Endocrinol. Metab.* **84**, 1483–6 (1999).

55. Farooqi, S. & O'Rahilly, S. Genetics of obesity in humans. *Endocr. Rev.* **27**, 710–18 (2006).

56. Shadiack, A. M., Sharma, S. D., Earle, D. C., Spana, C., & Hallam, T. J. Melanocortins in the treatment of male and female sexual dysfunction. *Curr. Top. Med. Chem.* **7**, 1137–44 (2007).

57. Ju, S. H., Cho, G.-B., & Sohn, J.-W. Understanding melanocortin-4 receptor control of neuronal circuits: toward novel therapeutics for obesity syndrome. *Pharmacol. Res.* **129**, 10–19 (2018).

58. Roxby, P. Gene mutation means paracyclist has no fat under skin. *BBC News* (2013). Available at: www.bbc.co.uk/news/health-22903537.

59. Fiorenza, C. G., Chou, S. H., & Mantzoros, C. S. Lipodystrophy: pathophysiology and advances in treatment. *Nat. Rev. Endocrinol.* **7**, 137–50 (2011).

60. Garg, A., Peshock, R. M., & Fleckenstein, J. L. Adipose tissue distribution pattern in patients with familial partial lipodystrophy (Dunnigan variety). *J. Clin. Endocrinol. Metab.* **84**, 170–4 (1999).

61. Garg, A. Acquired and inherited lipodystrophies. *N. Engl. J. Med.* **350**, 1220–34 (2004).

62. Oliveira, J., Freitas, P., Lau, E., & Carvalho, D. Barraquer-Simons syndrome: a rare form of acquired lipodystrophy. *BMC Res. Notes* **9**, 175 (2016).

63. Vigouroux, C., Caron-Debarle, M., Le Dour, C., Magré, J., & Capeau, J. Molecular mechanisms of human lipodystrophies: from adipocyte lipid droplet to oxidative stress and lipotoxicity. *Int. J. Biochem. Cell Biol.* **43**, 862–76 (2011).

64. Agarwal, A. K. *et al.* AGPAT2 is mutated in congenital generalized lipodystrophy linked to chromosome 9q34. *Nat. Genet.* **31**, 21–3 (2002).

65. Simha, V. & Garg, A. Phenotypic heterogeneity in body fat distribution in patients with congenital generalized lipodystrophy caused by mutations in the AGPAT2 or seipin genes. *J. Clin. Endocrinol. Metab.* **88**, 5433–7 (2003).

66. Shackleton, S. *et al.* LMNA, encoding lamin A/C, is mutated in partial lipodystrophy. *Nat. Genet.* **24**, 153–6 (2000).

67. Ersek, R. A., Bell, H. N., & Salisbury, A. V. Serial and superficial suction for steatopygia (Hottentot bustle). *Aesthetic Plast. Surg.* **18**, 279–82 (1994).

68. Parkinson, J. The significance of Sarah Baartman. *BBC News* (2016). Available at: www.bbc.co.uk/news/magazine-35240987.

69. Ahmadian, M. *et al.* PPARγ signaling and metabolism: the good, the bad and the future. *Nat. Med.* **19**, 557–66 (2013).

70. Carey, D. G. *et al.* Effect of rosiglitazone on insulin sensitivity and body composition in type 2 diabetic patients [corrected]. *Obes. Res.* **10**, 1008–15 (2002).

71. Miyazaki, Y. *et al.* Effect of pioglitazone on abdominal fat distribution and insulin sensitivity in type 2 diabetic patients. *J. Clin. Endocrinol. Metab.* **87**, 2784–91 (2002).

72. Rasouli, N. *et al.* Pioglitazone improves insulin sensitivity through reduction in muscle lipid and redistribution of lipid into adipose tissue. *Am. J. Physiol. Endocrinol. Metab.* **288**, E930–4 (2005).

73. Iwanishi, M. *et al.* Clinical characteristics and efficacy of pioglitazone in a Japanese diabetic patient with an unusual type of familial partial lipodystrophy. *Metabolism* **58**, 1681–7 (2009).

74. Simha, V., Rao, S., & Garg, A. Prolonged thiazolidinedione therapy does not reverse fat loss in patients with familial partial lipodystrophy, Dunnigan variety. *Diabetes. Obes. Metab.* **10**, 1275–6 (2008).

75. Wang, S., Dougherty, E. J., & Danner, R. L. PPARγ signaling and emerging opportunities for improved therapeutics. *Pharmacol. Res.* **111**, 76–85 (2016).

76. Maggi, P. *et al.* Cardiovascular risk and dyslipidemia among persons living with HIV: a review. *BMC Infect. Dis.* **17**, 551 (2017).

77. Stanley, T. L. & Grinspoon, S. K. Body composition and metabolic changes in HIV-infected patients. *J. Infect. Dis.* **205 Suppl.**, S383–90 (2012).

78. Pacenti, M. *et al.* Microarray analysis during adipogenesis identifies new genes altered by antiretroviral drugs. *AIDS* **20**, 1691–705 (2006).

79. de Waal, R., Cohen, K., & Maartens, G. Systematic review of antiretroviral-associated lipodystrophy: lipoatrophy, but not central fat gain, is an antiretroviral adverse drug reaction. *PLoS One* **8**, e63623 (2013).

80. Shlay, J. C. *et al.* The effect of individual antiretroviral drugs on body composition in HIV-infected persons initiating highly active antiretroviral therapy. *J. Acquir. Immune Defic. Syndr.* **51**, 298–304 (2009).

81. Rojo, L. E. *et al.* Metabolic syndrome and obesity among users of second generation antipsychotics: a global challenge for modern psychopharmacology. *Pharmacol. Res.* **101**, 74–85 (2015).

82. Correll, C. U., Lencz, T., & Malhotra, A. K. Antipsychotic drugs and obesity. *Trends Mol. Med.* **17**, 97–107 (2011).

83. Gonçalves, P., Araújo, J. R., & Martel, F. Antipsychotics-induced metabolic alterations: focus on adipose tissue and molecular mechanisms. *Eur. Neuropsychopharmacol.* **25**, 1–16 (2015).

84. Lett, T. A. P. *et al.* Pharmacogenetics of antipsychotic-induced weight gain: review and clinical implications. *Mol. Psychiatry* 17, 242–66 (2012).

85. Stojakovic, A., Espinosa, E. P., Farhad, O. T., & Lutfy, K. Effects of nicotine on homeostatic and hedonic components of food intake. *J. Endocrinol.* 235, R13–R31 (2017).

86. Glover, M., Breier, B. H., & Bauld, L. Could vaping be a new weapon in the battle of the bulge? *Nicotine Tob. Res.* 19, 1536–40 (2017).

87. Cochrane, C., Malcolm, R., & Brewerton, T. The role of weight control as a motivation for cocaine abuse. *Addict. Behav.* (1998). doi:10.1016/S0306-4603(97)00046-4

88. Ersche, K. D., Stochl, J., Woodward, J. M., & Fletcher, P. C. The skinny on cocaine: insights into eating behavior and body weight in cocaine-dependent men. *Appetite* (2013). doi:10.1016/j.appet.2013.07.011

89. Saunders, K. H., Umashanker, D., Igel, L. I., Kumar, R. B., & Aronne, L. J. Obesity pharmacotherapy. *Med. Clin. North Am.* 102, 135–48 (2018).

90. Mullard, A. Mediator scandal rocks French medical community. *Lancet* 377, 890–2 (2011).

91. Busquets-Garcia, A. *et al.* Dissecting the cannabinergic control of behavior: the where matters. *Bioessays* 37, 1215–25 (2015).

92. Horn, H., Böhme, B., Dietrich, L., & Koch, M. Endocannabinoids in body weight control. *Pharmaceuticals* 11, (2018).

93. Badowski, M. E. & Yanful, P. K. Dronabinol oral solution in the management of anorexia and weight loss in AIDS and cancer. *Ther. Clin. Risk Manag.* 14, 643–51 (2018).

94. Burke, L. K. & Heisler, L. K. 5-hydroxytryptamine medications for the treatment of obesity. *J. Neuroendocrinol.* 27, 389–98 (2015).

95. NHS. US weight-loss drug lorcaserin 'safe' but only modestly effective. (2018). Available at: www.nhs.uk/news/obesity/us-weight-loss-drug-lorcaserin-safe-only-modestly-effective/.

96. Bohula, E. A. *et al.* Cardiovascular safety of lorcaserin in overweight or obese patients. *N. Engl. J. Med.* 16, NEJMoa1808721 (2018).

97. Tak, Y. J. & Lee, S. Y. Anti-obesity drugs: long-term efficacy and safety: an updated review. *World J. Mens. Health* 38, (2020).

98. Divertie, G. D., Jensen, M. D., & Miles, J. M. Stimulation of lipolysis in humans by physiological hypercortisolemia. *Diabetes* 40, 1228–32 (1991).

99. Djurhuus, C. B. *et al.* Effects of cortisol on lipolysis and regional interstitial glycerol levels in humans. *Am. J. Physiol. Endocrinol. Metab.* 283, E172–7 (2002).

100. Manolopoulos, K. N., O'Reilly, M. W., Bujalska, I. J., Tomlinson, J. W., & Arlt, W. Acute hypercortisolemia exerts depot-specific effects on abdominal and femoral adipose tissue function. *J. Clin. Endocrinol. Metab.* 102, 1091–101 (2017).

101. Lee, M.-J., Pramyothin, P., Karastergiou, K., & Fried, S. K. Deconstructing the roles of glucocorticoids in adipose tissue biology and the development of central obesity. *Biochim. Biophys. Acta* 1842, 473–81 (2014).

102. Raglan, G. B., Schmidt, L. A., & Schulkin, J. The role of glucocorticoids and corticotropin-releasing hormone regulation on anxiety symptoms and response to treatment. *Endocr. Connect.* **6**, R1–R7 (2017).

103. Lanzino, G., Maartens, N. F., & Laws, E. R. Cushing's case XLV: Minnie G. *J. Neurosurg.* **97**, 231–4 (2002).

104. Cushing, H. The basophil adenomas of the pituitary body and their clinical manifestations (pituitary basophilism). 1932. *Obes. Res.* **2**, 486–508 (1994).

105. Yalcin, S. & Öberg, K. *Neuroendocrine Tumours: Diagnosis and Management.* Springer Berlin Heidelberg, 2015.

106. Hodgens, A. & Sharman, T. *Corticosteroids.* StatPearls, 2020.

107. Nieman, L. K. Cushing's syndrome: update on signs, symptoms and biochemical screening. *Eur. J. Endocrinol.* **173**, M33–8 (2015).

108. Geer, E. B. *et al.* MRI assessment of lean and adipose tissue distribution in female patients with Cushing's disease. *Clin. Endocrinol.* **73**, 469–75 (2010).

109. Rockall, A. G. *et al.* Computed tomography assessment of fat distribution in male and female patients with Cushing's syndrome. *Eur. J. Endocrinol.* **149**, 561–7 (2003).

110. Roerink, S. H. P. P. *et al.* Increased adipocyte size, macrophage infiltration, and adverse local adipokine profile in perirenal fat in Cushing's syndrome. *Obesity (Silver Spring)* **25**, 1369–74 (2017).

111. Laforest, S., Labrecque, J., Michaud, A., Cianflone, K., & Tchernof, A. Adipocyte size as a determinant of metabolic disease and adipose tissue dysfunction. *Crit. Rev. Clin. Lab. Sci.* **52**, 301–13 (2015).

112. Ferraù, F. & Korbonits, M. Metabolic comorbidities in Cushing's syndrome. *Eur. J. Endocrinol.* **173**, M133–57 (2015).

113. Chapman, A. B., Knight, D. M., & Ringold, G. M. Glucocorticoid regulation of adipocyte differentiation: hormonal triggering of the developmental program and induction of a differentiation-dependent gene. *J. Cell Biol.* **101**, 1227–35 (1985).

114. Lee, M.-J., Gong, D.-W., Burkey, B. F., & Fried, S. K. Pathways regulated by glucocorticoids in omental and subcutaneous human adipose tissues: a microarray study. *Am. J. Physiol. Endocrinol. Metab.* **300**, E571–80 (2011).

115. Pickering, R. T., Lee, M.-J., Karastergiou, K., Gower, A., & Fried, S. K. Depot dependent effects of dexamethasone on gene expression in human omental and abdominal subcutaneous adipose tissues from obese women. *PLoS One* **11**, e0167337 (2016).

116. Appel, B. & Fried, S. K. Effects of insulin and dexamethasone on lipoprotein lipase in human adipose tissue. *Am. J. Physiol.* **262**, E695–9 (1992).

117. Ottosson, M., Vikman-Adolfsson, K., Enerbäck, S., Olivecrona, G., & Björntorp, P. The effects of cortisol on the regulation of lipoprotein lipase activity in human adipose tissue. *J. Clin. Endocrinol. Metab.* **79**, 820–5 (1994).

118. Ottosson, M., Mårin, P., Karason, K., Elander, A., & Björntorp, P. Blockade of the glucocorticoid receptor with RU 486: effects in vitro and in vivo on human adipose tissue lipoprotein lipase activity. *Obes. Res.* **3**, 233–40 (1995).

119. Fried, S. K., Russell, C. D., Grauso, N. L., & Brolin, R. E. Lipoprotein lipase regulation by insulin and glucocorticoid in subcutaneous and omental adipose tissues of obese women and men. *J. Clin. Invest.* **92**, 2191–8 (1993).

120. Wang, Y. *et al.* The human fatty acid synthase gene and de novo lipogenesis are coordinately regulated in human adipose tissue. *J. Nutr.* **134**, 1032–8 (2004).

121. Gathercole, L. L. *et al.* Regulation of lipogenesis by glucocorticoids and insulin in human adipose tissue. *PLoS One* **6**, e26223 (2011).

122. Diraison, F. *et al.* Differences in the regulation of adipose tissue and liver lipogenesis by carbohydrates in humans. *J. Lipid Res.* **44**, 846–53 (2003).

123. Strawford, A., Antelo, F., Christiansen, M., & Hellerstein, M. K. Adipose tissue triglyceride turnover, de novo lipogenesis, and cell proliferation in humans measured with 2H2O. *Am. J. Physiol. Endocrinol. Metab.* **286**, E577–88 (2004).

124. Peckett, A. J., Wright, D. C., & Riddell, M. C. The effects of glucocorticoids on adipose tissue lipid metabolism. *Metabolism* **60**, 1500–10 (2011).

125. Exton, J. H. *et al.* Interaction of glucocorticoids with glucagon and epinephrine in the control of gluconeogenesis and glycogenolysis in liver and of lipolysis in adipose tissue. *J. Biol. Chem.* **247**, 3579–88 (1972).

126. van Raalte, D. H. *et al.* Low-dose glucocorticoid treatment affects multiple aspects of intermediary metabolism in healthy humans: a randomised controlled trial. *Diabetologia* **54**, 2103–12 (2011).

127. Weitzman, E. D. *et al.* Twenty-four-hour pattern of the episodic secretion of cortisol in normal subjects. *J. Clin. Endocrinol. Metab.* (1971). doi:10.1210/jcem-33-1-14

128. Samra, J. S. *et al.* Effects of morning rise in cortisol concentration on regulation of lipolysis in subcutaneous adipose tissue. *Am. J. Physiol.* **271**, E996–1002 (1996).

129. Chung, S., Son, G. H., & Kim, K. Circadian rhythm of adrenal glucocorticoid: its regulation and clinical implications. *Biochim. Biophys. Acta* **1812**, 581–91 (2011).

130. Chrousos, G. P. & Kino, T. Glucocorticoid action networks and complex psychiatric and/or somatic disorders. *Stress* **10**, 213–19 (2007).

131. Wang, M. The role of glucocorticoid action in the pathophysiology of the metabolic syndrome. *Nutr. Metab.* **2**, 3 (2005).

132. Boyar, R. M., Witkin, M., Carruth, A., & Ramsey, J. Circadian cortisol secretory rhythms in Cushing's disease. *J. Clin. Endocrinol. Metab.* **48**, 760–5 (1979).

133. Moreira, A. C., Antonini, S. R., & de Castro, M. Mechanisms in endocrinology: a sense of time of the glucocorticoid circadian clock: from the ontogeny to the diagnosis of Cushing's syndrome. *Eur. J. Endocrinol.* **179**, R1–R18 (2018).

134. Geiker, N. R. W. *et al.* Does stress influence sleep patterns, food intake, weight gain, abdominal obesity and weight loss interventions and vice versa? *Obes. Rev.* **19**, 81–97 (2018).

135. Debono, M., Ross, R. J., & Newell-Price, J. Inadequacies of glucocorticoid replacement and improvements by physiological circadian therapy. *Eur. J. Endocrinol.* **160**, 719–29 (2009).

136. Egol, K. A., Tolisano, A. M., Spratt, K. F., & Koval, K. J. Mortality rates following trauma: the difference is night and day. *J. Emerg. Trauma. Shock* **4**, 178–83 (2011).

137. Lee, M.-J. *et al.* Depot-specific regulation of the conversion of cortisone to cortisol in human adipose tissue. *Obesity (Silver Spring)* **16**, 1178–85 (2008).

138. Michailidou, Z. *et al.* Omental 11beta-hydroxysteroid dehydrogenase 1 correlates with fat cell size independently of obesity. *Obesity (Silver Spring)* **15**, 1155–63 (2007).

139. Masuzaki, H. *et al.* A transgenic model of visceral obesity and the metabolic syndrome. *Science* **294**, 2166–70 (2001).

140. Kershaw, E. E. *et al.* Adipocyte-specific glucocorticoid inactivation protects against diet-induced obesity. *Diabetes* **54**, 1023–31 (2005).

141. Morgan, S. A. *et al.* 11β-HSD1 is the major regulator of the tissue-specific effects of circulating glucocorticoid excess. *Proc. Natl. Acad. Sci. U. S. A.* **111**, E2482–91 (2014).

142. Bujalska, I. J., Kumar, S., & Stewart, P. M. Does central obesity reflect 'Cushing's disease of the omentum'? *Lancet* **349**, 1210–13 (1997).

143. Morgan, S. A., Hassan-Smith, Z. K., & Lavery, G. G. Mechanisms in endocrinology: tissue-specific activation of cortisol in Cushing's syndrome. *Eur. J. Endocrinol.* **175**, R83–9 (2016).

144. Jackson, S. E., Kirschbaum, C., & Steptoe, A. Hair cortisol and adiposity in a population-based sample of 2,527 men and women aged 54 to 87 years. *Obesity (Silver Spring)* **25**, 539–44 (2017).

145. Engeli, S. *et al.* Regulation of 11beta-HSD genes in human adipose tissue: influence of central obesity and weight loss. *Obes. Res.* **12**, 9–17 (2004).

146. Kannisto, K. *et al.* Overexpression of 11beta-hydroxysteroid dehydrogenase-1 in adipose tissue is associated with acquired obesity and features of insulin resistance: studies in young adult monozygotic twins. *J. Clin. Endocrinol. Metab.* **89**, 4414–21 (2004).

147. Paulsen, S. K., Pedersen, S. B., Fisker, S., & Richelsen, B. 11Beta-HSD type 1 expression in human adipose tissue: impact of gender, obesity, and fat localization. *Obesity (Silver Spring)* **15**, 1954–60 (2007).

148. Stomby, A., Andrew, R., Walker, B. R., & Olsson, T. Tissue-specific dysregulation of cortisol regeneration by 11βHSD1 in obesity: has it promised too much? *Diabetologia* **57**, 1100–10 (2014).

149. Li, X., Wang, J., Yang, Q., & Shao, S. 11β-Hydroxysteroid dehydrogenase type 1 in obese subjects with type 2 diabetes mellitus. *Am. J. Med. Sci.* **354**, 408–14 (2017).

150. Omar, H. R. *et al.* Licorice abuse: time to send a warning message. *Ther. Adv. Endocrinol. Metab.* **3**, 125–38 (2012).

151. World Health Organization. Depression—factsheet (2018). Available at: www.who.int/news-room/fact-sheets/detail/depression.

152. Remes, O., Brayne, C., van der Linde, R., & Lafortune, L. A systematic review of reviews on the prevalence of anxiety disorders in adult populations. *Brain Behav.* **6**, e00497 (2016).
153. Hryhorczuk, C., Sharma, S., & Fulton, S. E. Metabolic disturbances connecting obesity and depression. *Front. Neurosci.* **7**, 177 (2013).
154. Yau, Y. H. C. & Potenza, M. N. Stress and eating behaviors. *Minerva Endocrinol.* **38**, 255–67 (2013).
155. Tuulari, J. J. *et al.* Feeding releases endogenous opioids in humans. *J. Neurosci.* **37**, 8284–91 (2017).
156. Amir, S., Brown, Z. W., & Amit, Z. The role of endorphins in stress: evidence and speculations. *Neurosci. Biobehav. Rev.* **4**, 77–86 (1980).
157. Bodnar, R. J. Endogenous opiates and behavior: 2016. *Peptides* **101**, 167–212 (2018).
158. Adam, T. C. & Epel, E. S. Stress, eating and the reward system. *Physiol. Behav.* **91**, 449–58 (2007).
159. Brewis, A. A. Stigma and the perpetuation of obesity. *Soc. Sci. Med.* **118**, 152–8 (2014).
160. Leow, S., Jackson, B., Alderson, J. A., Guelfi, K. J., & Dimmock, J. A. A role for exercise in attenuating unhealthy food consumption in response to stress. *Nutrients* **10**, (2018).
161. Masih, T., Dimmock, J. A., Epel, E. S., & Guelfi, K. J. Stress-induced eating and the relaxation response as a potential antidote: a review and hypothesis. *Appetite* **118**, 136–43 (2017).
162. Bhatia, A., Sekhon, H. K., & Kaur, G. Sex hormones and immune dimorphism. *ScientificWorldJournal* **2014**, 159150 (2014).
163. dos Santos, R. L., da Silva, F. B., Ribeiro, R. F., & Stefanon, I. Sex hormones in the cardiovascular system. *Horm. Mol. Biol. Clin. Investig.* **18**, 89–103 (2014).
164. Anderson, L. J., Liu, H., & Garcia, J. M. Sex differences in muscle wasting. *Adv. Exp. Med. Biol.* **1043**, 153–97 (2017).
165. Khosla, S. & Monroe, D. G. Regulation of bone metabolism by sex steroids. *Cold Spring Harb. Perspect. Med.* **8**, (2018).
166. Diotel, N. *et al.* Steroid transport, local synthesis, and signaling within the brain: roles in neurogenesis, neuroprotection, and sexual behaviors. *Front. Neurosci.* **12**, 84 (2018).
167. Pulit, S. L., Karaderi, T., & Lindgren, C. M. Sexual dimorphisms in genetic loci linked to body fat distribution. *Biosci. Rep.* **37**, (2017).
168. Westergaard, D., Moseley, P., Sørup, F. K. H., Baldi, P., & Brunak, S. Population-wide analysis of differences in disease progression patterns in men and women. *Nat. Commun.* **10**, 666 (2019).
169. Avgerinos, K. I., Spyrou, N., Mantzoros, C. S., & Dalamaga, M. Obesity and cancer risk: emerging biological mechanisms and perspectives. *Metabolism* **92**, 121–35 (2019).
170. Wang, Y. *et al.* Sex differences in the association between diabetes and risk of cardiovascular disease, cancer, and all-cause and cause-specific mortality: a

systematic review and meta-analysis of 5,162,654 participants. *BMC Med.* 17, 136 (2019).

171. Johnson, J., Sharman, Z., Vissandjée, B., & Stewart, D. E. Does a change in health research funding policy related to the integration of sex and gender have an impact? *PLoS One* 9, e99900 (2014).

172. Becker, J. B. *et al.* Strategies and methods for research on sex differences in brain and behavior. *Endocrinology* 146, 1650–73 (2005).

173. Lee, S. K. Sex as an important biological variable in biomedical research. *BMB Rep.* 51, 167–73 (2018).

174. Bird, C. E. & Rieker, P. P. Gender differences in health. In *Gender and Health*, 16–53. Cambridge University Press, 2012. doi:10.1017/CBO9780511807305.003

175. Snow, R. C. Sex, gender, and vulnerability. *Glob. Public Health* 3 Suppl. 1, 58–74 (2008).

176. Bélanger, C., Luu-The, V., Dupont, P., & Tchernof, A. Adipose tissue intracrinology: potential importance of local androgen/estrogen metabolism in the regulation of adiposity. *Horm. Metab. Res.* 34, 737–45.

177. Mizutani, T. *et al.* Identification of estrogen receptor in human adipose tissue and adipocytes. *J. Clin. Endocrinol. Metab.* 78, 950–4 (1994).

178. Dieudonne, M. N., Pecquery, R., Boumediene, A., Leneveu, M. C., & Giudicelli, Y. Androgen receptors in human preadipocytes and adipocytes: regional specificities and regulation by sex steroids. *Am. J. Physiol.* 274, C1645–52 (1998).

179. Anderson, L. A., McTernan, P. G., Barnett, A. H., & Kumar, S. The effects of androgens and estrogens on preadipocyte proliferation in human adipose tissue: influence of gender and site. *J. Clin. Endocrinol. Metab.* 86, 5045–51 (2001).

180. Li, C., Ford, E. S., Zhao, G., Balluz, L. S., & Giles, W. H. Estimates of body composition with dual-energy X-ray absorptiometry in adults. *Am. J. Clin. Nutr.* 90, 1457–65 (2009).

181. Ijichi, N. *et al.* Estrogen-related receptor alpha modulates the expression of adipogenesis-related genes during adipocyte differentiation. *Biochem. Biophys. Res. Commun.* 358, 813–18 (2007).

182. Benvenuti, S. *et al.* Androgens and estrogens prevent rosiglitazone-induced adipogenesis in human mesenchymal stem cells. *J. Endocrinol. Invest.* 35, 365–71 (2012).

183. Newell-Fugate, A. E. The role of sex steroids in white adipose tissue adipocyte function. *Reproduction* 153, R133–49 (2017).

184. Machinal-Quélin, F., Dieudonné, M.-N., Pecquery, R., Leneveu, M.-C., & Giudicelli, Y. Direct in vitro effects of androgens and estrogens on ob gene expression and leptin secretion in human adipose tissue. *Endocrine* 18, 179–84 (2002).

185. Hong, S. C. *et al.* Correlation between estrogens and serum adipocytokines in premenopausal and postmenopausal women. *Menopause* 14, 835–40

186. Hickey, M. S. *et al.* Gender differences in serum leptin levels in humans. *Biochem. Mol. Med.* 59, 1–6 (1996).

187. Gavin, K. M., Cooper, E. E., Raymer, D. K., & Hickner, R. C. Estradiol effects on subcutaneous adipose tissue lipolysis in premenopausal women are adipose tissue depot specific and treatment dependent. *Am. J. Physiol. Endocrinol. Metab.* **304**, E1167–74 (2013).

188. Richelsen, B. Increased alpha 2- but similar beta-adrenergic receptor activities in subcutaneous gluteal adipocytes from females compared with males. *Eur. J. Clin. Invest.* **16**, 302–9 (1986).

189. Pedersen, S. B., Kristensen, K., Hermann, P. A., Katzenellenbogen, J. A., & Richelsen, B. Estrogen controls lipolysis by up-regulating alpha2A-adrenergic receptors directly in human adipose tissue through the estrogen receptor alpha. Implications for the female fat distribution. *J. Clin. Endocrinol. Metab.* **89**, 1869–78 (2004).

190. Koehler, K. F., Helguero, L. A., Haldosén, L.-A., Warner, M., & Gustafsson, J.-A. Reflections on the discovery and significance of estrogen receptor beta. *Endocr. Rev.* **26**, 465–78 (2005).

191. Dieudonné, M. N., Leneveu, M. C., Giudicelli, Y., & Pecquery, R. Evidence for functional estrogen receptors alpha and beta in human adipose cells: regional specificities and regulation by estrogens. *Am. J. Physiol. Cell Physiol.* **286**, C655–61 (2004).

192. Anwar, A. *et al.* Site-specific regulation of oestrogen receptor-alpha and -beta by oestradiol in human adipose tissue. *Diabetes. Obes. Metab.* **3**, 338–49 (2001).

193. Shin, J.-H. *et al.* The ratio of estrogen receptor alpha to estrogen receptor beta in adipose tissue is associated with leptin production and obesity. *Steroids* **72**, 592–9 (2007).

194. Pedersen, S. B. *et al.* Demonstration of estrogen receptor subtypes alpha and beta in human adipose tissue: influences of adipose cell differentiation and fat depot localization. *Mol. Cell. Endocrinol.* **182**, 27–37 (2001).

195. Gavin, K. M., Cooper, E. E., & Hickner, R. C. Estrogen receptor protein content is different in abdominal than gluteal subcutaneous adipose tissue of overweight-to-obese premenopausal women. *Metabolism* **62**, 1180–8 (2013).

196. Abdulnour, J. *et al.* The effect of the menopausal transition on body composition and cardiometabolic risk factors: a Montreal-Ottawa New Emerging Team group study. *Menopause* **19**, 760–7 (2012).

197. Ley, C. J., Lees, B., & Stevenson, J. C. Sex- and menopause-associated changes in body-fat distribution. *Am. J. Clin. Nutr.* **55**, 950–4 (1992).

198. Lovejoy, J. C., Champagne, C. M., de Jonge, L., Xie, H., & Smith, S. R. Increased visceral fat and decreased energy expenditure during the menopausal transition. *Int. J. Obes.* **32**, 949–58 (2008).

199. Abildgaard, J. *et al.* Menopause is associated with decreased whole body fat oxidation during exercise. *Am. J. Physiol. Endocrinol. Metab.* **304**, E1227–36 (2013).

200. Lundholm, L. *et al.* Key lipogenic gene expression can be decreased by estrogen in human adipose tissue. *Fertil. Steril.* **90**, 44–8 (2008).

201. Ijuin, H., Douchi, T., Oki, T., Maruta, K., & Nagata, Y. The contribution of menopause to changes in body-fat distribution. *J. Obstet. Gynaecol. Res.* **25**, 367–72 (1999).

202. Price, T. M. *et al.* Estrogen regulation of adipose tissue lipoprotein lipase--possible mechanism of body fat distribution. *Am. J. Obstet. Gynecol.* **178**, 101–7 (1998).

203. Tchernof, A. *et al.* Ovarian hormone status and abdominal visceral adipose tissue metabolism. *J. Clin. Endocrinol. Metab.* **89**, 3425–30 (2004).

204. Lapointe, A., Piché, M.-E., Weisnagel, S. J., Bergeron, J., & Lemieux, S. Associations between circulating free fatty acids, visceral adipose tissue accumulation, and insulin sensitivity in postmenopausal women. *Metabolism.* **58**, 180–5 (2009).

205. Piché, M.-E. *et al.* Regional body fat distribution and metabolic profile in postmenopausal women. *Metabolism.* **57**, 1101–7 (2008).

206. Chalouhi, S. Menopause: a complex and controversial journey. *Post Reprod. Heal.* **23**, 128–31 (2017).

207. Lock, M. M. *Encounters with Aging: Mythologies of Menopause in Japan and North America.* University of California Press, 1994.

208. Genazzani, A. R. & Gambacciani, M. Effect of climacteric transition and hormone replacement therapy on body weight and body fat distribution. *Gynecol. Endocrinol.* **22**, 145–50 (2006).

209. Yüksel, H. *et al.* Effects of postmenopausal hormone replacement therapy on body fat composition. *Gynecol. Endocrinol.* **23**, 99–104 (2007).

210. Munoz, J., Derstine, A., & Gower, B. A. Fat distribution and insulin sensitivity in postmenopausal women: influence of hormone replacement. *Obes. Res.* **10**, 424–31 (2002).

211. Lewis, C. E. & Wellons, M. F. Menopausal hormone therapy for primary prevention of chronic disease. *JAMA* **318**, 2187–9 (2017).

212. Hulley, S. *et al.* Randomized trial of estrogen plus progestin for secondary prevention of coronary heart disease in postmenopausal women. Heart and Estrogen/progestin Replacement Study (HERS) Research Group. *JAMA* **280**, 605–13 (1998).

213. Marjoribanks, J., Farquhar, C., Roberts, H., Lethaby, A., & Lee, J. Long-term hormone therapy for perimenopausal and postmenopausal women. *Cochrane Database Syst. Rev.* **1**, CD004143 (2017).

214. Cobin, R. H., Goodman, N. F., & AACE Reproductive Endocrinology Scientific Committee. American Association of Clinical Endocrinologists and American College of Endocrinology Position Statement on Menopause–2017 Update. *Endocr. Pract.* **23**, 869–80 (2017).

215. Newson, L. Menopause and cardiovascular disease. *Post Reprod. Heal.* **24**, 44–9 (2018).

216. El Khoudary, S. R. Gaps, limitations and new insights on endogenous estrogen and follicle stimulating hormone as related to risk of cardiovascular disease in women traversing the menopause: a narrative review. *Maturitas* **104**, 44–53 (2017).

217. Tom, S. E., Cooper, R., Wallace, R. B., & Guralnik, J. M. Type and timing of menopause and later life mortality among women in the Iowa Established Populations for the Epidemiological Study of the Elderly (EPESE) cohort. *J. Womens. Health (Larchmt).* **21**, 10–16 (2012).

218. Pannier, B. *et al.* Cardiovascular risk markers associated with the metabolic syndrome in a large French population: the 'SYMFONIE' study. *Diabetes Metab.* **32**, 467–74 (2006).

219. Cerhan, J. R. *et al.* A pooled analysis of waist circumference and mortality in 650,000 adults. *Mayo Clin. Proc.* **89**, 335–45 (2014).

220. Lobo, R. A. *et al.* Prevention of diseases after menopause. *Climacteric* **17**, 540–56 (2014).

221. Delitala, A. P., Capobianco, G., Delitala, G., Cherchi, P. L., & Dessole, S. Polycystic ovary syndrome, adipose tissue and metabolic syndrome. *Arch. Gynecol. Obstet.* **296**, 405–19 (2017).

222. Bozdag, G., Mumusoglu, S., Zengin, D., Karabulut, E., & Yildiz, B. O. The prevalence and phenotypic features of polycystic ovary syndrome: a systematic review and meta-analysis. *Hum. Reprod.* **31**, 2841–55 (2016).

223. Torchen, L. C. Cardiometabolic risk in PCOS: more than a reproductive disorder. *Curr. Diab. Rep.* **17**, 137 (2017).

224. Butler, M. G., McGuire, A., & Manzardo, A. M. Clinically relevant known and candidate genes for obesity and their overlap with human infertility and reproduction. *J. Assist. Reprod. Genet.* **32**, 495–508 (2015).

225. Escobar-Morreale, H. F. & San Millán, J. L. Abdominal adiposity and the polycystic ovary syndrome. *Trends Endocrinol. Metab.* **18**, 266–72 (2007).

226. Franik, G. *et al.* The effect of abdominal obesity in patients with polycystic ovary syndrome on metabolic parameters. *Eur. Rev. Med. Pharmacol. Sci.* **21**, 4755–61 (2017).

227. Glintborg, D., Petersen, M. H., Ravn, P., Hermann, A. P., & Andersen, M. Comparison of regional fat mass measurement by whole body DXA scans and anthropometric measures to predict insulin resistance in women with polycystic ovary syndrome and controls. *Acta Obstet. Gynecol. Scand.* **95**, 1235–43 (2016).

228. Cosar, E. *et al.* Body fat composition and distribution in women with polycystic ovary syndrome. *Gynecol. Endocrinol.* **24**, 428–32 (2008).

229. Martínez-García, M. Á. *et al.* Evidence for masculinization of adipokine gene expression in visceral and subcutaneous adipose tissue of obese women with polycystic ovary syndrome (PCOS). *J. Clin. Endocrinol. Metab.* **98**, E388–96 (2013).

230. Silvestris, E., de Pergola, G., Rosania, R., & Loverro, G. Obesity as disruptor of the female fertility. *Reprod. Biol. Endocrinol.* **16**, 22 (2018).

231. Moran, L. J. *et al.* Dietary composition in the treatment of polycystic ovary syndrome: a systematic review to inform evidence-based guidelines. *J. Acad. Nutr. Diet.* **113**, 520–45 (2013).

232. Blouin, K. *et al.* Androgen inactivation and steroid-converting enzyme expression in abdominal adipose tissue in men. *J. Endocrinol.* **191**, 637–49 (2006).

233. Tchoukalova, Y. D. *et al.* Sex- and depot-dependent differences in adipogenesis in normal-weight humans. *Obesity (Silver Spring)* **18**, 1875–80 (2010).

234. Blouin, K. *et al.* Effects of androgens on adipocyte differentiation and adipose tissue explant metabolism in men and women. *Clin. Endocrinol.* **72**, 176–88 (2010).

235. Gupta, V. *et al.* Effects of dihydrotestosterone on differentiation and proliferation of human mesenchymal stem cells and preadipocytes. *Mol. Cell. Endocrinol.* **296**, 32–40 (2008).

236. Chazenbalk, G. *et al.* Androgens inhibit adipogenesis during human adipose stem cell commitment to preadipocyte formation. *Steroids* **78**, 920–6 (2013).

237. Horenburg, S., Fischer-Posovszky, P., Debatin, K.-M., & Wabitsch, M. Influence of sex hormones on adiponectin expression in human adipocytes. *Horm. Metab. Res.* **40**, 779–86 (2008).

238. Nishizawa, H. *et al.* Androgens decrease plasma adiponectin, an insulin-sensitizing adipocyte-derived protein. *Diabetes* **51**, 2734–41 (2002).

239. Woodhouse, L. J. *et al.* Dose-dependent effects of testosterone on regional adipose tissue distribution in healthy young men. *J. Clin. Endocrinol. Metab.* **89**, 718–26 (2004).

240. Schiffer, L., Kempegowda, P., Arlt, W., & O'Reilly, M. W. Mechanisms in endocrinology: the sexually dimorphic role of androgens in human metabolic disease. *Eur. J. Endocrinol.* **177**, R125–R143 (2017).

241. Allan, C. A., Strauss, B. J. G., Burger, H. G., Forbes, E. A., & McLachlan, R. I. Testosterone therapy prevents gain in visceral adipose tissue and loss of skeletal muscle in nonobese aging men. *J. Clin. Endocrinol. Metab.* **93**, 139–46 (2008).

242. Emmelot-Vonk, M. H. *et al.* Effect of testosterone supplementation on functional mobility, cognition, and other parameters in older men: a randomized controlled trial. *JAMA* **299**, 39–52 (2008).

243. Frederiksen, L. *et al.* Testosterone therapy decreases subcutaneous fat and adiponectin in aging men. *Eur. J. Endocrinol.* **166**, 469–76 (2012).

244. Schroeder, E. T. *et al.* Effects of androgen therapy on adipose tissue and metabolism in older men. *J. Clin. Endocrinol. Metab.* **89**, 4863–72 (2004).

245. Nam, Y. S., Lee, G., Yun, J. M., & Cho, B. Testosterone replacement, muscle strength, and physical function. *World J. Mens. Health* **36**, 110–22 (2018).

246. Fink, J., Matsumoto, M., & Tamura, Y. Potential application of testosterone replacement therapy as treatment for obesity and type 2 diabetes in men. *Steroids* **138**, 161–6 (2018).

247. Gladyshev, T. V & Gladyshev, V. N. A disease or not a disease? Aging as a pathology. *Trends Mol. Med.* **22**, 995–6 (2016).

248. Elbers, J. M., Asscheman, H., Seidell, J. C., & Gooren, L. J. Effects of sex steroid hormones on regional fat depots as assessed by magnetic resonance imaging in transsexuals. *Am. J. Physiol.* **276**, E317–25 (1999).

249. Elbers, J. M., Asscheman, H., Seidell, J. C., Megens, J. A., & Gooren, L. J. Long-term testosterone administration increases visceral fat in female to male transsexuals. *J. Clin. Endocrinol. Metab.* **82**, 2044–7 (1997).

250. Van Caenegem, E. *et al.* Bone mass, bone geometry, and body composition in female-to-male transsexual persons after long-term cross-sex hormonal therapy. *J. Clin. Endocrinol. Metab.* **97**, 2503–11 (2012).

251. Klaver, M. *et al.* Changes in regional body fat, lean body mass and body shape in trans persons using cross-sex hormonal therapy: results from a multicenter prospective study. *Eur. J. Endocrinol.* **178**, 165–73 (2018).

252. Klaver, M. *et al.* Early hormonal treatment affects body composition and body shape in young transgender adolescents. *J. Sex. Med.* **15**, 251–60 (2018).

253. Elbers, J. M. H. *et al.* Effects of sex steroids on components of the insulin resistance syndrome in transsexual subjects. *Clin. Endocrinol.* **58**, 562–71 (2003).

254. Maraka, S. *et al.* Sex steroids and cardiovascular outcomes in transgender individuals: a systematic review and meta-analysis. *J. Clin. Endocrinol. Metab.* **102**, 3914–23 (2017).

255. Christou, G. A., Christou, K. A., Nikas, D. N., & Goudevenos, J. A. Acute myocardial infarction in a young bodybuilder taking anabolic androgenic steroids: a case report and critical review of the literature. *Eur. J. Prev. Cardiol.* **23**, 1785–96 (2016).

256. Achar, S., Rostamian, A., & Narayan, S. M. Cardiac and metabolic effects of anabolic-androgenic steroid abuse on lipids, blood pressure, left ventricular dimensions, and rhythm. *Am. J. Cardiol.* **106**, 893–901 (2010).

257. Christou, M. A. *et al.* Effects of anabolic androgenic steroids on the reproductive system of athletes and recreational users: a systematic review and meta-analysis. *Sports Med.* **47**, 1869–83 (2017).

258. Bautista, C. J., Martínez-Samayoa, P. M., & Zambrano, E. Sex steroids regulation of appetitive behavior. *Mini Rev. Med. Chem.* **12**, 1107–18 (2012).

259. Rubinow, K. B. *et al.* Circulating sex steroids coregulate adipose tissue immune cell populations in healthy men. *Am. J. Physiol. Endocrinol. Metab.* **313**, E528–E539 (2017).

260. Apostolova, G., Schweizer, R. A. S., Balazs, Z., Kostadinova, R. M., & Odermatt, A. Dehydroepiandrosterone inhibits the amplification of glucocorticoid action in adipose tissue. *Am. J. Physiol. Endocrinol. Metab.* **288**, E957–64 (2005).

261. Zhu, L. *et al.* Testosterone stimulates adipose tissue 11beta-hydroxysteroid dehydrogenase type 1 expression in a depot-specific manner in children. *J. Clin. Endocrinol. Metab.* **95**, 3300–8 (2010).

262. Navarro, G., Allard, C., Xu, W., & Mauvais-Jarvis, F. The role of androgens in metabolism, obesity, and diabetes in males and females. *Obesity (Silver Spring)* **23**, 713–19 (2015).

263. Rubinow, K. B. Estrogens and body weight regulation in men. *Adv. Exp. Med. Biol.* **1043**, 285–313 (2017).

264. Lean, M. E. J., Vlachou, P., Govan, L., & Han, T. S. Different associations between body composition and alcohol when assessed by exposure frequency

or by quantitative estimates of consumption. *J. Hum. Nutr. Diet.* **31**, 747–57 (2018).

265. Schütze, M. *et al.* Beer consumption and the 'beer belly': scientific basis or common belief? *Eur. J. Clin. Nutr.* **63**, 1143–9 (2009).

266. Kim, K. H. *et al.* Alcohol consumption and its relation to visceral and subcutaneous adipose tissues in healthy male Koreans. *Ann. Nutr. Metab.* **60**, 52–61 (2012).

267. Bergmann, M. M. *et al.* The association of lifetime alcohol use with measures of abdominal and general adiposity in a large-scale European cohort. *Eur. J. Clin. Nutr.* **65**, 1079–87 (2011).

268. Coulson, C. E. *et al.* Alcohol consumption and body composition in a population-based sample of elderly Australian men. *Aging Clin. Exp. Res.* **25**, 183–92 (2013).

269. Hagnäs, M. P. *et al.* Alcohol consumption and binge drinking in young men as predictors of body composition changes during military service. *Alcohol* **52**, 365–71 (2017).

270. Bendsen, N. T. *et al.* Is beer consumption related to measures of abdominal and general obesity? A systematic review and meta-analysis. *Nutr. Rev.* **71**, 67–87 (2013).

271. Bantle, J. P. Dietary fructose and metabolic syndrome and diabetes. *J. Nutr.* **139**, 1263S–1268S (2009).

272. Basaranoglu, M., Basaranoglu, G., Sabuncu, T., & Sentürk, H. Fructose as a key player in the development of fatty liver disease. *World J. Gastroenterol.* **19**, 1166–72 (2013).

273. Jegatheesan, P. & De Bandt, J.-P. Fructose and NAFLD: the multifaceted aspects of fructose metabolism. *Nutrients* **9**, (2017).

274. Ter Horst, K. W. & Serlie, M. J. Fructose consumption, lipogenesis, and non-alcoholic fatty liver disease. *Nutrients* **9**, (2017).

275. Qin, P. *et al.* Sugar and artificially sweetened beverages and risk of obesity, type 2 diabetes mellitus, hypertension, and all-cause mortality: a dose–response meta-analysis of prospective cohort studies. *Eur. J. Epidemiol.* (2020). doi:10.1007/s10654-020-00655-y

276. Bray, G. A. & Popkin, B. M. Dietary sugar and body weight: have we reached a crisis in the epidemic of obesity and diabetes?: health be damned! Pour on the sugar. *Diabetes Care* **37**, 950–6 (2014).

277. Deshpande, G., Mapanga, R. F., & Essop, M. F. Frequent sugar-sweetened beverage consumption and the onset of cardiometabolic diseases: cause for concern? *J. Endocr. Soc.* **1**, 1372–85 (2017).

278. Brunkwall, L. *et al.* Sugar-sweetened beverage consumption and genetic predisposition to obesity in 2 Swedish cohorts. *Am. J. Clin. Nutr.* **104**, 809–15 (2016).

279. Olsen, N. J. *et al.* Interactions between genetic variants associated with adiposity traits and soft drinks in relation to longitudinal changes in body weight and waist circumference. *Am. J. Clin. Nutr.* **104**, 816–26 (2016).

280. Haslam, D. E., McKeown, N. M., Herman, M. A., Lichtenstein, A. H., & Dashti, H. S. Interactions between genetics and sugar-sweetened beverage consumption on health outcomes: a review of gene-diet interaction studies. *Front. Endocrinol.* **8**, 368 (2017).

281. Arsenault, B. J., Lamarche, B., & Després, J.-P. Targeting overconsumption of sugar-sweetened beverages vs. overall poor diet quality for cardiometabolic diseases risk prevention: place your bets! *Nutrients* **9**, (2017).

282. Naude, C. E., Visser, M. E., Nguyen, K. A., Durao, S., & Schoonees, A. Effects of total fat intake on bodyweight in children. *Cochrane Database Syst. Rev.* **2**, CD012960 (2018).

283. Muka, T. *et al.* Dietary fat composition, total body fat and regional body fat distribution in two Caucasian populations of middle-aged and older adult women. *Clin. Nutr.* **36**, 1411–19 (2017).

284. Hooper, L. *et al.* Effects of total fat intake on body weight. *Cochrane Database Syst. Rev.* CD011834 (2015). doi:10.1002/14651858.CD011834

285. Katz, D. L. Competing dietary claims for weight loss: finding the forest through truculent trees. *Annu. Rev. Public Health* **26**, 61–88 (2005).

286. Green, C. J. & Hodson, L. The influence of dietary fat on liver fat accumulation. *Nutrients* **6**, 5018–33 (2014).

287. Hooper, L., Martin, N., Abdelhamid, A., & Davey Smith, G. Reduction in saturated fat intake for cardiovascular disease. *Cochrane Database Syst. Rev.* CD011737 (2015). doi:10.1002/14651858.CD011737

288. Bonaccio, M. *et al.* High adherence to the Mediterranean diet is associated with cardiovascular protection in higher but not in lower socioeconomic groups: prospective findings from the Moli-sani study. *Int. J. Epidemiol.* **46**, 1478–87 (2017).

289. Eslamparast, T., Tandon, P., & Raman, M. Dietary composition independent of weight loss in the management of non-alcoholic fatty liver disease. *Nutrients* **9**, (2017).

290. Seidelmann, S. B. *et al.* Dietary carbohydrate intake and mortality: a prospective cohort study and meta-analysis. *Lancet. Public Heal.* **3**, e419–e428 (2018).

291. Golubic, R. *et al.* The Cambridge Intensive Weight Management Programme appears to promote weight loss and reduce the need for bariatric surgery in obese adults. *Front. Nutr.* **5**, 54 (2018).

292. Harvie, M. N. *et al.* The effects of intermittent or continuous energy restriction on weight loss and metabolic disease risk markers: a randomized trial in young overweight women. *Int. J. Obes.* **35**, 714–27 (2011).

293. Antoni, R., Johnston, K. L., Collins, A. L., & Robertson, M. D. Intermittent v. continuous energy restriction: differential effects on postprandial glucose and lipid metabolism following matched weight loss in overweight/obese participants. *Br. J. Nutr.* **119**, 507–16 (2018).

294. Chao, A. M., Quigley, K. M., & Wadden, T. A. Dietary interventions for obesity: clinical and mechanistic findings. *J. Clin. Invest.* **131**, (2021).

295. Leslie, W. S., Taylor, R., Harris, L., & Lean, M. E. J. Weight losses with low-energy formula diets in obese patients with and without type 2 diabetes: systematic review and meta-analysis. *Int. J. Obes.* **41**, 96–101 (2017).

296. Kujala, U. M. Evidence on the effects of exercise therapy in the treatment of chronic disease. *Br. J. Sports Med.* **43**, 550–5 (2009).

297. Pedersen, B. K. & Saltin, B. Evidence for prescribing exercise as therapy in chronic disease. *Scand. J. Med. Sci. Sports* **16** Suppl. 1, 3–63 (2006).

298. Zaccardi, F. *et al.* Cardiorespiratory fitness and risk of type 2 diabetes mellitus: a 23-year cohort study and a meta-analysis of prospective studies. *Atherosclerosis* **243**, 131–7 (2015).

299. Kodama, S. *et al.* Cardiorespiratory fitness as a quantitative predictor of all-cause mortality and cardiovascular events in healthy men and women: a meta-analysis. *JAMA* **301**, 2024–35 (2009).

300. Bourbeau, K., Moriarty, T., Ayanniyi, A., & Zuhl, M. The combined effect of exercise and behavioral therapy for depression and anxiety: systematic review and meta-analysis. *Behav. Sci.* **10**, (2020).

301. Langleite, T. M. *et al.* Insulin sensitivity, body composition and adipose depots following 12 w combined endurance and strength training in dysglycemic and normoglycemic sedentary men. *Arch. Physiol. Biochem.* **122**, 167–79 (2016).

302. Tsuzuku, S., Kajioka, T., Sakakibara, H., & Shimaoka, K. Slow movement resistance training using body weight improves muscle mass in the elderly: a randomized controlled trial. *Scand. J. Med. Sci. Sports* **28**, 1339–44 (2018).

303. Mikkola, I. *et al.* Aerobic performance and body composition changes during military service. *Scand. J. Prim. Health Care* **30**, 95–100 (2012).

304. Thyfault, J. P. & Bergouignan, A. Exercise and metabolic health: beyond skeletal muscle. *Diabetologia* **63**, 1464–74 (2020). doi:10.1007/s00125-020-05177-6

305. Hens, W. *et al.* The effect of diet or exercise on ectopic adiposity in children and adolescents with obesity: a systematic review and meta-analysis. *Obes. Rev.* **18**, 1310–22 (2017).

306. Sabag, A. *et al.* Exercise and ectopic fat in type 2 diabetes: a systematic review and meta-analysis. *Diabetes Metab.* **43**, 195–210 (2017).

307. Hiuge-Shimizu, A. *et al.* Reduction of visceral fat correlates with the decrease in the number of obesity-related cardiovascular risk factors in Japanese with Abdominal Obesity (VACATION-J Study). *J. Atheroscler. Thromb.* **19**, 1006–18 (2012).

308. Albu, J. B. *et al.* Metabolic changes following a 1-year diet and exercise intervention in patients with type 2 diabetes. *Diabetes* **59**, 627–33 (2010).

309. Fabbrini, E. *et al.* Intrahepatic fat, not visceral fat, is linked with metabolic complications of obesity. *Proc. Natl. Acad. Sci. U. S. A.* **106**, 15430–5 (2009).

310. Bays, H. Central obesity as a clinical marker of adiposopathy; increased visceral adiposity as a surrogate marker for global fat dysfunction. *Curr. Opin. Endocrinol. Diabetes. Obes.* **21**, 345–51 (2014).

311. van der Heijden, G.-J. *et al.* A 12-week aerobic exercise program reduces hepatic fat accumulation and insulin resistance in obese, Hispanic adolescents. *Obesity (Silver Spring)* **18**, 384–90 (2010).

312. Benito, P. J. *et al.* Influence of previous body mass index and sex on regional fat changes in a weight loss intervention. *Phys. Sportsmed.* **45**, 450–7 (2017).

313. Serra, M. C. *et al.* Effects of weight loss with and without exercise on regional body fat distribution in postmenopausal women. *Ann. Nutr. Metab.* **70**, 312–20 (2017).

314. Chaston, T. B. & Dixon, J. B. Factors associated with percent change in visceral versus subcutaneous abdominal fat during weight loss: findings from a systematic review. *Int. J. Obes.* **32**, 619–28 (2008).

315. Merlotti, C., Ceriani, V., Morabito, A., & Pontiroli, A. E. Subcutaneous fat loss is greater than visceral fat loss with diet and exercise, weight-loss promoting drugs and bariatric surgery: a critical review and meta-analysis. *Int. J. Obes.* **41**, 672–82 (2017).

316. Singh, P. *et al.* Effects of weight gain and weight loss on regional fat distribution. *Am. J. Clin. Nutr.* **96**, 229–33 (2012).

317. Vispute, S. S., Smith, J. D., LeCheminant, J. D., & Hurley, K. S. The effect of abdominal exercise on abdominal fat. *J. Strength Cond. Res.* **25**, 2559–64 (2011).

318. Ramírez-Campillo, R. *et al.* Regional fat changes induced by localized muscle endurance resistance training. *J. Strength Cond. Res.* **27**, 2219–24 (2013).

319. Medrano, M. *et al.* Evidence-based exercise recommendations to reduce hepatic fat content in youth–a systematic review and meta-analysis. *Prog. Cardiovasc. Dis.* (2018). doi:10.1016/j.pcad.2018.01.013

320. Hashida, R. *et al.* Aerobic vs. resistance exercise in non-alcoholic fatty liver disease: a systematic review. *J. Hepatol.* **66**, 142–52 (2017).

321. Su, L. *et al.* Effects of HIIT and MICT on cardiovascular risk factors in adults with overweight and/or obesity: a meta-analysis. *PLoS One* **14**, e0210644 (2019).

322. Batacan, R. B., Duncan, M. J., Dalbo, V. J., Tucker, P. S., & Fenning, A. S. Effects of high-intensity interval training on cardiometabolic health: a systematic review and meta-analysis of intervention studies. *Br. J. Sports Med.* **51**, 494–503 (2017).

323. You, T. *et al.* Addition of aerobic exercise to dietary weight loss preferentially reduces abdominal adipocyte size. *Int. J. Obes.* **30**, 1211–16 (2006).

324. Barrès, R. & Zierath, J. R. The role of diet and exercise in the transgenerational epigenetic landscape of T2DM. *Nat. Rev. Endocrinol.* **12**, 441–51 (2016).

325. Rönn, T. *et al.* A six month exercise intervention influences the genome-wide DNA methylation pattern in human adipose tissue. *PLoS Genet.* **9**, e1003572 (2013).

326. Allen, J., Sun, Y., & Woods, J. A. Exercise and the regulation of inflammatory responses. *Prog. Mol. Biol. Transl. Sci.* **135**, 337–54 (2015).

327. Kirk, B., Feehan, J., Lombardi, G., & Duque, G. Muscle, bone, and fat crosstalk: the biological role of myokines, osteokines, and adipokines. *Curr. Osteoporos. Rep.* (2020). doi:10.1007/s11914-020-00599-y

328. Svendstrup, M. *et al.* Genetic risk scores for body fat distribution attenuate weight loss in women during dietary intervention. *Int. J. Obes.* **42**, 370–5 (2018).

329. Livingstone, K. M. *et al.* FTO genotype and weight loss: systematic review and meta-analysis of 9563 individual participant data from eight randomised controlled trials. *BMJ* **354**, i4707 (2016).

330. Furnham, A. & Levitas, J. Factors that motivate people to undergo cosmetic surgery. *Can. J. Plast. Surg.* **20**, e47–50 (2012).

331. Sharp, G., Tiggemann, M. & Mattiske, J. The role of media and peer influences in Australian women's attitudes towards cosmetic surgery. *Body Image* **11**, 482–7 (2014).

332. Sun, Q. Materialism, self-objectification, and capitalization of sexual attractiveness increase young Chinese women's willingness to consider cosmetic surgery. *Front. Psychol.* **9**, 2002 (2018).

333. Castle, H. E. XVI. Obesity and its surgical treatment by lipectomy. *Ann. Surg.* **54**, 706–10 (1911).

334. Glicenstein, J. Dujarier's case. *Ann. Chir. Plast. Esthet.* **34**, 290–2 (1989).

335. Bellini, E., Grieco, M. P., & Raposio, E. A journey through liposuction and liposculture: review. *Ann. Med. Surg.* **24**, 53–60 (2017).

336. Fischer, A. & Fischer, G. First surgical treatment for molding body's cellulite with three 5 mm incisions. *Bull Int Acad Cosmet Surg* **3**, 35 (1976).

337. Illouz, Y. G. Body contouring by lipolysis: a 5-year experience with over 3000 cases. *Plast. Reconstr. Surg.* **72**(5) 591–7 (1983). doi:10.1097/00006534-198311000-00001

338. Newman, J. Lipo-suction surgery: past—present—future. *Am. J. Cosmet. Surg.* **1**, 19–20 (1984).

339. Klein, J. A. The tumescent technique for lipo-suction surgery. *Am. J. Cosmet. Surg.* **4**, 263–7 (1987).

340. Scheflan, M. & Tazi, H. Ultrasonically assisted body contouring. *Aesthetic Surg. J.* **16**, 117–22 (1996).

341. Apfelberg, D. Laser-assisted liposuction may benefit surgeons and subjects. *Clin Laser Mon* **10**, 259 (1992).

342. Valizadeh, N., Jalaly, N. Y., Zarghampour, M., Barikbin, B., & Haghighatkhah, H. R. Evaluation of safety and efficacy of 980-nm diode laser-assisted lipolysis versus traditional liposuction for submental rejuvenation: a randomized clinical trial. *J. Cosmet. Laser Ther.* **18**, 41–5 (2016).

343. Kaoutzanis, C. *et al.* Cosmetic liposuction: preoperative risk factors, major complication rates, and safety of combined procedures. *Aesthetic Surg. J.* **37**, 680–94 (2017).

344. Klein, S. *et al.* Absence of an effect of liposuction on insulin action and risk factors for coronary heart disease. *N. Engl. J. Med.* **350**, 2549–57 (2004).

345. Martínez-Abundis, E., Molina-Villa, C. A., González-Ortiz, M., Robles-Cervantes, J. A., & Saucedo-Ortiz, J. A. Effect of surgically removing subcutaneous fat by abdominoplasty on leptin concentrations and insulin sensitivity. *Ann. Plast. Surg.* **58**, 416–19 (2007).

346. Hong, Y. G. *et al.* Impact of large-volume liposuction on serum lipids in orientals: a pilot study. *Aesthetic Plast. Surg.* **30**, 327–32

347. González-Ortiz, M., Robles-Cervantes, J. A., Cárdenas-Camarena, L., Bustos-Saldaña, R., & Martínez-Abundis, E. The effects of surgically removing

subcutaneous fat on the metabolic profile and insulin sensitivity in obese women after large-volume liposuction treatment. *Horm. Metab. Res.* 34, 446–9 (2002).

348. Geliebter, A., Krawitz, E., Ungredda, T., Peresechenski, E., & Giese, S. Y. Physiological and psychological changes following liposuction of large volumes of fat in overweight and obese women. *J. Diabetes Obes.* 2, 1–7 (2015).

349. Giugliano, G. *et al.* Effect of liposuction on insulin resistance and vascular inflammatory markers in obese women. *Br. J. Plast. Surg.* 57, 190–4 (2004).

350. Mohammed, B. S., Cohen, S., Reeds, D., Young, V. L., & Klein, S. Long-term effects of large-volume liposuction on metabolic risk factors for coronary heart disease. *Obesity (Silver Spring)* 16, 2648–51 (2008).

351. Seretis, K., Goulis, D. G., Koliakos, G., & Demiri, E. The effects of abdominal lipectomy in metabolic syndrome components and insulin sensitivity in females: a systematic review and meta-analysis. *Metabolism* 64, 1640–9 (2015).

352. Ramos-Gallardo, G. *et al.* Effect of abdominoplasty in the lipid profile of patients with dyslipidemia. *Plast. Surg. Int.* 2013, 861348 (2013).

353. Matarasso, A., Kim, R. W., & Kral, J. G. The impact of liposuction on body fat. *Plast. Reconstr. Surg.* 102, 1686–9 (1998).

354. Seretis, K., Goulis, D. G., Koliakos, G., & Demiri, E. Short- and long-term effects of abdominal lipectomy on weight and fat mass in females: a systematic review. *Obes. Surg.* 25, 1950–8 (2015).

355. Rinomhota, A. S. *et al.* Women gain weight and fat mass despite lipectomy at abdominoplasty and breast reduction. *Eur. J. Endocrinol.* 158, 349–52 (2008).

356. Benatti, F. *et al.* Liposuction induces a compensatory increase of visceral fat which is effectively counteracted by physical activity: a randomized trial. *J. Clin. Endocrinol. Metab.* 97, 2388–95 (2012).

357. Hernandez, T. L. *et al.* Femoral lipectomy increases postprandial lipemia in women. *Am. J. Physiol. Endocrinol. Metab.* 309, E63–71 (2015).

358. Tomkin, G. H. & Owens, D. The chylomicron: relationship to atherosclerosis. *Int. J. Vasc. Med.* 2012, 1–13 (2012).

359. Hernandez, T. L. *et al.* Fat redistribution following suction lipectomy: defense of body fat and patterns of restoration. *Obesity (Silver Spring)* 19, 1388–95 (2011).

360. Fabbrini, E. *et al.* Surgical removal of omental fat does not improve insulin sensitivity and cardiovascular risk factors in obese adults. *Gastroenterology* 139, 448–55 (2010).

361. Lima, M. M. O. *et al.* Visceral fat resection in humans: effect on insulin sensitivity, beta-cell function, adipokines, and inflammatory markers. *Obesity (Silver Spring)* 21, E182–9 (2013).

362. Andersson, D. P. *et al.* Omentectomy in addition to gastric bypass surgery and influence on insulin sensitivity: a randomized double blind controlled trial. *Clin. Nutr.* 33, 991–6 (2014).

363. Andersson, D. P. *et al.* Omentectomy in addition to bariatric surgery–a 5-year follow-up. *Obes. Surg.* 27, 1115–18 (2017).

364. Marcadenti, A. & de Abreu-Silva, E. O. Different adipose tissue depots: metabolic implications and effects of surgical removal. *Endocrinol. Nutr.* 62, 458–64 (2015).

365. American Society of Plastic Surgeons. New statistics reflect the changing face of plastic surgery (2015). (2016). Available at: www.plasticsurgery.org/news/press-releases/new-statistics-reflect-the-changing-face-of-plastic-surgery.

366. Alizadeh, Z., Halabchi, F., Mazaheri, R., Abolhasani, M., & Tabesh, M. Review of the mechanisms and effects of noninvasive body contouring devices on cellulite and subcutaneous fat. *Int. J. Endocrinol. Metab.* **14**, e36727 (2016).

367. Derrick, C. D., Shridharani, S. M., & Broyles, J. M. The safety and efficacy of cryolipolysis: a systematic review of available literature. *Aesthetic Surg. J.* **35**, 830–6 (2015).

368. Rzepecki, A. K., Farberg, A. S., Hashim, P. W., & Goldenberg, G. Update on noninvasive body contouring techniques. *Cutis* **101**, 285–8 (2018).

369. Toledo, L. S. Gluteal augmentation with fat grafting: the Brazilian buttock technique: 30 years' experience. *Clin. Plast. Surg.* **42**, 253–61 (2015).

370. Rapkiewicz, A. V *et al.* Fatal complications of aesthetic techniques: the gluteal region. *J. Forensic Sci.* **63**, 1406–12 (2018).

371. Mofid, M. M. *et al.* Report on mortality from Gluteal Fat Grafting: Recommendations from the ASERF Task Force. *Aesthetic Surg. J.* **37**, 796–806 (2017).

372. Cansancao, A. L., Condé-Green, A., David, J. A., & Vidigal, R. A. Subcutaneous-only gluteal fat grafting: a prospective study of the long-term results with ultrasound analysis. *Plast. Reconstr. Surg.* **143**, 447–51 (2019).

373. English, W. J. & Williams, D. B. Metabolic and bariatric surgery: a viable treatment option for obesity. *Prog. Cardiovasc. Dis.* (2018). doi:10.1016/j.pcad.2018.06.003

374. Colquitt, J. L., Pickett, K., Loveman, E., & Frampton, G. K. Surgery for weight loss in adults. *Cochrane Database Syst. Rev.* CD003641 (2014). doi:10.1002/14651858.CD003641.pub4

375. Pedroso, F. E. *et al.* Weight loss after bariatric surgery in obese adolescents: a systematic review and meta-analysis. *Surg. Obes. Relat. Dis.* **14**, 413–22 (2018).

376. Yan, Y. *et al.* Roux-en-Y gastric bypass versus medical treatment for type 2 diabetes mellitus in obese patients: a systematic review and meta-analysis of randomized controlled trials. *Medicine* **95**, e3462 (2016).

377. Fakhry, T. K. *et al.* Bariatric surgery improves nonalcoholic fatty liver disease: a contemporary systematic review and meta-analysis. *Surg. Obes. Relat. Dis.* (**2018**). doi:10.1016/j.soard.2018.12.002

378. Wei, Y., Chen, Q., & Qian, W. Effect of bariatric surgery on semen parameters: a systematic review and meta-analysis. *Med. Sci. Monit. Basic Res.* **24**, 188–97 (2018).

379. Kwong, W., Tomlinson, G., & Feig, D. S. Maternal and neonatal outcomes after bariatric surgery; a systematic review and meta-analysis: do the benefits outweigh the risks? *Am. J. Obstet. Gynecol.* **218**, 573–80 (2018).

380. Wang, Y. *et al.* Impact of gastric bypass surgery on body fat distribution in patients with metabolic syndrome. *Zhonghua Wei Chang Wai Ke Za Zhi* **15**, 32–5 (2012).

381. Abdesselam, I. *et al.* Time course of change in ectopic fat stores after bariatric surgery. *J. Am. Coll. Cardiol.* **67**, 117–19 (2016).

382. Gaborit, B. *et al.* Effects of bariatric surgery on cardiac ectopic fat: lesser decrease in epicardial fat compared to visceral fat loss and no change in myocardial triglyceride content. *J. Am. Coll. Cardiol.* **60**, 1381–9 (2012).

383. Toro-Ramos, T. *et al.* Continued loss in visceral and intermuscular adipose tissue in weight-stable women following bariatric surgery. *Obesity (Silver Spring)* **23**, 62–9 (2015).

384. Hao, Z. *et al.* Does gastric bypass surgery change body weight set point? *Int. J. Obes. Suppl.* **6**, S37–S43 (2016).

385. Albers, P. H. *et al.* Enhanced insulin signaling in human skeletal muscle and adipose tissue following gastric bypass surgery. *Am. J. Physiol. Regul. Integr. Comp. Physiol.* **309**, R510–24 (2015).

386. Severino, A. *et al.* Early effect of Roux-en-Y gastric bypass on insulin sensitivity and signaling. *Surg. Obes. Relat. Dis.* **12**, 42–7 (2016).

387. Adami, G. F., Scopinaro, N., & Cordera, R. Adipokine pattern after bariatric surgery: beyond the weight loss. *Obes. Surg.* **26**, 2793–801 (2016).

388. Trakhtenbroit, M. A. *et al.* Body weight, insulin resistance, and serum adipokine levels 2 years after 2 types of bariatric surgery. *Am. J. Med.* **122**, 435–42 (2009).

389. Aghamohammadzadeh, R. *et al.* Effects of bariatric surgery on human small artery function: evidence for reduction in perivascular adipocyte inflammation, and the restoration of normal anticontractile activity despite persistent obesity. *J. Am. Coll. Cardiol.* **62**, 128–35 (2013).

390. Miller, G. D., Nicklas, B. J., & Fernandez, A. Serial changes in inflammatory biomarkers after Roux-en-Y gastric bypass surgery. *Surg. Obes. Relat. Dis.* **7**, 618–24

391. Kratz, M. *et al.* Improvements in glycemic control after gastric bypass occur despite persistent adipose tissue inflammation. *Obesity (Silver Spring)* **24**, 1438–45 (2016).

392. Hagman, D. K. *et al.* The short-term and long-term effects of bariatric/metabolic surgery on subcutaneous adipose tissue inflammation in humans. *Metabolism.* **70**, 12–22 (2017).

393. Frikke-Schmidt, H., O'Rourke, R. W., Lumeng, C. N., Sandoval, D. A., & Seeley, R. J. Does bariatric surgery improve adipose tissue function? *Obes. Rev.* **17**, 795–809 (2016).

394. Laferrère, B. Bariatric surgery and obesity: influence on the incretins. *Int. J. Obes. Suppl.* **6**, S32–S36 (2016).

395. Holst, J. J. *et al.* Mechanisms in bariatric surgery: gut hormones, diabetes resolution, and weight loss. *Surg. Obes. Relat. Dis.* **14**, 708–14 (2018).

396. le Roux, C. W. *et al.* Gut hormone profiles following bariatric surgery favor an anorectic state, facilitate weight loss, and improve metabolic parameters. *Ann. Surg.* **243**, 108–14 (2006).

397. Ionut, V., Burch, M., Youdim, A., & Bergman, R. N. Gastrointestinal hormones and bariatric surgery-induced weight loss. *Obesity (Silver Spring)* **21**, 1093–103 (2013).

398. Roth, C. L. & Doyle, R. P. Just a gut feeling: central nervous effects of peripheral gastrointestinal hormones. *Endocr. Dev.* **32**, 100–23 (2017).

399. Hunt, K. F. *et al*. Differences in regional brain responses to food ingestion after Roux-en-Y gastric bypass and the role of gut peptides: a neuroimaging study. *Diabetes Care* **39**, 1787–95 (2016).

400. Nance, K., Eagon, J. C., Klein, S., & Pepino, M. Y. Effects of sleeve gastrectomy vs. Roux-en-Y gastric bypass on eating behavior and sweet taste perception in subjects with obesity. *Nutrients* **10**, (2017).

401. Makaronidis, J. M. *et al*. Reported appetite, taste and smell changes following Roux-en-Y gastric bypass and sleeve gastrectomy: effect of gender, type 2 diabetes and relationship to post-operative weight loss. *Appetite* **107**, 93–105 (2016).

402. Faria, S. L., Faria, O. P., Cardeal, M. de A., Ito, M. K., & Buffington, C. Diet-induced thermogenesis and respiratory quotient after Roux-en-Y gastric bypass surgery: a prospective study. *Surg. Obes. Relat. Dis.* **10**, 138–43.

403. Li, W. & Richard, D. Effects of bariatric surgery on energy homeostasis. *Can. J. Diabetes* **41**, 426–31 (2017).

404. Thursby, E. & Juge, N. Introduction to the human gut microbiota. *Biochem. J.* **474**, 1823–36 (2017).

405. Leung, C., Rivera, L., Furness, J. B., & Angus, P. W. The role of the gut microbiota in NAFLD. *Nat. Rev. Gastroenterol. Hepatol.* **13**, 412–25 (2016).

406. Canfora, E. E., Meex, R. C. R., Venema, K., & Blaak, E. E. Gut microbial metabolites in obesity, NAFLD and T2DM. *Nat. Rev. Endocrinol.* (2019). doi:10.1038/s41574-019-0156-z

407. Clapp, M. *et al*. Gut microbiota's effect on mental health: the gut-brain axis. *Clin. Pract.* **7**, 987 (2017).

408. Pickard, J. M., Zeng, M. Y., Caruso, R., & Nunez, G. Gut microbiota: role in pathogen colonization, immune responses, and inflammatory disease. *Immunol. Rev.* **279**, 70–89 (2017).

409. Han, H. *et al*. Gut microbiota and type 1 diabetes. *Int. J. Mol. Sci.* **19**, (2018).

410. Gallagher, J. Why a faecal transplant could save your life. *BBC News* (2018). Available at: www.bbc.co.uk/news/health-43815369

411. Palleja, A. *et al*. Roux-en-Y gastric bypass surgery of morbidly obese patients induces swift and persistent changes of the individual gut microbiota. *Genome Med.* **8**, 67 (2016).

412. Magouliotis, D. E., Tasiopoulou, V. S., Sioka, E., Chatedaki, C., & Zacharoulis, D. Impact of bariatric surgery on metabolic and gut microbiota profile: a systematic review and meta-analysis. *Obes. Surg.* **27**, 1345–57 (2017).

413. Graessler, J. *et al*. Metagenomic sequencing of the human gut microbiome before and after bariatric surgery in obese patients with type 2 diabetes: correlation with inflammatory and metabolic parameters. *Pharmacogenomics J.* **13**, 514–22 (2013).

414. Guo, Y. *et al*. Modulation of the gut microbiome: a systematic review of the effect of bariatric surgery. *Eur. J. Endocrinol.* **178**, 43–56 (2018).

415. Hundt, M. & John, S. *Physiology, Bile Secretion*. StatPearls, 2018.

416. So, S. S. Y., Yeung, C. H. C., Schooling, C. M., & El-Nezami, H. Targeting bile acid metabolism in obesity reduction: a systematic review and meta-analysis. *Obes. Rev.* **21**, e13017 (2020).

417. Wang, C. *et al*. Role of bile acids in dysbiosis and treatment of nonalcoholic fatty liver disease. *Mediators Inflamm*. **2019**, 7659509 (2019).

418. Albaugh, V. L., Banan, B., Ajouz, H., Abumrad, N. N., & Flynn, C. R. Bile acids and bariatric surgery. *Mol. Aspects Med*. **56**, 75–89 (2017).

419. Mertens, K. L., Kalsbeek, A., Soeters, M. R., & Eggink, H. M. Bile acid signaling pathways from the enterohepatic circulation to the central nervous system. *Front. Neurosci*. **11**, 617 (2017).

420. Browning, M. G., Pessoa, B. M., Khoraki, J., & Campos, G. M. Changes in bile acid metabolism, transport, and signaling as central drivers for metabolic improvements after bariatric surgery. *Curr. Obes. Rep*. **8**, 175–84 (2019).

421. Fouladi, F., Mitchell, J. E., Wonderlich, J. A., & Steffen, K. J. The contributing role of bile acids to metabolic improvements after obesity and metabolic surgery. *Obes. Surg*. **26**, 2492–502 (2016).

422. Andersen, A., Lund, A., Knop, F. K., & Vilsbøll, T. Glucagon-like peptide 1 in health and disease. *Nat. Rev. Endocrinol*. **14**, 390–403 (2018).

423. Velapati, S. R. *et al*. Weight regain after bariatric surgery: prevalence, etiology, and treatment. *Curr. Nutr. Rep*. **7**, 329–34 (2018).

424. Gilbertson, N. M. *et al*. Bariatric surgery resistance: using preoperative lifestyle medicine and/or pharmacology for metabolic responsiveness. *Obes. Surg*. **27**, 3281–91 (2017).

425. Gómez-Ambrosi, J. *et al*. Cardiometabolic profile related to body adiposity identifies patients eligible for bariatric surgery more accurately than BMI. *Obes. Surg*. **25**, 1594–603 (2015).

426. Eriksson Hogling, D. *et al*. Body fat mass and distribution as predictors of metabolic outcome and weight loss after Roux-en-Y gastric bypass. *Surg. Obes. Relat. Dis*. (2018). doi:10.1016/j.soard.2018.03.012

427. Divoux, A. *et al*. Fibrosis in human adipose tissue: composition, distribution, and link with lipid metabolism and fat mass loss. *Diabetes* **59**, 2817–25 (2010).

428. Abdennour, M. *et al*. Association of adipose tissue and liver fibrosis with tissue stiffness in morbid obesity: links with diabetes and BMI loss after gastric bypass. *J. Clin. Endocrinol. Metab*. **99**, 898–907 (2014).

429. Nielsen, M. S. *et al*. Predictors of weight loss after bariatric surgery—a cross-disciplinary approach combining physiological, social, and psychological measures. *Int. J. Obes*. (2020). doi:10.1038/s41366-020-0576-9

430. Adami, G. F., Carbone, F., Montecucco, F., Camerini, G., & Cordera, R. Adipose tissue composition in obesity and after bariatric surgery. *Obes. Surg*. **29**, 3030–8 (2019).

431. McCarty, T. R., Echouffo-Tcheugui, J. B., Lange, A., Haque, L., & Njei, B. Impact of bariatric surgery on outcomes of patients with nonalcoholic fatty liver disease: a nationwide inpatient sample analysis, 2004-2012. *Surg. Obes. Relat. Dis*. **14**, 74–80 (2018).

432. Nickel, F. *et al*. Bariatric surgery as an efficient treatment for non-alcoholic fatty liver disease in a prospective study with 1-year follow-up: BariScan Study. *Obes. Surg*. **28**, 1342–50 (2018).

433. Casagrande, D. S. *et al*. Incidence of cancer following bariatric surgery: systematic review and meta-analysis. *Obes. Surg*. **24**, 1499–509 (2014).

434. Winder, A. A., Kularatna, M., & MacCormick, A. D. Does bariatric surgery affect the incidence of breast cancer development? A systematic review. *Obes. Surg.* 27, 3014–20 (2017).

435. Winder, A. A., Kularatna, M., & MacCormick, A. D. Does bariatric surgery affect the incidence of endometrial cancer development? A systematic review. *Obes. Surg.* 28, 1433–40 (2018).

436. Schauer, D. P. *et al.* Bariatric surgery and the risk of cancer in a large multisite cohort. *Ann. Surg.* (2017). doi:10.1097/SLA.0000000000002525

437. Reges, O. *et al.* Association of bariatric surgery using laparoscopic banding, Roux-en-Y gastric bypass, or laparoscopic sleeve gastrectomy vs usual care obesity management with all-cause mortality. *JAMA* 319, 279–90 (2018).

438. Gulliford, M. C. *et al.* Costs and outcomes of increasing access to bariatric surgery: cohort study and cost-effectiveness analysis using electronic health records. *Value Heal.* 20, 85–92 (2017).

8
Conclusion

The Start of a New Relationship

Fat has played a critical role in the emergence and evolution of the human race as well as nearly every organism on the planet. As we have learned, the emergence of fat droplets and adipose tissue represent milestones in evolutionary history that allowed our ancestors to uncouple themselves from their environment by conferring the ability to store immediately available calories for use at a later time. Such a critical occurrence opened the door to the development of more complex organisms capable of movement, locomotion, and migration, as well as provided an opportunity for human intelligence to evolve as a weapon in the fight to survive and thrive in their hostile environment. This process also resulted in fat coming to occupy a central role that links energy metabolism to numerous biological phenomena. This link, however, is being pushed beyond its limit by the monolithic global obesity epidemic that has manifested since the 1970s, with more than a third of the world's population now being overweight or obese, with no country or age group proving immune.[1]

The weight of the obesity crisis bearing down on the world has the potential to cause the collapse of our healthcare infrastructure as the cases of obesity-related metabolic and cardiovascular disease, cancer, and osteoarthritis surge,[2] and treatment of communicable diseases, most notably COVID-19,[3,4] become far more complicated. It remains to be seen how global obesity will affect the success of vaccination efforts for the current pandemic,[5] but it is likely that they will be negatively affected based on prevailing vaccine data for other infectious diseases, such as the flu.[3,6] The obesity crisis isn't just bad for our health though. It represents a massive drain on work productivity and personal earnings, and to the world's economies more generally.[7] In addition to its deleterious effects on our health and wealth, our future as a species might also be in jeopardy as obesity represents one of the biggest threats to male[8] and female[9] fertility. Fat's effects on human life and society do not end there though. The expansion of the world's waistline has not only provided clear evidence of fat tissue's crucial role in numerous, seemingly disparate, biological processes, but it has also generated some intriguing situations that challenge prevailing assumptions.

The global obesity crisis has provided clear evidence of the health risks associated with the accumulation of excessive amounts of fat (particularly in conjunction with low amounts of lean mass). However, there is a notable paradox in that 'not all obese people have metabolic disease, and not all metabolic disease patients are obese.' Astute observation of a group of rare individuals has highlighted a striking similarity in which people who have hardly any adipose tissue—such as those with a congenital lipodystrophy[10]—become very ill and develop metabolic and cardiovascular diseases usually associated with people who are obese. To reconcile this paradox, we have to cast away any preconceived notions that fat is a passive, homogenous layer of blubber under our skin that simply exists to make our jeans feel tight. As *Waisted* has repeatedly emphasized, we must look at the issue with fresh eyes.

Based on a substantial and compelling evidence base generated as a result of extensive research efforts in various disciplines, fat is clearly far more complex and important than many currently believe. From this more detailed knowledge, it has become apparent that the world is not just experiencing an obesity crisis, but a *central* obesity crisis (in which lower body fat accumulation, in contrast, confers protection). This striking relationship between body shape and health is underpinned by the fact that not all fat tissue is the same. Differences in fat biology manifest at various levels, ranging from blood flow at the macromolecular/tissue level to fatty acid handling, adipocyte hypertrophy/hyperplasia, insulin sensitivity, extracellular matrix turnover, inflammation, and gene expression at the cellular and molecular levels. Assimilating this multitude of data from *in vitro* and *in vivo* studies has advanced our understanding of how different fat depots play complementary but distinct roles within the multi-faceted 'adipose organ',[11] and enabled the identification of potential mechanisms underpinning the striking relationships between overall and regional fat mass with health.

By integrating the information regarding the relationships between body shape, size, and composition with the depot-specific biology of fat, an intriguing picture has emerged. It appears that (excessive) upper body fat accumulation, which often manifests as central obesity, is not necessarily the underlying cause of various obesity-related diseases. Instead, dysfunctional subcutaneous adipose tissue filled beyond capacity appears to be a key contributor. The seemingly idiosyncratic relationship between how much weight people can put on before they develop various diseases has prompted the notion of the 'personal fat threshold.'[12] Arguably representing a modern scientific interpretation of the historical concept of embonpoint and ancient preferences for bodily constitutions that sat 'midway between thin and corpulent,' these data also raise questions about how we measure and define overweight and obesity. Combined with the concept of 'expandability' in conjunction with the depot-specific properties of adipose tissue,[13] it has become possible to rationalize some of the seemingly paradoxical relationships between fat mass and distribution in the context of health.

While providing a neat, broad explanation for why these relationships between certain body shapes and health outcomes may exist, much work remains to be done to provide the requisite substance and detail for this conceptual framework. Perhaps in the future we will be able to predict an individual's personal fat threshold (e.g., using biomarkers based on circulating stem cells[14]), as well as identify and measure what factors determine 'adipose expandability.' Such knowledge could inform targeted preventative action (e.g., diet and exercise interventions) in addition to helping devise novel treatment options which strike to the core of the pathogenic mechanisms linking fat accumulation to various diseases. While the gynoid pattern of fat distribution protects against cardiovascular and metabolic disease, simply carving our bodies into that shape is not sufficient. The evidence indicates that achieving and maintaining good health involves an integrated, whole-body approach that requires vigilance throughout life, although it need not be an all-consuming endeavour. Attaining a greater understanding of the mechanisms that control the regional accumulation and function of fat represents a massive opportunity for developing new interventions to improve various aspects of human health, with the collective desire for a successful response to the COVID-19 pandemic also providing a particularly strong impetus to shrink the world's bulging waistline.

What the modern face of obesity and metabolic disease therapy will look like remains an exciting and unpredictable prospect. Perhaps modulation of the immune system,[15] the extracellular matrix,[16] epigenetics,[17,18] or (local) sex steroid[19] action will be involved. In a somewhat ironic twist, obesity-related metabolic and cardiovascular disease might be treated via fat or stem cell transplantation[20] to artificially enhance an individual's personal fat threshold. It is also possible that harnessing brown fat[21] will enable us to shed those dangerous excess calories without breaking a sweat (albeit perhaps feeling pleasantly warm). In identifying potential leads, genetic data suggest that the cause of obesity may reside in our brains whereas body fat distribution is driven by (regional) adipose biology and development.

Despite the wealth of data and knowledge accumulated in the laboratories and clinics around the world over the past hundred years or so, the data raise many more questions than they answer. However, advances in molecular technology (including genetic sequencing), imaging techniques, and computing power mean that we have some of the most powerful analytical tools known to humanity at our disposal. These technological advances are providing new insights and types of data that are revolutionizing not only how biomedical research is conducted, but also how we think about adipose tissue. Obtaining a truly comprehensive understanding of fat requires studying it from multiple angles and levels with various approaches though; obtaining a richer working knowledge of adipose biology will only be possible by combining our molecular and biochemical paradigms with anthropometric measures and imaging techniques to reinforce the 'bench to bedside and back again' loop that drives biomedical research forward. This should be complemented by interdisciplinary efforts that examine the role of social and cultural factors in adipose biology and the phenomena associated with its dysfunction. Evidence and knowledge are our greatest weapons in determining how to spend our time, energy, and finite resources effectively to stand a chance of slowing, stopping, or even reversing the onward march of the global central obesity crisis.

Obesity and metabolic disease will always be problems in society, but the alarming prevalence we are currently experiencing arguably represents the manifestation of the human body's ancient foundations' incompatibility with the modern world it developed and currently occupies. We have arrived at this situation through the coalescing of many distinct but interrelated factors that have together conspired to shift society's energy balance in favour of fat accumulation. The excessive consumption of calorie-dense food in conjunction with an increasingly sedentary lifestyle[22] are exacerbated by structural factors relating to socio-economic inequality[23] and stress,[24] and then reified by political short-sightedness. Given the colossal scale of this crisis which affects all countries and people of all ages, new ways of thinking about addressing obesity[25] must be embraced, given that current efforts have been largely ineffectual. Individual choices need to be supported by proportionate, sustainable policies that provide an environment in which such choices are possible, meaningful, and result in beneficial outcomes. There is no good reason why the debate about how our obesogenic environment and lifestyles contribute to poor long-term health should not be discussed in the same manner used to consider (and limit) the dangers of heavy drinking to the liver and brain, or the damage that smoking causes to our lungs and heart; we deserve much better than we are currently receiving, and should demand far more from the governments and food industries that serve us, as well as from ourselves. The stakes are too high to maintain the collective ignorance, apathy, or complicity under-pinning today's obesogenic status quo.

The public are increasingly fascinated with food and the notion of healthy eating, yet the actions of a significant majority belie these sentiments as the consumption of snacks, fast food, and sugar-sweetened beverages remains high, particularly among adolescents[26]—despite their clear association with adverse health outcomes.[27] Increasingly hectic lifestyles with limited opportunities for home-cooking coupled with wages stretched to breaking point for many and limited dietary options in inner-city 'food deserts' pro-vide the perfect conditions for many to choose the cheaper, more processed option. This narrowing of options has been exacerbated by lockdowns im-plemented to stem the spread of COVID-19 which have resulted in greater inactivity and fast food consumption around the world.[28] Overwhelming evidence indicates that increased consumption of sugar-sweetened drinks (many of which can contain more than a person's recommended daily al-lowance in a single serving) is strongly associated with the development of central obesity as well as metabolic and cardiovascular disease in people of all ages.[29]

There is more than enough solid data currently available to identify what constitutes a good diet for the vast majority of people.[30] That is not to say there is nothing more to be learned, far from it, but there is a risk that the quest for the 'ideal' diet for any specific demographic is simply distracting from the fact that overall energy intake, regardless of macronutrient com-position, plays the major role in determining one's body mass and compos-ition.[31,32] The nutritional quality of the world's collective diet is also ripe for improvement too. While it may be unpalatable to consider and will con-tinue to be met with furious resistance by various vested interests, getting the world out of its (central) obesity rut likely necessitates changing our nutritional environment in a meaningful way through legislation, educa-tion, and changing practices to enable as many people as possible to ob-tain a healthy diet produced in an environmentally sustainable manner.[33] Addressing the global obesity crisis will also involve getting everyone, particularly children, more physically active as the world is well on the way to becoming dangerously sedentary.[34]

As the average person's frame changes, seemingly irrevocably, it has become clear that we are not just dealing with the health and economic ramifications of society's physical transformation. Reviewing the wide range of biological phenomena underpinned or influenced by adipose tissue also represents a prime opportunity to re-appraise our social attitudes towards fat. There has been highly public pressure on the media and across the fashion worlds to represent a wider spectrum of body shapes and sizes to better reflect the global population's expanding waistline. The 'body positivity/acceptance' and 'fat pride' movements[35] have gained significant momentum and influence over recent years, but it is important that the pendulum does not swing too far the other way as overweight and obesity are responsible for many serious, chronic, preventable illnesses and premature deaths around the world. Instead, it is hoped that a greater appreciation of adipose biology facilitates constructive dialogue to identify and portray what constitutes a healthy, attractive, and attainable body without normalizing pathological states or encouraging behavioural extremes.

Both individually and collectively, the chapters within this book lay the foundation for a broader perspective on and appreciation of fat. The case presented herein should provide food for thought about the many important functions of adipose tissue, as well as the instrumental role it has played, and continues to play, in humanity's history. Understanding our fat and treating it with the respect it deserves will be necessary for devising solutions to slim the world's waistline and improve both our individual and collective health. How we achieve such a vital result remains to be seen, but understanding the problem means we've taken a step closer to solving it. In the meantime, my hope is that this volume will encourage a more nuanced and inclusive conversation around fat, one that is grounded in a deeper appreciation of this incredible organ and one that will leave its readers never looking at a bum or tum in the same way again.

References

1. Ng, M. *et al.* Global, regional, and national prevalence of overweight and obesity in children and adults during 1980–2013: a systematic analysis for the Global Burden of Disease Study 2013. *Lancet* **384**, 766–81 (2014).
2. Blüher, M. Obesity: global epidemiology and pathogenesis. *Nat. Rev. Endocrinol.* **15**, 288–98 (2019).

3. Kwok, S. *et al.* Obesity: a critical risk factor in the COVID-19 pandemic. *Clin. Obes.* **10**, e12403 (2020).

4. Sattar, N., McInnes, I. B., & McMurray, J. J. V. Obesity is a risk factor for severe COVID-19 infection. *Circulation* **142**, 4–6 (2020).

5. Ryan, D. H., Ravussin, E., & Heymsfield, S. COVID-19 and the patient with obesity—the editors speak out. *Obesity (Silver Spring)* **28**, 847 (2020).

6. Neidich, S. D. *et al.* Increased risk of influenza among vaccinated adults who are obese. *Int. J. Obes.* **41**, 1324–30 (2017).

7. Finkelstein, E. A. *et al.* Obesity and severe obesity forecasts through 2030. *Am. J. Prev. Med.* **42**, 563–70 (2012).

8. Kahn, B. E. & Brannigan, R. E. Obesity and male infertility. *Curr. Opin. Urol.* **27**, 441–5 (2017).

9. Silvestris, E., de Pergola, G., Rosania, R., & Loverro, G. Obesity as disruptor of the female fertility. *Reprod. Biol. Endocrinol.* **16**, 22 (2018).

10. Fiorenza, C. G., Chou, S. H., & Mantzoros, C. S. Lipodystrophy: pathophysiology and advances in treatment. *Nat. Rev. Endocrinol.* **7**, 137–50 (2011).

11. Cinti, S. The adipose organ. *Prostaglandins. Leukot. Essent. Fatty Acids* **73**, 9–15 (2005).

12. Taylor, R. & Holman, R. R. Normal weight individuals who develop type 2 diabetes: the personal fat threshold. *Clin. Sci.* **128**, 405–10 (2015).

13. Carobbio, S., Pellegrinelli, V., & Vidal-Puig, A. Adipose tissue function and expandability as determinants of lipotoxicity and the metabolic syndrome. *Adv. Exp. Med. Biol.* **960**, 161–96 (2017).

14. Sen, S. Adult stem cells: beyond regenerative tool, more as a bio-marker in obesity and diabetes. *Diabetes Metab. J.* **43**, 744–51 (2019).

15. Gerner, R. R., Wieser, V., Moschen, A. R., & Tilg, H. Metabolic inflammation: role of cytokines in the crosstalk between adipose tissue and liver. *Can. J. Physiol. Pharmacol.* **91**, 867–72 (2013).

16. Williams, A. S., Kang, L., & Wasserman, D. H. The extracellular matrix and insulin resistance. *Trends Endocrinol. Metab.* **26**, 357–66 (2015).

17. Pigeyre, M., Yazdi, F. T., Kaur, Y., & Meyre, D. Recent progress in genetics, epigenetics and metagenomics unveils the pathophysiology of human obesity. *Clin. Sci.* **130**, 943–86 (2016).

18. Sharma, S. & Taliyan, R. Histone deacetylase inhibitors: future therapeutics for insulin resistance and type 2 diabetes. *Pharmacol. Res.* **113**, 320–6 (2016).

19. Newell-Fugate, A. E. The role of sex steroids in white adipose tissue adipocyte function. *Reproduction* **153**, R133–R149 (2017).

20. Payab, M. *et al.* Stem cell and obesity: current state and future perspective. *Adv. Exp. Med. Biol.* **1089**, 1–22

21. Marlatt, K. L., Chen, K. Y., & Ravussin, E. Is activation of human brown adipose tissue a viable target for weight management? *Am. J. Physiol. Regul. Integr. Comp. Physiol.* (2018). doi:10.1152/ajpregu.00443.2017

22. Hruby, A. & Hu, F. B. The epidemiology of obesity: a big picture. *Pharmacoeconomics* **33**, 673–89 (2015).

23. Bilger, M., Kruger, E. J., & Finkelstein, E. A. Measuring socioeconomic inequality in obesity: looking beyond the obesity threshold. *Health Econ.* **26**, 1052–66 (2017).

24. Geiker, N. R. W. *et al.* Does stress influence sleep patterns, food intake, weight gain, abdominal obesity and weight loss interventions and vice versa? *Obes. Rev.* **19**, 81–97 (2018).

25. Lee, B. Y. *et al.* A systems approach to obesity. *Nutr. Rev.* **75**, 94–106 (2017).

26. Beal, T., Morris, S. S., & Tumilowicz, A. Global patterns of adolescent fruit, vegetable, carbonated soft drink, and fast-food consumption: a meta-analysis of global school-based student health surveys. *Food Nutr. Bull.* **40**, 444–59 (2019).

27. Mullee, A. *et al.* Association between soft drink consumption and mortality in 10 european countries. *JAMA Intern. Med.* **179**, 1479 (2019).

28. Ruíz-Roso, M. B. *et al.* Changes of physical activity and ultra-processed food consumption in adolescents from different countries during Covid-19 pandemic: an observational study. *Nutrients* **12**, (2020).

29. Deshpande, G., Mapanga, R. F., & Essop, M. F. Frequent sugar-sweetened beverage consumption and the onset of cardiometabolic diseases: cause for concern? *J. Endocr. Soc.* **1**, 1372–85 (2017).

30. Katz, D. L. Competing dietary claims for weight loss: finding the forest through truculent trees. *Annu. Rev. Public Health* **26**, 61–88 (2005).

31. Emadian, A., Andrews, R. C., England, C. Y., Wallace, V., & Thompson, J. L. The effect of macronutrients on glycaemic control: a systematic review of dietary randomised controlled trials in overweight and obese adults with type 2 diabetes in which there was no difference in weight loss between treatment groups. *Br. J. Nutr.* **114**, 1656–66 (2015).

32. Sacks, F. M. *et al.* Comparison of weight-loss diets with different compositions of fat, protein, and carbohydrates. *N. Engl. J. Med.* **360**, 859–73 (2009).

33. Kc, K. B. *et al.* When too much isn't enough: does current food production meet global nutritional needs? *PLoS One* **13**, e0205683 (2018).

34. Guthold, R., Stevens, G. A., Riley, L. M., & Bull, F. C. Global trends in insufficient physical activity among adolescents: a pooled analysis of 298 population-based surveys with 1.6 million participants. *Lancet Child Adolesc. Heal.* **4**, 23–35 (2020).

35. Cherry, K. What is body positivity? *VeryWell Mind* (2020). Available at: www.verywellmind.com/what-is-body-positivity-4773402.

Index

For the benefit of digital users, indexed terms that span two pages (e.g., 52–53) may, on occasion, appear on only one of those pages.

Tables and figures are indicated by *t* and *f* following the page number
vs. indicates a comparison.

abdominal computed tomography 145–46
abdominal fat 54, 55*f*
1-acylglycerol-3-phosphate
    O-acyltransferase 2 gene 202
adenosine triphosphate (ATP) 47
    generation 98–99, 99*f*
AdipoChaser mouse 162
adipocyte hypertrophy 170–71
    Cushing's disease 209
adipocytes 53–54
    generation *see* adipogenesis
    inflammatory signalling 175–76
    size 171–72
    turnover of 171
adipogenesis 178–80, 179*f*
    gene expression 183
    glucocorticoids 210
    oestrogen 218
adipokines 75
    polycystic ovary syndrome 222
adipose tissue
    blood flow 163, 164*f*, 165
    bone marrow *see* bone marrow
        adipose tissue
    breasts 16
    brown *see* brown adipose tissue (BAT)
    connections to 163–65
    distribution *see* adipose tissue distribution
    extracellular matrix and 173
    fatty acid uptake 165
    femoral fat 54, 55*f*
    hyperplasia 170–71
    inflammation in Cushing's disease 209
    measurement *see* body fat measurement
    metabolic disease 168–70, 169*f*
    visceral *see* visceral adipose tissue
    see also body fat

adipose tissue distribution 197–270
    bariatric surgery 240
    drugs 204–7
    exercise & diet 226–32
    female form 217–22
    genetics 197–204
    glucocorticoids 207–16
    hormone replacement therapy 220
    male form 222–23
    sex steroids 216–25
    stress response 215–16
    surgery 232–44
adrenaline 166
adults
    brown adipose tissue 92*f*, 92–93
    obesity prevalence 1
advertising 30–31
aerobic exercise, resistance exercise and 231
Afghanistan 27
Africa 149
agouti gene 200–1
agouti mice 200–1
agouti-related protein (AgRP) 201
AGPAT2 gene 202
alcohol consumption 274–75
    adipose tissue distribution 226
aldosterone 71–72
all-cause mortality 145–46
alpha-melanocyte-stimulating hormone
    (α-MSH) 200–1
American Medical Association (AMA) 2
American Society of Liposuction 234
amphetamines 206
androgen receptors 217
androgens 216
    bodybuilding 225
android shape 125–26

animal trials, beta-3 adrenoceptor
    activators 96
anorexia nervosa 12–13, 108
antipsychotic medications 205–6
anti-retroviral drugs 205
apartheid, female ideal and 25
apolipoproteins 58
appetite regulation, fat deposits 75–76
appetite suppressant drugs 206, 207
Asia 124t
atherosclerosis 72–75, 236–37
atherosclerotic plaques 73
Atkin, Robert 67
Atkins diet 67
ATP see adenosine triphosphate
    (ATP)
ATP synthase 98–99
attractiveness 17–18
    geographical variation 20–21
axillary adipose tissue 161–62

Baartman, Sarah 203
Bangladesh 24
bariatric surgery 239f, 239–41
    definition 239–40
Barraquer–Simons syndrome 201–2
BAT see brown adipose tissue (BAT)
beauty 17–35
beer gut 226
behavioural modification programmes 229
benfluorex 206
beta-3 adrenoceptor activators 96
beta-adrenoceptors 65
bile 56
bile acids
    cholesterol 71–72
    metabolism of 242–43
bioelectrical impedance analysis
    (BIA) 133–34
bipedalism 8–9
birth
    bipedalism 9
    early foetal development 9–10
bladder cancer 204–5
Bloch, Felix 132
blood flow, adipose tissue 163, 164f, 165
blood glucose levels, type 2 diabetes 52
BMD see bone mineral density (BMD)
BMI see body mass index (BMI)
body asymmetry 19
bodybuilding

androgens 225
2,4-dinitrophenol 101
body composition
    exercise effects 230
    fat distribution and 147–49
    health vs. 135–42
    quantification 148–49
    sex-specific differences 216–17
body dysmorphic disorder 33–34
body fat
    compartments 145–47
    evolution 7–8
    fertility and 12–13, 77–78
    mobilization 63–64
    re-distribution in Cushing's
        disease 209f, 209
    see also adipocytes; adipose tissue; lower
        body fat
body fat accumulation
    evolution 13
    oestrogen 13
body fat distribution 54, 125
    body composition and 147–49
    post-menopause 218–19
    sex-specific 125–26
body fat measurement 121–35
    method choice 134–35
    see also bioelectrical impedance analysis
        (BIA); body mass index (BMI);
        computed tomography (CT); dual-
        energy X-ray absorptiometry (DXA);
        magnetic resonance imaging (MRI);
        waist-to-hip ratio (WHR)
body frame
    changes in 276
    mass and 125
    weight appropriateness 125
body mass, frame appropriateness 125
body mass index (BMI) 121–25
    attractiveness geographical variation 20
    calculation of 124f
    categories 124t
    central obesity 144
    development of 121
    drawbacks to 142
    epidemiological studies 135–36
    fat mass percentage vs. 137–38
    fractures vs. 105
    limitations 123–25
    men & women differences 147
    obesity/overweight 135–36

waist circumference *vs.* 142–43
waist-to-hip ratio *vs.* 142–43
body modification 223–25, 224*f*
body proportionality 19
body shape
    culture 2–3
    evolution 7–10
    historical aspects 2–3, 7–45
    societal views 19
    white adipose tissue 109–10
bone
    fractures 106–7, 204–5
    structure & waist-hip ratio 127–28
bone health
    metabolic health and 105
    type 2 diabetes 106–7
bone marrow adipose tissue 104–9
    body shape 108–9
    diet and 106
    functions 107
bone mineral density (BMD)
    bone marrow adipose tissue 104–5
    dual-energy X-ray absorptiometry 128
bony ridges, face 10
brain size
    starvation in 66
    upper limit 9–10
Brazilian butt lift 238
breasts 14–17
    attractiveness & geographical
        variation 20
    attractiveness measure 19
    biomechanics 14
    composition 16
    development 15–17
    evolution 14–15
    fat 54, 55*f*
    nutritional store signs 18
    size & function 16
    visual signal as 16–17
    see also lactation
Brillat-Savin, Jean Anthelme 33
brown adipose tissue (BAT) 91–103
    activation of 94–95
    adipogenesis 179–80
    circadian rhythm 102–3
    distribution 91–93, 92*f*
    evolutionary role 93–94
    females *vs.* males 95–96
    heat production 93–94, 95–98
    innervation 96

    white adipose tissue and 94
Brown, Michael S. 71–72
buttocks 8

calorie-dense food 274–75
Cameron, John 128
cancer 136–37
carbohydrates 48*f*, 48–51
    metabolism 67–70
cardiovascular disease
    BMI 137
    cholesterol 73–74
    corticosteroids 211
    fat fibrosis 173–74
    fatty acids 71
    liposuction effects 235
    lower body fat 144
    menopause 221
    upper body fat accumulation 143
carotid atherosclerosis 141–42
Castle, H. E. 232–33
catecholamines 96, 163–64
CCAAT/enhancer-binding protein
        family 178–79
cell membrane 71
cellular stress 227
central nervous system (CNS)
        199–200
central obesity 144, 272
    metabolic disease 105–6, 168
    mouse models 161–62
CGL1 (congenital generalized lipodystrophy
        type 1) 202
chemotherapy 104
chewing 54–56
children, obesity prevalence 1
China 21–23
    historical female ideal 21–22
    male ideal 22–23
    modern female ideal 22
cholesterol 56, 71–75
chromatin 182
chronic inflammation 175–77
chylomicrons 58, 164–65
Clostridium difficile 242
clothes 31–32
CNS (central nervous system) 199–200
cocaine 206
cold, brown adipose tissue
        activation 94–95
compartments, body fat 145–47

computed tomography (CT) 130*f*, 130–31
  abdomen 145–46
  development 131
  disadvantages 131
  radiation dose 131
congenital generalized lipodystrophy 77
congenital generalized lipodystrophy type 1
  (CGL1) 202
congenital lipodystrophy disorders 201–
  2, 272
Cormack, Allan 131
coronary heart disease 136–37, 220–21
corticosteroids 212, 213*f*
cortisol 71–72
  anorexia nervosa 108–9
  Cushing's disease 208
  fat mobilization/accumulation 210–11
  stress 78
  24-hour cyclicity 211
cosmetic surgery
  Afghanistan 27
  Westernized ideal form 33
COVID-19 pandemic 2, 79, 271–72,
  273, 275
cryolipolysis 237–38
CT *see* computed tomography (CT)
culture
  attractiveness 20–21
  body shape 2–3
Cushing's disease 208, 209*f*, 210, 214
Cuvier, Georges 203–4

Damadian, Raymond 132
de novo lipogenesis (DNL) 68–69, 210
diabetes mellitus 51
  type 1 *see* type 1 diabetes
  type 2 *see* type 2 diabetes
diabetic ketoacidosis 66–67
diet
  adipose tissue distribution 226–32
  bone marrow adipose tissue and 106
  liposuction *vs.* 235
dietary cholesterol 72
dietary fat 228–29
  absorption 57*f*, 57–58
  consumption 228–29
  digestion 54–57, 57*f*
  restriction 60
  taste 54
dietary sugars 227–28

dieting 229
2,4-dinitrophenol (DNP) 100–2
DNA methylation 181–82
drugs, adipose tissue distribution 204–7
dual-energy X-ray absorptiometry
  (DXA) 128–30, 129*f*
  adipose tissue distribution 198
  body fat compartments 146
  development 128
  fat in body compartments 138
  lean mass 139–40
  pre-surgery 243
  radiation doses 128
Dubin, Louis I. 122–23
Dujarier, Charles 232–33

eating disorders 33–34
eating patterns 102–3
ectopic fat mass, exercise and 230
embonpoint 170
Endo, Akira 74–75
endotrophin 174–75
energy stores 47
  mobilisation 64–65
epicardial fat 109
epigenetics 180–84, 181*f*, 273–74
  chromatin 182
  DNA methylation 181–82
  histone modifications 182
  microRNAs 182–83
essential fatty acids 70
ethnicity
  attractiveness 20–21
  body composition 149
Europe 123–25, 124*t*
European Prospective Investigation into Cancer
  and Nutrition (EPIC) study 144–45
exercise
  adipose tissue distribution 226–32
  advantages of 65
  benefits of 229
  fatty acid mobilization 166
  hitting the wall 64–65
  lactic acid accumulation 64–65
  liposuction *vs.* 235
  support of 64–65
expandability 170
extracellular matrix 172–75, 273–74
  adipose tissue and 173
  turnover of 174–75

face
    evolution of 10–12
    sexual selection and 11–12
    symmetry 19
fad diets 34
familial hypercholesterolaemia (FH) 74
familial partial lipodystrophy of the
        Dunnigan variety (FPLD) 201–3
famine 11
fashion 31, 32–33
fat
    body fat *see* adipose tissue; body fat
    dietary fat *see* dietary fat
    functions of *see* functions of fat
fat droplets 52–53
fat mass estimates 123
fat mass percentage, BMI *vs.* 137–38
fatty acids 48*f*, 48–49, 52–54, 70–71
    generation of 68–69
    metabolism in liver 68–69, 69*f*
    mobilization 166
    release of 65
    structure 53*f*, 54
    uptake by adipose tissue 165
fatty livers 69–70
fatty streaks 73
feeding behaviour, leptin 75–76
female form
    adipose tissue distribution 217–22
    Afghanistan ideals 27
    artistic representations 3
    Chinese ideals 22
    historical ideals 23, 24, 28–29
    Japanese ideals 23–24
    modern ideals 22, 23–24, 27, 29
    Pacific Island ideals 28–29
    South African ideals 24
femoral fat 54, 55*f*
fertility 12–14
    body fat and 18, 77–78
    leptin 76
    oestrogen 15
    reduction in 12–13
fibrosis 173
fight-or-flight response 65
Fiji 28–30
fluid retention, thiazolidinediones 204–5
foam cells 73
Framingham Heart Study of Cardiovascular
        Risk 123

free fatty acids
    fat digestion 56–57
    metabolism 64
fructose 227
FTO gene 198–99, 231–32
fullness, neuronal signals 242
functional magnetic resonance imaging
        (fMRI) 133
functions of fat 47–89
    appetite regulation 75–76
    immunity 78–80
    metabolism 47–54
    sexual development & function 75–76
    stress 78
    warmth 75

Galen 32–33
gall bladder 56
gallstones 56, 220–21
Galvani, Luigi 133–34
gastric bypass surgery 240
gastrointestinal tract 241–43
gene expression
    adipogenesis 183
    mouse models 161–62
genetics
    adipose tissue distribution 197–204
    exercise and 231–32
    regional fat accumulation 148
    upper body fat accumulation 143
genetic sequencing 274
genome-wide association studies
        (GWAS) 137, 198–99
global obesity crisis 1
glucocorticoids
    adipogenesis 210
    adipose tissue distribution 207–16
    bone marrow adipose tissue 107–8
    metabolism by fat 78
gluconeogenesis 66
glucose 49
    homeostasis 50*f*, 50
    release from liver 50–51
    starvation 66
    structure 48*f*
gluteal fat 54, 55*f*
Glybera 60–61
glycerol 56–57, 64
glycogen 48*f*, 49
glycyrrhetic acid 214–15

Goldstein, Joseph L. 71–72
gut hormones 241
gut microbiota 242
GWAS (genome-wide association
    studies) 137, 198–99
gynaecomastia 225
gynoid shape 125–26, 273

Hadza tribe 20
Hawaii 28–29
HDLs (high-density lipoproteins) 72–73
head 10
health
    body composition vs. 135–42
    obesity/overweight 2, 272
    status assessment 18–19
    subcutaneous abdominal fat and 167–68
healthy body weight see normal/healthy
    body weight
healthy eating 275
heart, energy demand 62
Heart and Estrogen/Progestin Replacement
    Study (HERS) 220–21
heart attacks 73–74, 141–42
heart disease 139, 204–5
heritability 197–98
    studies 199
high-density lipoproteins (HDLs) 72–73
high-intensity focused ultrasound 237–38
high-intensity interval training
    (HIIT) 231
hips 144–45
    health status 18–19
    nutritional store signs 18
histone modifications 182
HIV infection/AIDS 25, 79–80
HMG-CoA reductase 74–75
Hoorn study (Netherlands) 144–45
hormone replacement therapy
    (HRT) 219, 220–21
Hounsfield, Geoffrey 131, 132–33
HRT (hormone replacement
    therapy) 219, 220–21
hunger 65–67
11β-hydroxysteroid dehydrogenases
    (HSDs) 212–15
hyperplasia, adipose tissue 170–71

imaging techniques 274
immune system 175–77, 273–74

immunity 78–80
    energy metabolism and 79–80
India 148–49
infertility 78
inflammation
    chronic 175–77
    obesity/overweight 79
inguinal pads, mouse models 161–62
insulin
    adipose tissue connections 163–64
    fat mobilization 63
    glucose homeostasis 50
    lipoprotein lipase promotion 59
    resistance 52
    sensitivity see insulin sensitivity
    subcutaneous fat deposition 168–70
    type 1 diabetes 51
insulin-sensitive obese individuals 141
insulin sensitivity
    adipose tissue and 172
    bariatric surgery 240–41
    post-surgery 243–44
insurance companies, BMI use 122
INTERHEART study 144
Iran 28
Israel 28
Itsenko, Nikolai 208

Jamaica 26–27
Japan 20, 23–24
jaws 10

ketogenesis 66
ketogenic diets 67
ketone bodies 66
Keys, Ancel 123
Khoisan tribe 203
kidneys 62
Klein, Jeffrey 234

lactation
    energy cost 12, 16
    oestrogen 15
    see also breasts
lactic acid 64–65
LDLs (low-density lipoproteins) 68–
    69, 72–73
lean mass 139–40
    measurement 139–40
    waist-hip ratio 127–28

leptin
    bone marrow adipose tissue 107–8
    feeding behaviour control 75–76
    oestrogen 218
    puberty & fertility 76
lifestyle 34, 275
linoleic acid 53f, 70
α-linoleic acid 53f, 70
lipectomy 232–33
lipodystrophy 109–10, 177
lipomas 131
lipoprotein lipase (LPL) 59
    glucocorticoids 210
    non-functionality 59–60
lipoproteins 58, 72–75
liposuction 232–36, 234f
    disease effects 235
    exercise/diet vs. 235
    safety 235
    ultrasound and 234–35
liver
    cholesterol synthesis 72
    fatty acid metabolism 68–69, 69f
    glucose formation 50–51
    glucose release 50–51
liver fat 146
liver fat mass 230
Lock, Margaret 220
locomotion, bipedalism 8–9
lorcaserin 207
lovastatin 74–75
low-density lipoproteins (LDLs) 68–
    69, 72–73
lower body fat
    accumulation 13, 20
    disease and 144
    fatty acid mobilization 166
    post-menopause 218–19
low-level laser therapy 237–38
LPL see lipoprotein lipase (LPL)
lymphatic system 58

magnetic resonance imaging
    (MRI) 130f, 132–33
    development 132
    safety 133
male form
    adipose tissue distribution 222–23
    artistic representations 3
    attractiveness variation 20

fat distribution 14
modern Chinese ideal 22–23
modern Japanese ideal 23–24
sex differences 222
sex-specific roles 11
white adipose tissue 55f
Mansfield, Peter 132
marijuana 206–7
M C4R gene 201
media 1, 30–31
    bariatric surgery 240
melanocyte receptors (MCRs) 201
Mendel, Gregor 197
Mendelian randomization studies 137
menopause 148, 218–19, 221
metabolically healthy obesity
    (MHO) 140–41
metabolic balance 48
metabolic disease
    adipose tissue 168–70, 169f
    bone health and 105
    bone marrow adipose tissue 105
    central obesity 105–6, 168
    corticosteroids 211
    lower body fat 144
    obesity/overweight and 94
    upper body fat accumulation 143
metabolic flexibility 63
metabolic obesity 139
metformin 205–6
MHO (metabolically healthy
    obesity) 140–41
microRNAs 182–83
Middle East 27–28
mineralocorticoids 71–72
mirabegron 97
missing heritability 199
mitochondria 98–99, 99f
mono-unsaturated fat 228–29
mortality, waist circumference vs. 142–43
mouse models 161–62, 162f
MRI see magnetic resonance
    imaging (MRI)
multi-cultural society 30–31
muscle see skeletal muscle
muscle weakness 140

NAFLD (non-alcoholic fatty liver
    disease) 69
Nbedele tribe 24

Nepal 24
neuronal signals, fullness 242
newborns 91–92, 92*f*
nicotine 206
nitric oxide 163–64
non-alcoholic fatty liver disease
 (NAFLD) 69
non-alcoholic liver disease 228–29
non-essential fatty acids 53*f*, 70
non-essential unsaturated fatty acids 70
non-invasive fat reduction
 technologies 237–38
noradrenaline 96, 163–64
normal/healthy body weight 122
normal weight obesity 177
North America 123–25
nucleoside reverse transcription
 inhibitors 205

obesity
 bone health 106
 health risks 272
 infertility 78
 measure by BMI 137–38
 metabolic disease and 94
 post-WWII 123
 social aspects 2–3
obesity crisis 271–72
oestradiol 217
oestrogens 71–72, 216
 adipogenesis 218
 fat accumulation 13
 fertility & lactation 15
 leptin 218
 male-to-female transsexuals 223–25
 receptors 217, 218
oleic acid 53*f*
omentectomy 237
orlistat 56–57
osteoporosis 108

Pacific Islands 28–30
palmitoleate 167
pancreas 51, 57–58
PCOS (polycystic ovary syndrome) 221–22
pelvis
 bipedalism 8
 evolution 8
 sex-specific differences 10
perilipins 63–64, 65

peroxisome proliferator-activated receptor
 gamma (PPARG) 178
persistence hunting 8–9
personal earnings, obesity/
 overweight 271–72
personal fat threshold 168–70, 273
The Physiology of Taste (Brillat-Savin) 33
polycystic ovary syndrome (PCOS) 221–22
Polynesia 148–49
poly-unsaturated fat 228–29
positron emission tomography
 (PET) 92–93
post-menopause fat distribution 218–19
post-natal development 9–10
PPARG (peroxisome proliferator-activated
 receptor gamma) 178
preadipocytes 53–54
 visceral 173
pregnancy
 bipedalism 9
 energy cost 12
pre-operative body composition 243
pre-receptor metabolism,
 corticosteroids 212, 213*f*
protease inhibitors 205
protein 63–64
psychiatric disorders 211
psychological stress 215
puberty
 average age of 77
 body composition 148
 leptin 76
Purcell, Edward 132

Quetelet, Adolphe 121
Quetelet index 121–22

*Recherches sur le poids de l'homme aux
 différent âges* (Quetelet) 121–22
recreational drugs 206
regional fat genetics 148
regional fat mass 129–30
reproductive capacity 11, 18–19
reproductive health 240
resistance exercise, aerobic exercise
 and 231
respiratory disease 136–37

sarcopenic obesity 140
saturated fats 228–29

Savacool, Julia 27
sedentary lifestyle 274–75
selective pressures 17–18
sex hormones 71–72
sex-reassignment hormone therapy 223–
   25, 224*f*
sex steroids 216–25, 273–74
sexual advertising 17–18
sexual development 75–76
sexual selection 11
SGLT2 inhibitors 101–2
shift workers 103
single slice imaging 135, 136*f*
skeletal muscle
   structure 62
   temperature regulation 98
   testosterone 223
skinfold measurement 126
sleep 63
small intestine, fat digestion 54–56
social aspects, obesity 2–3
social media 32
society
   body shape 19
   sex-specific differences 217
   sex-specific roles 11
socioeconomic status 228–29
Sorenson, James 128
South Africa 20, 24–26
South Asia 149
Spain 149
spot reduction 230–31
starvation 65–66
   bone marrow adipose tissue 107–8
statins 74–75, 205–6
stearic acid 53*f*
steatohepatitis 69
steatopygia 203–4
steroids 71–72
stomach, fat digestion 54–56
strength training, type 2 diabetes 140
stress 78, 215
   adipose tissue distribution 215–16
stroke 136–37
stromovascular fraction
   (SVF) 53–54
subcutaneous abdominal fat
   computed tomography 131
   fatty acid mobilization 166
   fibrosis 173–74

health and 167–68
inflammation 176
subcutaneous adipose tissue 54, 145–46
   all-cause mortality *vs.* 145–46
   blood flow 163, 164*f*
   fat deposition 168–70
   free fatty acids 165
   removal of 236–37
sub-scapular fat 54
sugar-sweetened beverages 227–28
surgery
   adipose tissue distribution 232–44
   historical aspects 232–33

TAG *see* triacylglycerol (TAG)
Tanzania 20
taste, fat 54
TBX5 gene 180
teeth evolution 10
television shows 34
temperature regulation, skeletal muscle 98
testosterone 14, 71–72, 216
   female-to-male transsexuals 223–25
   skeletal muscle 223
thiazolidinediones (TZDs) 106–7
   adipose tissue distribution 204
   adverse effects 204–5
thighs 18
thoracic duct 58
thromboembolism 220–21
thyroid hormones 95–96
Tonga 28–29
transcription factors, adipogenesis 178
trans-fats 70–71
transgenic mice 212–15
transplant studies, preadipocytes 173
transsexuals 223–25, 224*f*
triacylglycerol (TAG) 54
   generation 58
   protein 63–64
triglycerides 48*f*
tropical disease, South Africa 25
24-hour cyclicity
   cortisol 211
   obesity/overweight 103
twin studies 197–98
type 1 diabetes 52
type 2 diabetes 2, 52
   agouti mice 200–1
   body mass index 137

type 2 diabetes (*cont.*)
  bone health 106–7
  bone marrow adipose tissue 105
  fat fibrosis 173–74
  fatty acids 71
  gender distribution 148
  liposuction effects 235
  metabolic obesity 139
  muscle weakness 140
  risks of 141–42
  upper body fat accumulation 143
TZDs *see* thiazolidinediones (TZDs)

ultrasound
  high-intensity focused
    ultrasound 237–38
  liposuction and 234–35
uncoupling protein 1 (UCP-1) 98, 99–100
United Kingdom 30–32
United States 30–32
upper body fat accumulation 142–43
  post-menopause 218–19

Vague, Jean 125
vascular function, bariatric surgery 241
very low-density lipoproteins
    (VLDLs) 68–69
visceral adipose tissue 54, 145–46
  bone marrow adipose tissue and 105
  computed tomography 131
  CT/MRI 134–35
  exercise effects 230
  fibrosis 173–74
  inflammation 176
  liver fat 146
  post-menopause 219
visceral pericardium 109
vitamin D 71–72
VLDLs (very low-density lipoproteins) 68–69

waist circumference
  BMI *vs.* 142–43
  health status 18–19
  hormone replacement therapy 220
  mortality *vs.* 142–43
waist-to-hip ratio (WHR) 125–28
  adipose tissue distribution 198
  attractiveness 18–19, 20
  BMI *vs.* 142–43
  development of 125
  health outcomes 145
  hormone replacement therapy 220
  limitations 127–28
  measurement of 126–27, 127*f*
  pre-surgery 243
  sex-specific cut-offs 126–27
warmth, fat deposits 75
weight loss industry 32–33
Westernized ideal form 30–32
  poor definitions & confusion 32–33
white adipose tissue 49
  adipogenesis 179–80
  body shape 109–10
  brown adipose tissue and 94
  human anatomy 55*f*
white blood cells 79
WHR *see* waist-to-hip ratio (WHR)
Winckelmann, Johann
    Joachim 34–35
women
  bone marrow adipose tissue 104–5
  fat distribution 147
  reproductive capacity 11
  sex-specific roles 11
  white adipose tissue 55*f*
work productivity, obesity/
    overweight 271–72
World Health Organization (WHO) 1,
    126–27